CANCEROL(

CANCEROLOGY

the fight for YOUR life

Lawrence Wray

ISBN: 9798775884222

CANCEROLOGY – THE FIGHT FOR YOUR LIFE

The information contained in this book is intended to be advice for dealing with the journey through cancer and the associated treatment based on the personal experience of Lawrence Wray. It should not be used as a substitute for professional medical advice.

If you obtain information from this book which motivates you to do something in relation to your health, you must seek professional medical advice before implementation.

The only treatment recommended by this book is conventional treatment administered by a professional medical practitioner. For the purposes of clarification, conventional treatment for cancer is accepted to be, but not limited to, surgery, chemotherapy, immunotherapy, radiotherapy, and any other treatment carried out as standard protocol by National Health Service Hospitals in the United Kingdom.

This book may include words, brand names and other descriptions of products that are or are asserted to be proprietary names or trademarks. No judgement concerning the legal status of such words is made or implied thereby. Their inclusion does not imply that they have acquired, for legal purposes, a non-proprietary or general significance nor any other judgement concerning their legal status.

Any statistics quoted are up to date at the date of publication, but should you need to quote or refer to any of them, you should check the web for information on current figures.

Any links to websites are for information and clarification purposes only and are up to date at the date of publication but may have changed in the interim.

First Edition – November 2021

Cover Design – Edenderry Print – Alan Kirkpatrick

This book is dedicated to the memory of Ruth Potts

Ruth was one of the team from

Cancer Focus NI (previously The Ulster Cancer Foundation)

who helped me through my Stem Cell Transplant.

She was one of a kind. Caring, compassionate and understanding.

Sadly, cancer claimed my friend in the end.

Gone but not forgotten.

These pages are dedicated to those responsible for me still being here.

A big thanks to…

Rosehall Surgery

Whiteabbey Hospital

Dr Rodgers and all the team.

(Ultrasound and endoscopy)

Antrim Area Hospital

Dr Anne Kyle (my consultant)

Dr Phillip Burnside

Dr Francis Turtle

Dr Christine Lee

Dr Petrina Davies

Dr Whiteside

All the staff in Laurel House, especially Bernie (my chemo nurse) and the other nurses.

All the staff in wards B1 and B2.

Cleaners, catering, ward clerks, auxiliaries, nurses, doctors, phlebotomists, lab staff, radiographers for Ultra-Sound, CT, and MRI scanners, pharmacy staff, newsagents, the hospital Chaplin, the ambulance drivers for that one occasion, and all the casualty staff.

(Non-Hodgkin Lymphoma treatment including CHOP, ESHAP and IVE as well as ongoing check-ups)

CANCEROLOGY

Belfast City Hospital

Dr Kettle

Dr Mary Drake

Susan Piggott (Transplant Coordinator)

All the nurses and doctors on 10 North who looked after me.

(Stem Cell Transplant)

Mr Keane

Mr Hagan

All the staff in Level 3 North and South.

(Bladder and Kidney Cancer Treatment)

Dr Chris Hill

(Kidney Cancer)

Royal Hospital

Barbara, Ann, Terri and Chris in the Department of Nuclear Medicine

(PET Scanner)

If not for professionals like these to rely on, where would we be?

Please forgive me if I missed anyone, it wasn't intentional.

Table of Contents

Contents

CANCEROLOGY

CANCEROLOGY

CANCEROLOGY

More than just a book

When I had Cancerology nearly finished, I thought, 'if I was going to buy this book, what would I want?'

Well, I'd want the book, but I'd want more. I'd want a website, I'd want to be able to see the guy who wrote the book in a video, I'd like some exclusive content… put bluntly, I'd want as much as possible (after all, I've got cancer).

So, with that in mind, here's what I came up with.

Lifetime access

Lifetime access to exclusive online material to help you through your journey.

Updates

Don't you hate it when you buy a book and then it's updated? Sometimes you get the updated version if it's an eBook, but as it doesn't say where the updates are, you have to read the whole thing again, and even then, you might miss something.

With Cancerology, you get the updates before they're even uploaded. Just the updates, not the whole book.

Free printable PDF files

Fluid charts, weight charts, blood pressure records, output charts, medicine timetable, puzzles to do in hospital, etc.

Free MP3 files

Simply download to your computer or phone and listen to visualisation exercises, meditation sessions, pre-procedure relaxation sessions, etc.

Free articles

As and when I find news, you'll be the first to know.

Free videos

Any new videos I upload about cancer or treatment, you get access first, and some of the videos are exclusive and not available on YouTube or anywhere else.

Free exercises to help with chemo-brain

Chemo-brain ruins your memory, but only if you let it. Easy exercises help you to not only understand the problem, but cope with it and strengthen your memory muscle.

"I don't write what people want to hear; I write what they need to hear." ~ Lawrence Wray

Knock, knock

Cancer doesn't politely knock on your door one day and say, "Would now be a good time?"

No, cancer walks up to your door, kicks it in and says, "Ta Da. I've arrived. I'm here to kill you. Deal with it."

It's a fact that one in two people will get cancer at some point in their lives, yet, until it arrives, nobody believes they're going to be in the 50% who get it, then, when it turns up, they don't know what to do. I was in that category as well. Everybody is.

I've been told I had cancer seventeen different times.

I've been through all different treatments, and although I know how many cancers I've had and the treatments I've been given, I couldn't begin to count the number of mistakes I've made that were easy to avoid, yet nobody tells you about them. The thing about making mistakes is, the more you make, the more you learn. The more you learn, the better you get at avoiding them next time, because you don't make the same mistakes twice.

You can learn from my mistakes.

The cancerology survey

On 23rd and 24th July 2021, two friends went into Belfast City centre (Northern Ireland) with clipboards to ask passers-by a series of questions using the following script.

"Hello, could you help me by answering six quick questions for an advertising campaign?"

"Great, all you have to do is say the first word that comes into your head when I say a word. Six one word questions, six one word answers?"

I told them to practise the questions so that once the answers started, they could speed up to reduce thinking time.

"Okay, first word?"

"Up." (A: Down) *Most popular answers shown in brackets.*

"Left." (A: Right)

"In." (A: Out)

"Top." (A: Bottom)

"Black." (A: White)

"Cancer." (What would you have said?)

Once they had fifty answers each, they were finished.

Exactly eighty-four people said 'Death, dead, or dying' when they heard the word 'Cancer', which was the only question I wanted answered.

The clipboards each had a dictation machine recording the answers and I was able to listen to them afterwards, and the sixteen who didn't answer 'death' said the following:

One said, "That's not fair."

One cried. (Yeah, that one sucked.)

One said, "Fuck off."

One said, "You're kidding, I'm not answering that."

One said, "Vomiting."

One said, "Being sick."

Two said, "No hair."

Two walked away.

Three said, "No."

Three said, "Bald."

Interestingly, when the cancer question was asked, most people had a hesitation I could detect in the recordings, but it seemed that as the brain was committed to quick answers, it was out before they realised. Some tried to change their answers afterwards, but we were after a knee-jerk reaction—the first thing they thought of.

Quick answers with no thought. The truth.

Most people (84/100) thought of death when they heard the word cancer, so I think it would be fair to assume that most people expect death as a result of a diagnosis, whether that be them or someone else.

This has to change, because it's wrong, and not only that, the perception has the power to transform into a self-fulfilling prophecy.

I should be dead.

I've had cancer seventeen times.

I should definitely be dead.

But I'm not. (obviously)

Some of you may be thinking—with immense optimism—he's going to tell us a secret.

He's got some extraordinary power.

He knows something the rest of us don't know.

And in a way, that last part, (he knows something the rest of us don't know) is true.

It's very true.

I know something the rest of you don't know about cancer, and I found out through experience.

You could say, I learnt the hard way.

The good news is you don't have to.

What got me through cancer was medicine, doctors, nurses, professionalism, consultants and oncologists and haematologists, radiographers, and phlebotomists, and on, and on.

What got me through cancer was an attitude where I would do anything and everything to beat it.

I know that's not what you want to hear, and I know from experience I can't make it rosy for you.

It's a hard battle.

But what I can say is, it's far from impossible, and I can definitely make it easier.

You're listening to someone who has done it over and over; you're listening to someone who was given three days to live at one point, and you're listening to someone who made so many mistakes on the journey; someone who learned from them and avoided them next time.

In order to be successful in business, you emulate successful people; in order to get through cancer treatment, you emulate people who have done it and made mistakes, and you listen when they tell you how to avoid them.

When I had my first cancer and beat it, I thought; I'm glad that's over.

When I had my second, I thought; I had that one for my wife, so she's okay now.

Of course, I accept that life doesn't work like that, but it was a coping mechanism, an attempt, to rationalise why I got it again. In the end, there was no harm in it, and it made me feel good.

When I had my third, that one was for my daughter.

My fourth time was for my son.

Seventeen times in total.

I ran out of people to have it for.

"You cannot have life experiences that can help other people and not share them." ~ Lawrence Wray

Here's a question

What would you say if I invited you to take part in a race where—if you won—you would be cured of cancer forever?

You would probably say, "Yeah, bring it on."

But what would you say if you had to beat 40,000,000 other competitors to win? Yes, that's forty million.

Chances are you would give up before it even started.

The odds of winning are just so small it wouldn't be worth even trying.

One in forty million?

But here's the thing. You've already won that race.

One sperm is needed to fertilise an egg, and a healthy male can ejaculate between forty million and one point two billion sperm, yet here you are.

You're already a winner.

You're one out of forty million at the lower end, or one out of 1.2 billion at the higher end.

Boy did you beat the odds.

So now cancer has knocked on your door.

The chances of survival vary depending on the prognosis.

It's a hard fight, but it's one hell of a lot easier if you can get your mind around it.

"Success is often achieved by those who don't know that failure is inevitable." ~ Coco Chanel

The Drowning Man

A guy was walking along a seaside cliff when he slipped and fell into the sea.

A passer-by witnessed this and threw a life-ring into the water.

The guy shouted back, "No thanks, my God will save me."

Another passer-by called the coastguard.

A rowboat appeared and came over, but the guy shouted back, "No thanks, my God will save me."

By this time the coastguard appeared, but again, the guy shouted back, "No thanks, my God will save me."

Eventually, a helicopter arrived and dropped a rope ladder, but the guy in the water refused to grab it and shouted back, "No thanks, my God will save me."

Not unexpectedly, he drowned.

On the other side he demanded to see his God immediately.

"Why did you let me die?"

"But I sent you a life-ring, a rowboat, the coast guard and a helicopter. What happened?"

"From the day you receive your diagnosis, you're already in a ring facing an opponent who doesn't just want to win, they want to kill you; and it doesn't matter that by winning they die as well, that's how bad cancer is." ~ Lawrence Wray

Silly little big things

You have done it. I've done it. We've all done it at some stage. You say something and it's just a throwaway comment, something that seems insignificant, and you forget about it, then hours, or weeks, or months, or even years afterwards, somebody tells you that what you said changed their life, made an impact, made a difference, and you think back and shake your head wondering just what it was you said.

Several years ago I was waiting for my bladder cancer chemo when an elderly man came out of the treatment room having just been given his. (Turned out he was seventy-nine and his wife was eighty.) He sat down beside her and was exceptionally grumpy; it was hard not to hear him complaining. There were two other patients in the waiting room, and we listened to him and his wife as he complained and she tried to placate him. Eventually, he caught my eye and said, "You don't realise how bad this is. Every time I get chemo, I bleed like hell."

I replied, "Yes, I know, but that's how treatment is."

Then he said, "This is my third cancer. You wait till you get to this stage and you'll see how bad it can get. Every time I pee, it takes me at least ten minutes because it's so painful. It's like pissing razorblades and I have to stop and start over and over as the pain is so bad, and by the time I'm finished, I need to go again."

I'm not the type of person who will modify my feelings to satisfy somebody else, so I simply smiled rather than say something I would probably regret.

His wife noticed me smiling and said, “You don’t seem too concerned. How many times have you had cancer?”

Again, I smiled, then replied, “This is my thirteenth time.”

She said, “Oh.” But it wasn’t in the same tone of voice she had used for the question.

He then said, “Thirteen times?”

I said, “Yes,”

“…and do you bleed?”

“Yeah, of course.”

He said, “It’s awful, isn’t it?”

I said, “Depends how you look at it.”

He said, “What’s that supposed to mean?”

I paused, took a deep breath and it just came out; no thinking required.

“Three things. First one is, yes, it’s awful, but if you don’t take treatment, you’re probably going to die. Second one is when you’re bleeding, it shows the chemotherapy is working, it’s taking out some of the lining of the bladder and taking out the cancer cells, so it’s all good. The more you bleed and the more cancer cells you pee out, the better chance you have of surviving. It’s when you’re not bleeding you should be worried. The third thing is when you pee, you constantly stop as it’s painful, but if you count to four the pain goes. One, it’s excruciating, two, it’s even worse, three, you feel it subside, four; just let it flow and it’s not a problem, but if you stop, you have to start over.”

He grunted and I was called to have my chemo. As I was lying on the table, I thought I had been a bit sharp with him—considering his age—and decided to take time to explain things better, but when I came back, they were gone. I didn’t think about it again until I encountered them at the next chemo appointment.

As I was walking out of the elevator, they were coming out of the ward. His wife had seen me before I noticed them and I heard her say, "There he is." She hurried towards me, threw her arms around me and said, "He's a new man. You really helped him."

It was my turn to say, "Oh."

Then he came towards me, hand held out. I was about to apologise when he said, "After the last chemo I pissed blood for two days." Only this time it wasn't a complaint, it was a boast. He was smiling, nodding and proud. He leant towards me and whispered, "What you said…" I nodded, expecting to be told off, but instead he said, "…it was hard to listen to, but I needed it. I needed someone who wasn't scared to tell-it-like-it-is, to point me in the right direction."

One brief exchange that I thought too direct, changed his attitude.

A silly little thing to me turned out to be something big in his journey through treatment. Simply understanding why he was bleeding changed it from a problem to an achievement.

Sometimes, making someone's life easier is as simple as telling how you went through the same process and explaining the shortcuts and tricks you learnt on the way that made it easier. That's what Cancerology is all about.

As I wrote this book, I learned things about myself, about my journey, and yes, I'm biased, but I can honestly say that if this book had been available when I was first diagnosed, it would have made life so much easier.

Understanding what I could expect, why, and how to deal with it would have changed my whole experience. It would probably have saved my marriage, and it would definitely have saved other relationships that didn't survive.

I couldn't have written a book after just one cancer, or two, or even three, as I didn't have enough experience, and I wouldn't be so arrogant to assume I was qualified, but when life throws cancer at you seventeen times, you start to take notice, and as experience accumulates, you realise you just might have something worth sharing.

Where are the chapters?

As you go through this book, you will notice that traditional chapter structures are not used, and the reason is concentration, which is a problem when you've just been diagnosed and especially when you're on chemotherapy.

I have tried to keep the sections as short and to the point as possible. Of course, there are some long sections where a more detailed explanation is essential, but if you find them too long, you should be able to bookmark the relevant sections you think you may need to re-visit and read in short bursts.

Memory is also a problem, so if you read a section and think it's relevant to you, it's a good idea to make a note in your diary or journal. It doesn't have to be a long and detailed note, but something that will trigger the point you want to remember. If you do forget, forgive yourself as it's not you, it's a combination of diagnosis and treatment.

"*If you can dream it, you can do it.*" ~ Walt Disney

A book about cancer?

Yes, it's another book about cancer, but it's different, honestly. I've read a lot of books on the subject over the years and even more while researching this book, and most start with a misdiagnosis, then treatment and out the other side. Some are motivational, but none I found examined the potential problems with treatment or offer solutions. I'm different. I've been there, done that, bought the t-shirt, been sick, lost my hair, had depression, tried suicide, and had problems with everything along the way. If I had only had cancer once, I wouldn't have dared to write a book on the subject, but I've had seventeen cancers since 2002, so I do have a lot of experience dealing with the short and long term problems of treatment. If you want to know what it takes to fight cancer and how to avoid some of the pitfalls, this book is for you.

I can't promise you an ideal outcome, but I can promise you we'll grab cancer by the throat and see what happens.

I've already done it.

I've made the mistakes.

I've had cancer in my spleen, liver, heart, colon, lymphatic system, kidney, and bladder.

I have heard the phrase, 'I'm sorry, but you have cancer', seventeen times.

I've been given several estimated dates for my demise.

But... I'm not a doctor, so it follows I'm not an expert on cancer, but I am an expert on the cancer experience.

You ready?

How it started

In 2002, after being misdiagnosed for approximately two years, it was finally confirmed I had Non-Hodgkin Lymphoma, stage four, grade four, aggressive. The disease had progressed into the spleen, liver, and heart, and initially, I was given six months to live, and when it returned the following year, I was given three months. The fourth and last time Non-Hodgkin Lymphoma called in 2004, it decided to pay my colon a visit. My wife was told on a Wednesday I wouldn't see the weekend. At this stage, I was on palliative care and a hospice had already been contacted for end-of-life care.

During all four visits by Non-Hodgkin Lymphoma, I accepted the diagnosis each time, but I never accepted the prognosis I would die within a specific time. I was sick, and I accepted that, but in my mind, it wasn't my time to go. I was (and still am) a long way from maturity and a long way from being a grown up; even though I was married with kids and forty-one years old at the time of the original diagnosis.

Maybe it was the kid in me; the adult that still considered himself a teenager. At only age forty-one (which was probably around eighteen/nineteen in my mind), I was outraged at the diagnosis. Bloody angry. What the hell is going on? It ain't gonna happen. Die? Get real.

Do guys ever grow up? Maybe that's what saved me; the outrage at the potential early departure before having achieved anything worth remembering.

What I did know was I would do everything possible to beat it. Everything the doctors told me to do I would do and more, and I would research my disease and find other things to help.

My dad always asked me, "What do you want to be *if* you grow up?" It was a joke between us; always *if* and not *when*. I'm still waiting to find out.

In 2010, I was diagnosed with the first of what was to be twelve visits from bladder cancer.

In 2016, I was diagnosed with kidney cancer and had my left kidney removed on my birthday (25th Oct).

On 7th July 2017 I was told I had six months to a year to live, so my estimated date of demise was 7th July 2018.

It's now 2021+ (Depending when you're reading to this.) and I'm still here.

I've had cancer in my spleen, liver, heart, lymphatic system, colon, bladder, and one kidney, yet I continue to live, irrespective of cancer's best efforts to bring about my demise.

So yes, I feel qualified to talk about the journey, and I warn you now, there are sections you might find too frank or too opinionated, but if reading this book shocks you into action, hits you with reality and potentially saves your life, then irrespective of what you think of me, it's all good and... it's done with the best intentions.

Why this book?

The bottom line is I am fed up with people dying due to cancer. Friends, relatives, acquaintances, neighbours, and people I hardly know.

Those of you with sharp eyes will notice that in the previous sentence I used the words 'dying due to cancer' and not 'dying from cancer', and the reason for this is I'm fed up with people dying from their *attitude* towards cancer and not the disease itself. Don't get me wrong, I'm not suggesting the power of the mind will cure cancer, and some people have suggested that the word 'fight' in the sub-title suggests this, but in the context of the book it is the right word as it's meant to convey that conventional treatment such as chemotherapy is a fight in itself. The side effects can be hard to tolerate, and this is where the fight comes into the equation with the acceptance you will have side effects, and determination you will prepare for them, accept them, and fight through the process. In effect, your fight will mostly be with yourself, forcing you to do things you need to do, but you won't want to do.

The phrase, 'The fight against cancer', is still used, but its meaning has thankfully changed from the original when doctors took complete control of the treatment; which meant that irrespective of the patient's wishes, whatever treatment was deemed necessary was carried out. Initially, it was used by surgeons who thought that by cutting away as much tissue as possible surrounding a tumour, any spread would also be removed. In fairness, this proved to be right (to a degree), and with modern techniques we can do this with accuracy, but back then it meant butchery. For example, in breast cancer it was normal to not only remove the breasts, but also some ribs, bones, lymph nodes, pectoralis muscles, surrounding skin, and even arms in some cases.

A similar phrase was made popular in the 70s when Richard Nixon declared the US would wage 'war on cancer' and eradicate it within two years (which, of course, didn't happen) by throwing approximately $1.5b into finding a cure.

Two things are worth noting:

(1) US Presidents have a habit of promising to find a cure to beat cancer once elected, even though they have no idea about the disease, and it's never happened.

Bill Clinton. "In fact, it is now conceivable that our children's children will know the term cancer only as a constellation of stars."

George W Bush. "For the first time in human history. We can say with some measure of confidence that the war on cancer is winnable."

Barack Obama. "For the loved ones we've all lost, for the family we can still save, let's make America the country that cures cancer once and for all."

Donald Trump. "We will come up with the cures to many, many problems, to many, many diseases—including cancer."

Joe Biden. "I promise you if I'm elected president, you're going to see the single most important thing that changes America. We're gonna cure cancer."

(2) The $1.5b Nixon raised might not sound like a lot, but allowing for inflation it is estimated to be around $9.4b in today's money. Not exactly a drop in the ocean.

On my journey through treatment, I've listened to people complaining that the chemo is worse than the cancer and wondering why they bother with it. The fact is, cancer is almost always way worse than the treatment. Some have stopped treatment altogether with inevitable results. Cancer kills, and yes, treatment is hard, but it's better than the alternative.

I started writing this book on 8th May 2017, which was a day I was again diagnosed with bladder cancer. At the time, my brother—who was fifteen years older than me—was also battling cancer. He had been diagnosed only a couple of weeks before and I had told him I would write a book that would help him get to grips with the fight he would be facing, both with the cancer and the treatment. I printed out pages from the internet and wrote some myself, but the more I talked to him, the more I realised I was wasting my time. He wouldn't try to fight. Maybe it was his age (72), or maybe it was because he was from an era where it was accepted doctors always knew best; so if they predicted a bad outcome, that was considered fact and not opinion, and he hadn't been given the best news at diagnosis. And, no, I'm not suggesting doctors don't know best, rather the interpretation of what they say can be misconstrued by the patient. (I explain it later in the Nocebo section)

From experience I know the appetite goes when you're having chemotherapy, and you've no energy and don't feel like exercising, but taking into consideration the other option, I also know you must force yourself to do things you don't feel like doing.

I visited every day and tried to get him to eat, drink, go for a walk, meditate, do something; anything towards beating his cancer, but although he talked a good talk, it seemed he was resigned to dying, which he did on 31st May 2017: the day before I was due to go for another bladder operation.

From diagnosis to death he lasted approximately six weeks.

When he received the hospital appointment for the official diagnosis and treatment plan, he asked me to go with him. We talked on the way and I told him I had been given several serious results with grim predictions, but not to worry about what diagnosis he was given and be prepared for a major life change. We walked into the hospital and I asked him if he wanted to take the lift or use the stairs; thankfully, we ran up the two flights and he went in, chin held high. But when we left, he needed the lift to go down as he decided it was too strenuous to walk in his condition. That day was the day he died, even though every part of him was alive, in his mind he was already dead. A total and complete change in attitude in less than twenty minutes based on nothing more than a talk with his consultant and a diagnosis that wasn't as bad as initially expected.

A bad attitude can make the difference between life and death; and that's not an opinion, it's a fact based on my observations of other patients and their outcome. Horrible, but true.

I visited him at home the next day and he was lying on the settee. He said he was too tired to exercise (even though the previous day he had raced me up the hospital stairs), hadn't eaten much and hadn't drunk anything; and this was before treatment had even started. Every time I visited, he was lying on the settee, and later, he had a bed moved downstairs and lay on that. In my mind, he had given up when he received the diagnosis. Nothing I or anyone else could say would change that or get him into fight mode. He simply lay down and didn't get up again.

He lay on a settee, then a bed, then in a coffin. (that's couch, bed, and casket for my American friends)

Yes, I know it's blunt, but cancer isn't something you delegate to someone to fight for you. It's your fight and nobody can fight, except you.

Unfortunately, or possibly fortunately—depending on your point of view—I'm not one of those people who have a great deal of empathy for, or sympathy with others with cancer who are constantly using phrases such as *poor me*, or *why me?* or *this isn't fair* or *I don't deserve this* or whatever other pitiful phrases they choose to complain with. I can understand it, sure, but the fact is you've got it. Suck it up. Own it. Deal with it. Yes, it is a harsh attitude, but if you get stuck in poor me mode, the battle will be all one way (the wrong way).

You have two choices. You can let it walk all over you (which it will take great pleasure in doing), or you can fight.

If you do the former, it won't just walk on you, it'll jump up and down, then it'll punch and kick, then gouge your eyes out. It's a nasty piece of work with no moral compass. The worst thing you think it's capable of doesn't even scratch the surface.

Bottom line? It will try its hardest to kill you. To end your life. To expedite your demise from this mortal coil. And not only will it try its hardest, but it will do it in a particularly gruesome and painful way.

When you get a cancer diagnosis, and without ever being asked, you are in The Fight For Your Life. There is no other way to describe it.

I started writing this book for my brother, but I finished it for you.

After he died, I was left with my writing; some finished pages, some ideas, some headings, etc., but as I had started the writing to motivate him and he wouldn't read it or do anything, was there any point in continuing? Of course, another friend got cancer and I said, "I have some stuff written, would you like it?" … and here we are.

She survived and said that what I had given her had helped her through treatment and motivated. Yes, that's what she said; it had motivated, so I thought about how many people get cancer every day and how many I could potentially help and decided to finish it. So, ultimately, I wrote this book for you. Just you. I don't even know you, but if you have cancer, I can help and I want to help.

When I decided on the title 'Cancerology', I thought I was clever. I thought I had invented a neologism—a new word or expression—and I was really chuffed; however, the word already existed and means, *the study of cancer*, so not so clever after all. Then I thought that by the use of a subtitle, I could define it more precisely, so I tried, *The Fight of Your Life*, then, *The Fight for Life*; but on reflection, neither was right as although it is an undertaking, the ultimate result can be death, so I changed it to, *The Fight For Your Life*, which is exactly what it is. A one-time-only chance to get it right.

You can set out to write a nice book, or you can write an honest book where you share your experiences and opinions without the restrictions of worrying what the reader might ultimately think, and that's what I've done. It's no use telling anyone about potential side effects and then not explaining how they affected you when you had them, so in a way the book could, or should, be embarrassing to me, but it's not, it's the truth, and if you're embarking on the journey through cancer or know someone who is, it will definitely help.

I accept there are cancers detected too late, or ones that are simply too aggressive to fight, or, for example, an advanced inoperable tumour growing in the middle of a brain; but unless you are rendered unconscious, you can fight and see what happens. Seriously, what have you got to lose?

You need to have an attitude where you will at least take on the fight. If you don't already have a fight attitude, get one. Get one now.

Some ask me how they are expected to get a fight attitude; well, it's the same as someone saying they can't stop smoking, or lose weight, or learn a language, or jog, or… it's simply a realisation that doing what you're doing isn't going to work and accepting the solution is a change of mindset. Instead of poor me, stand in front of a mirror, smile, then say, Fuck Cancer, in a determined voice (I don't care if you don't normally swear, and in fact, it has an even greater impact if you don't. Make an exception or just mouth the words. You're gonna love the section 'Fuck, fuck, fuckety-fuck' later, and yes, it does make sense.). Say it out loud. Mean it. Repeat it often and see your face change. Fuck… Cancer. Yes, it sounds silly, but it's a simple and effective form of brain training.

The biggest problem in the fight against cancer is the word itself. People get diagnosed with all types of cancer, but in a lot of cases the patient only hears the word cancer. Nothing else registers.

You might have one of the most straightforward cancers to cure, one that can be sorted quickly and won't kill you, but it's the word, the 'C' word. The word probably kills as many people as the disease itself.

As a result of preconceived notions, the brain seems to malfunction in the translation of two things it hears when you are told you have cancer.

When you find yourself sitting across a table from a consultant and they say, "I'm sorry to have to tell you, but you've got cancer," the brain translates it into, "I'm gonna die." The second is the word itself which gets translated from *cancer* into the word *death*. It doesn't seem to matter the letters aren't simply re-arranged, but totally disregarded, and this is normally the biggest problem with receiving a cancer diagnosis. It's the perception and the expectation that can cause a major problem.

If we can change - “you’ve got cancer,” into “I’m going to have to really fight this,” and change - “cancer” into “I’m sick,” then we’re well on the way to tackling the problem without the associated baggage that can turn out to be a self-fulfilling prophecy.

If you expect the worst, you generally won’t be disappointed, but if you expect the best, your brain will do its utmost to fulfil your expectations.

The biggest weapon in the fight against cancer is your state of mind, as it determines your attitude to everything involved in tackling the disease.

When I was first diagnosed, I used to go into the waiting room and see people sitting with their chins firmly wedged against their chest. I thought they must be really sick until one of the nurses told me my diagnosis was much worse than anyone else in the room. Yeah, go me.

Why then were they all looking like they had already died?

I never understood it at the time, but I do now, and with this book, so will you.

I can’t say I ever looked forward to the chemo, but I knew it was the best way to beat the cancer, so bring it on. I’ll take all you got with knobs on.

At the start of this book you may have wondered why the joke was there. You may have thought a book about something as serious as cancer shouldn’t start with a joke; but think about it for a minute. A life ring, a rowboat, the coastguard, and a helicopter? All of which could have saved his life.

Surgery, chemotherapy, radiotherapy, immunotherapy, etc. All used effectively to cure cancer, yet some people refuse them or rely on alternative treatments that have been proven to be ineffective. And yes, some people do say, “No thanks, my God will save me.” Yeah, that one always works—until it doesn’t.

Everyone is on your side, but you must be there as well.

You can suffer cancer, or you can fight cancer. You choose.

Help is available

In the world of business, there are lots of books, YouTube videos, podcasts and professional speakers that will give ideas on how to improve your business and your attitude towards success. If you listen to them, you'll find the ideas do work; but with cancer, I don't think there is any similar idea to explain the journey through treatment. There is a multitude of books and websites that claim to have the elusive *magic cure* big pharma and governments don't want to give you, and at the end of this book, I've looked at most of the alternative cures offered and debunked them.

When you hear those three words, "You've got cancer," your heart sinks and you're basically left to get on with it. Except, you're not. Help is everywhere.

Sometimes you'll get booklets or a chat with a nurse, and while both are helpful, there isn't usually anyone who has been-there-done-that to talk to—yet.

Along your cancer journey there will be numerous things you need advice on, and hopefully, this book will help to fill in some of the gaps, but you will also meet other patients on the same journey when you're getting treatment, so talk to them. Ask them what you can expect, what experience they had, and what advice they have for a first-timer. You'll find everyone has different problems and solutions; but discussing them isn't just knowledge, it's power, it's preparation, it's gold.

I have no doubt I'll have more visits from cancer in the future, but I doubt it will kill me. It's just not on the cards. I'm one of those curious people that will probably die from an ingrown toenail or hiccups, but not cancer.

Two types of positive

There are two types of positive cancer patients. Being positive you're going to fight it (cancer) and win, or being positive it's going to beat you and you're gonna die. If you're positive in the negative, then go ahead and buy yourself as many packets of cigarettes as you want and smoke yourself to death. Even if you don't smoke, what have you got to lose? Light one up. It's your life and you can do what you want. After watching my brother give up, commit suicide, fail, waste his life, accept his fate, I'm not going to try and convince you that you shouldn't, and if you have negative vibes, then stay away. You're big enough to make your own decisions, so don't bother reading anymore, just go and have a happy death. Yes. I did say that. If I shock you into realisation, that's good. I will help if I can, but if you don't want it, that's okay too. If, however, you're of the opinion you're going to fight and win, then read on.

But… what I will say is this. There is nothing worse, and I really, really mean nothing on this planet, worse than deciding, for whatever reason, to let cancer have its way and then once it takes hold you change your mind. Yeah, when it's too late, when medical intervention won't help and you realise, if only. Think about it. You're now dying with the knowledge that if you had only fought in the beginning like you want to now, everything might be different. It's torture.

I've beaten it seventeen times so far.

I've had it so often I put it down on questionnaires as one of my hobbies.

Every time it appears, I fight like my life depends on it, which it does.

I have an anger that no person would ever want to be on the receiving end of.

Will you do the same? Please say yes and commit to a fight right now.

Realistically, the possibility is it might not work irrespective of what you do, but if you don't try, you're dramatically reducing your chances of a successful outcome.

When someone is told they have cancer, there are usually one of two questions asked; "How long have I got?" or "How are we going to fix this?" The wording may vary, but essentially, these are the two most popular questions.

You will recall I mentioned my brother earlier, and at the time of diagnosis the first question he asked was about the time he had left. Both the consultant and I argued he shouldn't be thinking like that, but to no avail.

I've asked several consultants about this scenario and they all say the same thing: The response to the diagnosis is an early indicator of how the patient will progress.

"How long have I got?" displays a resignation you're not going to beat it and don't expect to.

"How are we going to fix this?" shows an acceptance that something can be done, irrespective of how tenuous the possibility of a good outcome may be, they're willing to try.

For me, it was always the second one. Always. The first one didn't even exist.

"One must not forget that recovery is brought about not by the physician, but by the sick man himself. He heals himself, by his own power, exactly as he walks by means of his own power, or eats, or thinks, breathes or sleeps." ~ Georg Groddeck

A Positive Mental Attitude and Cancer

I read an article in the paper that said new research indicated a positive mental attitude had no effect on the outcome of cancer treatment. I beg to differ. You only have to look at my brother's history to see the effect attitude can have, and unfortunately, there have been too many others.

I have spoken extensively about this to consultants, doctors, and nurses, and let's not forget they are the people at the front line of the treatment, seeing it day in, day out, and without exception, all of them have noticed that patients with a positive mental attitude accept the treatment better, deal with the side effects better, and have better overall results.

I knew I would beat it. I knew it was just one of those curve balls life throws at you, and my attitude was bring it on, right from the start. I was forty-one, but in my mind, I was still in my teens and much too young to die, so it must be a mistake, and I was meant to fight it and beat it.

Now I'm not saying that if you are worried and can't get yourself into a positive frame of mind, you will get worse. I'm just saying you have a lot less worry if you are positive you are going to beat it.

There are no guarantees either way, but I've already proven attitude can make a huge difference, so you don't need to look far to find a success story, so if I can do it, you can too. From reading this book you also know I've made many mistakes, done things I regret, things that can't be undone, so you just have to do your best and forgive yourself along the way. Always try to improve. Accept the fight and come out swinging.

Don't forget the slogan, 'I cancer-vive' pronounced I CAN SURVIVE. Make it your daily mantra.

Some recent trials have shown very positive results in cases where patients visualise their bodies fighting the cancer and visualise the chemotherapy destroying the cancerous cells. For me, I know this process helped, but others say it has no effect. Irrespective, the fact you feel yourself participating in the process has a feel-good factor no medicine can induce.

I think it's wise to point out the human race is wonderfully talented and has invented some amazing things; but when it comes to understanding the workings of our brains, we are hopelessly inadequate.

Believe what you will, but I recommend a positive mental attitude. Six estimated dates of demise (EDOD), all proved wrong has to mean something… and no, it doesn't mean the doctors got it wrong, it means I choose to ignore and got it right. You'll find more relevant information in The Fabulous Nocebo Effect section.

Top ten things you need to sort now

1) **Smoking**

The number one cause of cancer is smoking.

The smoke from the end of a cigarette contains hundreds of toxic chemicals and over seventy have been identified as carcinogenic (having the potential to cause cancer).

Passive smoking can be even worse, so if you hang around others who routinely smoke and you inhale it, stop.

Cigars are worse as they emit around the same amount of second-hand smoke as an entire pack of cigarettes.

2) **Obesity**

Being overweight produces excess amounts of estrogen and other hormones that can stimulate cell growth and proliferation, and the more often cells divide and multiply, the greater the risk that cancer cells develop.

Obesity can also cause chronic inflammation which can damage DNA, which triggers cells to multiply.

3) **Diet**

According to Cancer Research UK, maintaining a healthy diet could prevent 1 in 20 cancers.

Diet is not only important to control weight, but a healthy diet rich in fruits and vegetables with high fibre can reduce the risk of cancer.

A high fibre diet increases the size of your poo and dilutes the contents. It also helps gut bacteria to produce chemicals that help in the processing of the food.

Processed foods such as ham, bacon, salami, sausages, etc., have been found to increase the risk of cancer.

Red meat, minced or frozen beef, lamb or pork, etc., all contain chemicals that are a natural part of the meat, but other chemicals which are produced when preserved or cooked have been found to promote the growth of cancer.

You should consider reducing your meat and processed food intake and replacing it with white meat such as chicken and fish, which are not linked with an increased risk of cancer.

4) **Exposure to the sun**

Skin cancer is on the rise, but something as simple as the correct sunscreen applied correctly can help protect you.

Use factor 30 or higher and aim to use about a shot glass (or as much as you can hold in one hand) and apply it thirty minutes before going into the sun to allow it to bind to your skin.

Irrespective of whether it is claimed to be waterproof, always reapply after swimming.

Make sure to include the top of the ears, feet, back of hands, and not just legs, face, and stomach.

If you're in a hot climate and it's overcast, don't think you are safe as up to 40% of ultraviolet radiation still penetrates, even on a completely cloudy day.

5) **Salt/Salty foods**

If you crave salt, you should substitute it with a safer alternative, or ideally, stop using it altogether.

Not only is it linked to high blood pressure, but it damages the lining of the stomach when ingested causing inflammation which makes the lining sensitive to cancer causing chemicals.

You should also try to avoid salt-preserved foods.

6) **Alcohol**

Regardless of whether it's wine, beer or spirits; alcohol is bad for you as it increases your risk of mouth, upper throat, oesophageal (food pipe), bowel and breast cancers.

It is estimated that 3% of cancers are caused by alcohol, and we're not talking about alcoholics, rather anyone who occasionally indulges.

Alcohol is converted into a toxic chemical called acetaldehyde, which has been found to cause cells to turn cancerous. It specifically causes the cells in the liver to grow faster than normal, which makes them more likely to divide and turn cancerous. It also increases the levels of some hormones which give the cells instructions to divide. DNA damage also occurs when alcohol causes Reactive Oxygen Species molecules to be produced that can have a negative effect on the DNA.

Alcohol causes one in thirteen cases of breast cancer

In a report published 4th October 2018 by Public Health England, it stated that over 55,100 people are diagnosed with breast cancer every year in the UK with alcohol being the cause in one out of every thirteen cases.

Drinkaware and Public Health England (PHE) are encouraging women of all ages to cut down on how much they are drinking by taking more drink free days to reduce their risk of developing breast cancer and a range of other health conditions including liver and heart disease.

7) **Sunbeds**

The ultraviolet (UV) rays from sunbeds increase your risk of skin cancer, as many of the tanning methods used in tanning salons give out much greater doses of UV rays than the midday tropical sun (up to 10 times stronger).

The World Health Organisation's International Agency for Research on Cancer has classified tanning devices as carcinogenic to humans.

In a study by Massachusetts General Hospital in 2008, the authors concluded that safe tanning with ultraviolet rays from a sunbed may be a physical impossibility.

Researcher Dr. Simon Lergenmuller, an epidemiologist at the University of Oslo, identified a link between squamous cell carcinoma (SCC), which is a form of skin cancer that develops when UV light makes cells in the skin reproduce quicker than normal.

Using sunbeds between the age of 25 and 35 increases the risk of skin cancer by 50%, and below the age of 25 the risk is increased to 75%.

In the UK, The Sunbeds (Regulation) Act 2010 makes it illegal for any business to allow anyone under 18 to use a sunbed.

Melanoma (skin cancer) is one of the largest causes of cancer deaths in 15-34 year-olds in the UK.

In the US, over 400,000 cases of skin cancer can be attributed to sunbeds.

There's no benefit having a nice tan when you're in a coffin.

8) **Sedentary lifestyle**

You need to get moving more and stop sitting in front of a TV or computer. (I smiled at this one when I was sitting at my desk. As a writer, it's a way of life.)

In an analysis of four million people and 70,000 cancer cases conducted in Germany, it was found that an additional two hours a day of sedentary behaviour was linked to an 8% increase in colon cancer, a 10% increase in endometrial cancer, and a 6% increase in lung cancer.

These findings were across the board and included people otherwise physically active.

If you find yourself sitting for long periods, make a point of taking an exercise break every hour. Something as simple as a short walk or running up a flight of steps could make all the difference.

9) **Fast Food**

Several reasons spring to mind, the first one being the calorie content. I recently looked at a menu at a fried chicken restaurant and a lunch box contained 1280 calories. Just for lunch?

Another reason is the glycemic index and glycemic load fast food contains which significantly increases the risk of endometrial cancer.

Basically, you're eating a mix of foods high in fat, starch, salt, and sugar content.

Sometimes I go months without fast food, but occasionally I cheat, but only once and then weeks pass—and everyone needs the occasional treat—but make up for it afterwards with exercise and good food.

10) **Sex**

I'm guessing there's no way you expected this to be on the list, but there are some sexually transmitted diseases such as hepatitis viruses, the human papillomavirus (HIV), and others that contribute to the development of certain cancers.

If you have a new partner, use protection until everyone is confirmed clean.

"Everybody's gotta die, it doesn't mean you deserve to die, and it doesn't mean it's your time now. Just because you have cancer doesn't mean it's time to go, it could mean it's your time to start living." ~ Lawrence Wray

How do I keep beating it?

Simple. I do absolutely everything the doctors tell me to do, and I have an extremely positive attitude. I suppose it doesn't do any harm I'm a guy, which means I'll never be anywhere near as developed as a female. Guys never grow up. They define Peter Pan. The male brain seems to be designed to remain as young and juvenile as possible for as long as possible. That's probably why—at the age of forty-one—when I was first diagnosed, I was outraged that someone so young could be facing the possibility of death, and why I was determined I wouldn't be a mortality statistic. Give me a one percent survival rate and I'll place myself firmly in that category, thank you very much.

Girls reading the above paragraph might be thinking, 'Well then, what chance have I got as I am a mature adult?' which, in itself is the answer. Guys got one thing, girls another. No two people are the same. At its most basic, it doesn't matter who or what you are; the ability to accept the situation and do whatever is necessary is in everyone.

As with anything in my life, the more times I do it, the easier it becomes, and that's not to say it isn't annoying when another diagnosis appears, it is, but my attitude is, 'I've beat it before, and I'll beat it again.

And yes, I know it depends on the diagnosis, but *knowledge is power, and experience teaches you a lot, and if you've been given an Estimated Date of Demise (EDOD) before and are still here, then human nature dictates you aren't going to pay too much attention to them. But if it's your first time being told you have a specific number of months left, it's scary, but you only have to look at me to realise it's just a guess, a figure plucked out of midair based on the experience of previous patients, who were not you, cuz you're reading this and know better.

*Knowledge actually is power, when you use it. Knowledge that isn't used is just a waste of brain space. Don't learn and ignore, learn and implement.

Wouldn't it be great to be rich?

Yes, it would, and if you have cancer and you're a millionaire, you could simply call your chauffeur to pick you up, your secretary to organise the Gulfstream jet and quickly follow that with a call to the best doctors in the world to organise the best medical treatment available. Money can buy you everything: the best doctors, the best hospital, the best room, the best view, the best surgeons, everything you could possibly need to fight cancer, period.

Sounds good—but is it?

As tends to be the way with rich people, they're used to getting their own way. They simply think they can click their fingers, throw money at it and everything will turn out tickety-boo; however, cancer isn't something that can be beaten simply by having cash. You can't buy an attitude. You either have it already or you develop it, but money can't buy it.

Too many patients are looking for the millionaire cure, and by that, I mean we're so used to popping pills for whatever ails us that some people think cancer can be cured the same way.

It's a fact that doctors can give you pills and treatment, but they won't normally be with you when you don't want to eat or drink or exercise, and that's where it becomes your fight.

Cancer is one of those diseases that will literally take your life if you delegate responsibility for the cure to the doctors and nurses. You have to actively participate in beating it yourself; otherwise, you're wasting what little time you have left. You have to participate in your own cure.

It takes determination and cooperation to beat it. When the doctors say jump, not only do you say, "how high?" but you double it and do it standing on your head.

If I was a millionaire.

The previous section came about as a result of a question from my son, and like everyone else, I can answer a question and carry on a conversation without pausing to think; but given time, I can also come up with a better response than one given on the spur of the moment. We all do it, when asked that question that deserves a clever and well thought out answer. Ten minutes later you know what you should have said, and ten minutes after that, you have an even better answer. But just this one time in my life, I gave an answer that was very relevant. After I said it, I thought, *where the hell did that come from*?

When I was going through treatment with my first visit from Non-Hodgkin Lymphoma, my son was only eight years old. His dad had lost a lot of weight and for some reason had no hair, no eyebrows, no eyelashes, and no energy. One day he said, "Dad, wouldn't it be great if we were millionaires and could go to America and get the best doctors in the world?"

I immediately replied, "No."

He looked at me like I was mad and asked why.

Again, I replied immediately and said, "If I was a millionaire, I would be used to people doing what I wanted just because of the money, so I would expect them to cure me and would just click my fingers and demand that as I was paying for it, they should just do it. I wouldn't be fighting myself, so it wouldn't work."

He looked at me, confused.

Hell, I was confused. Where had that come from?

The more I thought about it, the more it made sense, and that's where my phrase, 'You have to participate in your own cure,' comes from. And, yes, I realise the word 'own' should be removed, but I decided it emphasises the fact that you as a patient have potential ownership of the eventual outcome, so it stays.

You can't just assign responsibility for your cure to others. You have to be there. Take part. Fight your own fight. Not lie down. Not give up. At the very least, fighting will make you feel better.

Am I making it clear just what my thoughts are on how you should proceed with your treatment?

Cancer isn't something you can delegate to others to take care of; it doesn't work like that. You have to be positive about the outcome, you have to participate in your own cure and not just rely on the doctors and assume it will be cured for you. (…and yes, I'm repeating myself, but it needs to become second nature in your thought process. So forgive me.)

You're in The Fight For Your Life. Right now. This minute.

The phrase, 'Win some, lose some', can't be used with cancer. If you lose, you die. Game over.

This is a fight you *have* to try to win.

Nobody can fight for you.

Own it, beat it, and move on.

If you know you won't or can't beat it, or won't try, then don't be selfish. Stop treatment, say goodbye, throw a party, organise your funeral, do your bucket list, or simply lie back and wait for the inevitable; but I have to ask, why?

What's to lose?

If you fight and lose, that's life; but if you fight it and win?

Now, you may think, 'why is he labouring this, I'm ready to fight?' The potential problem is once treatment is started, you change your mind, and honestly, I need to make you understand that it is going to be hard, but numerous others have done it before you; it is not impossible. You need to understand that your mind will tell you it's not worth the trouble, it's too hard, what's the point? Get determined now, forgive yourself when thoughts are not positive, realise them for what they are and refocus.

Quality of life is frequently given as a reason to avoid treatment, but there is no quality of life in the final stages anyway.

Some people say they can't do treatment because it would take too long, so let me try and contextualise it for you.

Let's say you're 25 years old; would you give 1.38% of the life you've already lived to stay alive? (These figures are not 100% accurate to a decimal, but are accurate enough to illustrate.)

If you were 50 years old, would you give 0.69% of your life to stay alive?

And if you were a 60-year-old, would you happily give 0.57% to stay alive?

I think most people would say yes without hesitation.

Let me explain the figures so far.

A 25-year-old has lived 1300 weeks and basing it on six chemotherapy sessions three weeks apart, we get 18 weeks or 1.38% of the twenty-five years, but out of those six sessions, you're only going to feel sick for around a week for every treatment.

So rather than basing it on 18 weeks of treatment, it's really only six, which reduces the figure to 0.46%.

Jumping back to the 50-year-old at 0.69%, it reduces to 0.23%.

For the 60-year-old, it's now down to 0.19%.

All of the three examples are all less than half-of-one percent? It's a blink.

My calculations are based on time already lived, which isn't how life works; so you're having to spend the time as you go rather than somebody removing it from time already lived.

Irrespective, when you think about it, it's only a tiny percentage of your life.

It's hard to get your head around at diagnosis with treatment looming large, but it's far from impossible.

Don't think of treatment as a mountain to climb; think of it as a percentage of your life and it's minuscule.

An inconvenience you don't need, sure, but one you can handle.

I was initially given six months to live, then a couple of years later on a Wednesday morning they said I wouldn't see the weekend. My thoughts both times are unprintable, but basically 'rubbish' might be appropriate to sum up my feelings about my potential demise.

If I had accepted the weekend as my deadline, you probably wouldn't be reading this now.

Throughout my journey I have met other sufferers, and the one thing I notice is the change in their attitude when I tell them I've been where they are and beat it.

Money/health is wealth? Which one?

I have a friend who says that money is wealth. Every time I say, your health is your wealth, he counters it with, "no your wealth is your health because if anything goes wrong, you can get the best doctors," which seems to me to be a really stupid statement because if your health is your wealth, and your healthy, you're not going to need doctors in the first place. So while he's sitting there, puffing 40+ cigarettes per day, coughing all the time, and looking sick. He's under the impression that because he has money, and lots of property, if anything goes wrong, he can buy his way out of it, and it's one of those times where there is no talking to him. I can't convince him. His wife tries to convince him as she used to smoke but stopped. Friends try to convince him, but he is of the opinion that he is right. Some people, irrespective of the best will in the world, you just can't help.

Update

It would be fair to say I don't know the exact date I wrote the previous section, but I'm going to estimate two months, and during that time it turns out that wealth is health, did turn out to be total nonsense because during the time he was saying this, he had already been diagnosed with terminal inoperable lung cancer and didn't even tell his wife, but was quite happy to sit out the back having a barbecue and smoking 40+ cigarettes a day. He always said the more cigarettes he smoked, the better he could breathe.

I attended his funeral three days ago.

I spoke to his wife about his inclusion in the book and she said, "If it could stop just one person smoking, or make one person wise up, then maybe his death would mean something. So, yes, you have my blessing."

I knew the guy for about 10 years and he was a really straightforward honest nice guy, but smoking took over his life, arrogance took over his life, and ultimately, both took his life.

"A positive attitude may not solve all your problems, but it will annoy enough people to make it worth the effort."

~ Herm Albright

Four-minute mile

When Roger Bannister broke the four-minute mile on 6th May 1954, the time was confirmed as 3:59.4. Six-tenths of a second confirmed that after experts said the human body was not capable of breaking the four-minute barrier, they were wrong.

Relevance? I hear you ask.

Someone had done what they said couldn't be done, with the result that within six weeks of the record being set, John Landy shattered it in a time of 3:57.9 on 21st June 1954, which was only forty-six days later.

Attitude made all the difference, and I suspect if either man had been diagnosed with cancer, they wouldn't have considered it a death sentence, but a challenge.

The current record for a mile is 3:43.13, which is nearly sixteen seconds faster than Roger Banister's record, which at the time was amazing and (it was claimed) would never and could never be beaten.

Some scientists attribute the number of runners breaking the barrier to the reticular activating system (RAS) that helps the brain to focus on relevant information. The fact the record was broken meant other runners knew it could be done, so they did it, over and over.

The reticular activating system is an interesting brain development that I won't go into in too much detail, but the easiest way to explain it is the brain's ability to choose what it concentrates on. A good example is you've just purchased something really special, like a new car, coat, or watch, then everywhere you look someone else has exactly the same item; it's not that everyone just went out and purchased the same item, they've always been there, but your brain chooses to ignore them, then, when you have what you want, it unveils the real world. It's a type of protective mechanism as you can't cope with all the information in the world at once, so the brain filters out what might cause stress and can be ignored.

Moving back to cancer again, the fact is that when you meet someone who has already completed your journey and came out the other side, you know it's possible, and just knowing can make all the difference. The difference between acceptance and outrage; between life and death.

One of the methods Mr Banister used was visualisation. In his mind he did the run over and over, each time achieving what his body had been incapable of, but in his mind, he was a winner every time. When he attempted the run for real, his thinking was that he had already done it over and over with success, so his body and mind expected the outcome. Later in the book we will look at how visualisation can be used to make the journey through cancer much easier. It was one of the things I used extensively.

Tony Robbins tells about a basketball team who were all tested on their ability to get the ball in the net, then they were split into three groups. One group had to practice an exact number of shots each day, then stop. Another group were told to forget about basketball and relax. The third group were told to sit in a chair and practice getting the ball in every time in their mind. Now, which group do you think improved the most? Unlikely it's going to be the relax and forget group, which only leaves the ones who did practice and the ones who played in their mind. Surprisingly, the group with the biggest improvement were the mind players, the ones who visualised, the ones who never missed in their mind. When it came to actually doing it, they were so conditioned to never missing and expecting just that, they improved way more than those who did practice.

If you condition your mind to see yourself with a smile on your face celebrating your victory over cancer, it's way more powerful than if you just cross your fingers and hope.

Motivation can come from surprising places

Early on in my journey I was in Tesco's, shopping. At this stage I had maybe two treatments, and I had no hair, no eyebrows, and no eyelashes, so it was very clear I was either suffering from severe alopecia or had cancer. I remember it very clearly because it had a huge impact on my life at the time. I was standing at the counter waiting to be served when I felt a tap on my shoulder, I turned and there was a small elderly lady wearing a headscarf. At first glance I knew she had cancer when there were no eyebrows, then she looked up at me, smiled and said, "Don't worry big lad. I've had it twice and if I can do it at my age, you can do it too."

In a different section of this book I talk about the effect chemo can have on your emotions and specifically crying for no reason, so understandably, when you do have a reason—like someone older encouraging you—the tears start. I can remember people looking at me, but I didn't care, because ultimately, that lady give me something money can't buy, and that is hope and the realisation you're not in the fight on your own. She had already did it and was a lot older; I was younger, stronger, and determined. What chance did cancer have?

I can remember after she walked away, I said to my wife, "If she can do it, I can definitely do it."

By now, you already know how many times I've had cancer, so if I can do it? The next words out of your mouth (or going through your mind) should be, so can I.

Encouragement comes from strange and unexpected sources, but you have to participate in your own cure.

"When you have exhausted all possibilities, remember this: You haven't." ~ Thomas Edison

Okay, let's get started

In this book, we will be looking at ways of dealing with everything that appears in the cancer journey, from the initial diagnosis (and the effect it has on your mental state), throughout treatment, and afterwards.

You don't need to read this book in chronological order. You can dip in and out of the sections that interest you, but from my point of view, just writing this book made a difference to my understanding of the cancer journey. If it helped me, I have no doubt you will benefit from it as well.

What you don't want to do is look for a solution to a problem you might have avoided if you had read from start to finish, so although some sections might seem irrelevant, cancer has a way of surprising.

Irrespective of your diagnosis, you are reading a book written by a guy who has been diagnosed with multiple cancers and told several times he wouldn't live beyond a certain date. If nothing else, this should prove to you that it can be beaten, and now you've met someone who has done it, so if I can...

There are several types of patients when it comes to cancer.

The 'No-Treatment' Patient

Some people choose not to have any treatment due to their age or medical history or for other reasons. The outcome is predictable, but sometimes (rarely) the outcome is positive.

The 'Cure Me' Patient

I've got cancer and I don't want to know anything about it. Just cure me.

This is where the patient puts all responsibility on the doctors and sits back to see what happens.

The fact is, the treatment is what cures you, so if it's going to work there's nothing more you need to do, but relying on it alone and not joining in the fight is not something I would recommend.

If you adopt a positive attitude where you do everything you possibly can in addition to the chemo/treatment to beat your cancer, then the feel-good factor alone sets you up for a positive outcome, and the more you do, the more you want to do.

Conventional therapy on its own, without you eating, hydrating, and exercising, will probably kill you, irrespective of the cancer.

The 'fight' attitude is what will make you eat, drink, and exercise when you don't want to.

The 'Let's Fight This' Patient.

Okay, tell me what's involved? How did I get this? What's the survival rate? What chemotherapy will I be on and can I get more? Give me books on it. What else can I do to help myself?

For me, this is the ideal way to tackle cancer; it defines me. Frequently this group will force themselves to do everything the doctors recommend and more. They make use of therapies, exercise, meditate, eat well, hydrate themselves and maintain a positive attitude. They get into trouble if they walk in front of a mirror in a public place. They force themselves to places they've never experienced before. Doctors love this group as everyone is on the same team constantly working towards a positive outcome.

The 'I've Got A Better Way' Patient.

Alternative therapies are rife on the internet with more outrageous claims being made for the effectiveness of one miracle drug or another that the government/medical professionals won't tell you about. If any of these worked, they would be adopted for mainstream use.

Let me ask Dr Google

Almost all patients contact Dr Google or some other internet search engine to see if there is some new cure the doctors don't yet know about, and sometimes you will find something relevant that you can discuss with your consultant, but not often. (When I say not often, I mean, 'never'.)

Macmillan Cancer Support reports that surveys carried out revealed forty-two percent of people diagnosed with cancer, looked up their disease online. Personally, I think it's probably a lot higher.

You enter your particular cancer and are immediately inundated with results.

I typed in 'bladder cancer' and was given 9,910,000 results to view. Yes, nearly ten million websites relevant to bladder cancer.

Modify it to 'bladder cancer cure' and it returns 1,120,000 results.

Page one has all the recognised cancer sites such as government, research, hospitals, and the major charities, but I only needed to click to page two and halfway down I found the first of the 'quack' sites offering alternative therapies that don't work.

I found one called 'The Truth About Cancer', which opens as an informative page with a brief description of bladder cancer, some impressive pictures and then the 'magic cure' is wheeled out.

The article is attributed to Mr Ty Bollinger and he states the following:

"Not surprisingly, the "allopathic" (conventional) treatment options are surgery, chemotherapy, and radiation (the "Big 3"). If I were diagnosed with ANY TYPE OF CANCER, I would NEVER choose this "cut, poison, burn" protocol. In my opinion, it is barbaric."

In my opinion, Mr Bollinger hasn't had cancer and isn't qualified in any relevant way to comment on conventional medicine, but it's the internet and anyone can have an opinion, dangerous or not.

Further down the page he provides a helpful link to interviews with doctors that have been interviewed in what he calls 'The Global Quest Series', some of whom have been discredited as quacks with dubious qualifications.

My advice is be extremely careful about anything you find on the internet that claims to cure cancer, but if something does grab your attention, don't just take it at face value; research it exhaustively and if it still looks promising, seek further advice from qualified medical professionals.

There's an app for that.

Thousands of cancer sufferers all over the world have embraced technology and downloaded one of the many apps that claim to have the 'silver bullet' in the fight against cancer, but now, medical experts have called for the tech companies to act more responsibly as a lot of the apps are marketing unproven claims to beat cancer that simply don't work.

Tech giants such as Google and Apple have made many millions from apps such as Lifesum, which has been downloaded by more than 200,000 people in Britain alone in the last eighteen months and has more than twenty-five million users worldwide. Their website had an article titled, 'Adding a ketogenic to your cancer-fighting arsenal,' which claimed, 'Not only can the diet accelerate weight loss, but it's also been known to combat cancer.'

According to an estimate by app analyst Apptopia, the website has generated in excess of $7.7 million in revenue for the company since 2017.

After being contacted by The Times newspaper, they removed the article and issued a statement: 'Our official page for the ketogenic diet — and in-app content — makes no reference to the ongoing debate on the role of nutrition in cancer avoidance or treatment. However, we have removed a blog post in which we referenced some of the arguments being presented by those who advocate the diet as we feel it did not accurately reflect the complexity of the ongoing research.'

The fact is there have been no clinical trials in humans to substantiate any claim the ketogenic diet has any effect on cancer, and medical experts have warned that following a diet which restricts carbohydrates may have serious consequences as weight loss is likely to increase the side-effects of chemotherapy as you simply don't have enough energy.

Ben Goldacre, a senior clinical research fellow at the medical sciences division at Oxford University stated, "There is a sudden overwhelming tide of quackery in software," and "there needs to be more regulation in the app market."

Of course, there is a plethora of other apps that claim their cure is the best, which include the quack alternative cures known to either have no proven effect or actually make matters worse.

If there is money to be made, irrespective of the outcome, someone will step in to make a buck. The fact is they don't care whether you live or die; it's just about the money.

Another app called, The Ketodiet, claimed, 'A very low-carb ketogenic diet has been shown to help manage and even treat health conditions such as Alzheimer's, Parkinson's, and even Cancer.' When contacted by The Times regarding the claim they issued a statement: 'We actively discourage people from using the ketogenic diet itself as treatment for any conditions, and we always urge our users to contact medical professionals;' which would seem to contradict the initial claim.

If you find an app that offers a cure, be very wary, and if you consider using it, talk to your doctor first and seek advice.

The internet

I get it.

I did it.

I was persuaded to try the macrobiotic diet—which has absolutely no effect on cancer and can be detrimental to your health during treatment.

I've watched others do it.

You think you're dying, and you're trying to find a solution by searching the internet, because that's where the companies that make the real cure are hiding. Seriously?

The internet is great. There are lots of cancer sites that can help, and you already know who they are. Every major cancer charity has invested serious money in their web presence. They have online chat facilities with trained professionals waiting to help, and information sheets on every type of cancer, including yours. The doctors and nurses at your treatment centre can recommend lots of legitimate sites for you to browse, and occasionally, they'll point you in the direction of other helpful sites that aren't well known but are good.

If you're on FaceBook, there are groups for your cancer, but check the site first before you sign up and never give them your email address. Look for the number of members/followers and take your time. Once you find a group you can start to ask questions to other sufferers/survivors, and you will find them very helpful.

But then it happens. You get frustrated because you want the cure. The one that's hidden on the 'dark web' or recommended by a friend who has researched it.

You look at it and it seems professional. All you have to do is give them your email address and money every month and they'll do what the best medical minds in the world can't do. They'll cure you. Wow. How good is that?

Don't take my word for it. Sign up, and when you start getting little pills made of recycled shoes from Nigeria (the medical centre of excellence in the world of cancer), you can chew on them and think how lucky you are, and you'll also welcome all the emails you will be bombarded with that will definitely make your life better. On the bright side, there's also a fair chance someone will contact you and tell you you've won a lottery and all you have to do is send them an administration fee to claim it.

If you have cancer, or you're trying to help someone who has; realise the sufferer is emotionally weakened, and their guard is down, and that's a recipe criminals love. Don't do anything without thinking long and hard beforehand.

The cure for cancer does exist, but it's just for rich people.

I'm not going to try to convince you a magic cure doesn't exist, although that's what I believe; instead I'm going to give you a scenario and let you make up your own mind. You bought this book, so obviously you read, you're intelligent and open to ideas, so let's give it a go and see where we end up.

A guy working in a research lab finds the cure for cancer. He's tested it on every conceivable type of cancer, and it cures them all. What do you think he's going to do? It's his Eureka moment. He tells all his colleagues, he celebrates, he c it to his boss, but the boss tells him to keep quiet about it as the company is making too much money from cures that don't work.

Do you really think human nature works like this?

Months later, in a cruel twist of fate, one of his relatives or friends or spouse has cancer—a life-threatening cancer—and he has a guaranteed cure, but he can't tell anyone as he's signed a Non-Disclosure Agreement with the company. Do you really think he's going to keep quiet? Would you? Do you think he's not going to find a way to synthesise the cure somewhere else and cure his brother, mother, father or friend, or just tell the media?

If it has already been found could it be that Big Pharma has a group of researchers held somewhere on a remote island so that the rest of the world won't find out?

The magic cure (as yet) doesn't exist, or if it does, only rich people and celebrities can get it, like Steve Jobs, or Paul Allen… No, wait, they're both dead. Both were billionaires. I've already mentioned Steve Jobs elsewhere in this book, but Paul Allen, co-founder of Microsoft, died 15th October 2018 as a result of septic shock when naturally produced chemicals to fight infections in the bloodstream caused severe inflammation. Yes, he had Non-Hodgkin Lymphoma, same as me. He wasn't a millionaire, he was a billionaire, worth over $20 billion. Any funds necessary for any treatment that could conceivably have cured him wasn't a problem. He could easily have thrown several billion at it and it still wouldn't have made a dent. So, believe me, the magic cure rumoured to exist for rich people, celebrities, and heads of state, doesn't exist.

The cure is a combination of your determination and the doctors' best efforts with what we currently have available. No, it's not perfect. No, it's not guaranteed to cure you. No, realistically, there isn't an alternative, yet.

Putting coffee up your bum or eating almond seeds or drinking any amount of witch-doctor-tea will not make a difference.

Every day we're getting better, and yes, every time something new comes along it costs; but it costs a huge amount to develop these drugs. Some are tested and found to be unusable after millions have been invested; and some work, but if we want to progress, further research has to be done on a continuous basis, which costs money, and the cancer funding fairy hasn't been seen in years, so the companies at the cutting edge of cancer research have to not only recoup their investment, but invest even more in search of the ultimate cure.

In America, health care does cost a huge amount of money, but a lot of countries provide free health care, so it's not the fault of pharmaceutical companies, it's the fault of government.

You can't invest in research if you're giving the medicine away.

It's not ideal, but it is realistic.

I have no doubt that the Eureka moment will come, and when it does, short of killing everyone with knowledge of the cure, nobody is going to keep it quiet. Nobody can. In today's connected world, it's going to get out.

Until that time comes, the best option is real medicine administered by real doctors. It's not perfect, but it's the best we have.

I plead with you not to go down the alternative medicine route and believe the hype and moo-cow-poo people make a fortune from. They aren't the ones gambling with their lives. You die, they don't care.

Tim Minchin hit it on the head when he said, "What do they call alternative medicine that works? Medicine."

If it works, we use it and it's adopted worldwide once proven.

Seriously, do you really believe a cure for the biggest disease on the planet could be kept quiet?

This is where I've either convinced you or not. Either way, I've done my best.

Cancer Myths and Facts

When diagnosed with cancer—and irrespective of what your consultant tells you—the usual place to research your problem is the internet, and although it contains a wealth of accurate information, there are many more sites that will scare you with ideas that have been scientifically proven to be wrong. Many of them will make perfect sense in the context presented, but they can do more harm than good.

Cancer is a death sentence

Nope, this is wrong. I could go into all sorts of cancer statistics and produce evidence that survival rates are increasing, but you don't have to go any further than the author of this book (me) to know cancer is not (necessarily) a death sentence. Throughout the world cancer survival rates are on the increase due to advancements in treatment.

Sugar gives you cancer

No, it doesn't. This myth is based on the fact that a PET scan is dependent on a small amount of radioactive tracer—typically a form of glucose—to locate the cancer cells. When this is injected, the cancer cells light up, so it was thought that sugar or glucose feeds the cells and causes cancer.

The fact is, sugar doesn't make cancer cells grow any faster or slower. The reason cancerous tissue absorbs more of the tracer is because cancer cells develop faster than normal cell tissue.

Consuming large amounts of sugar can be associated with an increased risk of cancer due to obesity and diabetes, but not feeding cells or turning regular cells into cancerous ones.

All cells prefer to use sugar for fuel, but can also use fat and protein, so cutting out sugar from your diet will not starve the cancer cells as the body will substitute the sugar with glucose anyway.

To completely exclude sugar from your diet you would have to stop eating bread, cereal, rice, pasta, milk, yoghurt, custard, fruit, potatoes, corn, soft drinks, fruit juice, etc. To get to the level required to cause cell death, you would also be killing the cells keeping you alive, and it's impossible anyway as you would already be dead.

Artificial Sweeteners cause cancer

No. Initially studies on rats tested in the early 70s linked certain substances used in artificial sweeteners to the development of cancer, but subsequent carcinogenicity studies have concluded there is no evidence of the same happening to humans.

Acidic foods cause cancer

As cancer thrives in an acidic environment, it was thought you could slow the growth or eradicate the cancer by eating an 'alkaline' diet; however, regardless of changes in diet, the body controls its own pH level.

If you could alter your blood pH level, your normal cells would not be able to survive and you would die anyway.

Surgery or biopsy causes the spread of cancer to other tissue

Technically, this is possible, but extremely rare. During biopsies and procedures, surgeons take steps to prevent any possibility of this by using different tools for each area and a high standard of hygiene. Realistically, nothing is ever perfect, but modern medicine is as near as you can get.

Cancer gets worse if exposed to air

No. Air has no effect on cancer cells.

Mobile/Cell Phones cause cancer

Cell phones do not cause cancer. Cancer is caused by genetic mutations and not by the low-frequency energy that cell phones emit. The fact brain tumour rates haven't changed much since the introduction of mobile phones over twenty years ago would tend to support this conclusion as mobile use has increased dramatically. But… I will admit to being dubious about 5G as there seems to have been little testing done, and no definitive studies as to the potential effects of the signal which is much stronger. I guess this one is going to be a wait and see scenario, but I suspect it will turn out okay.

Of course, I could be talking rubbish, because when I sent the book out to my beta readers, one, in particular, came back very aggressively and said she had seen a video showing three mobile phones sitting around an uncooked egg and after sixty-five minutes the egg was cooked solid.

I said, "That can't happen," but just to be sure, I did a search and found the relevant video. It was a hoax attributed to Charles Ivermee who put it on the web because of the concern people had about their brain being fried from using a mobile phone. He found it all a bit silly, so thought he would add to the silliness.

The guy seems to have the same sense of humour I have. If somebody thinks something stupid, I would either—depending on the seriousness—prove them right or prove them wrong. The problem with this is of course it's too important.

People stop using mobile phones because they think radiation will fry their brain. It was also shown that mobile phones can make corn pop. The problem with that video was it was found to be nothing more than clever editing with the exploding corn nothing more than a digital erase and the subsequent popcorn nothing more than someone above physically dropping it into the picture.

CANCEROLOGY

In October 2005, the television program Brainiac tried to cook an egg by placing it under a pile of 100 cell phones. At the end of it when they checked the egg, it was completely uncooked, cold, and no different from before the test.

Putting it in simple terms, you could probably cook an egg with a hairdryer, as it produces heat. I checked the specs for a cheap hairdryer, and they are available from 1000 watts to 2500 watts. A phone produces 0.25 watt when it's on, so for just 1000 watts you would need 4000 mobile phones, but unlike a hairdryer where the energy is focused on the egg, the phones are dispersing the energy all around, so it's impossible to cook an egg with a phone.

Power lines cause cancer

No. Power lines emit electric energy (which is shielded and weakened by walls and other objects) and magnetic energy (which is a low-frequency form of radiation) has no effect on genes.

My mum/dad/brother/sister had cancer, so I'll get it as well

Five to ten percent of cancers can be passed down, but thankfully, it's not guaranteed. If there is a history of cancer in your family, it's worthwhile mentioning it to your doctor to see if any tests need to be carried out.

Nobody in my family has had cancer, so I can't get it

Sorry, but this is incorrect. 1 in 2 people will get it at some point in their lives. Environmental factors such as your work or exposure to tobacco and radiation can have an impact on your health, irrespective of your family history.

Antiperspirants or deodorants cause breast cancer

Tests on the chemicals used have been conducted and no evidence has been found to link the use to cancer.

Hair dye causes cancer

No. During normal use, there is no risk; however, exposure to large quantities of hair dye and other chemical products used at a hairdresser or barbers' shop may increase the risk of bladder cancer.

Good people don't get cancer

New-born babies can have cancer. Enough said.

Microwave ovens cause cancer

No. Providing the microwave isn't leaking, they are safe.

Microwaving plastic containers and wraps causes cancer

No. Provided the containers and wraps are microwave-safe products, there is no risk.

Containers not intended for use in microwaves can melt and leak chemicals into the food.

Cancer is contagious

No, cancer isn't contagious in the normal scheme of things, but in the case of an organ or tissue transplant, in theory, this is possible; however, testing the tissue before transplant should ensure this doesn't happen as anyone with a history of cancer is not eligible to be a donor.

If you're living with or working with someone who has cancer, there is no chance of contracting it from them in the normal scheme of things.

Viruses are contagious and can lead to the development of cancer.

The HPV (Human Papillomavirus) can be transmitted through sexual intercourse and can lead to cervical and some other forms of cancer.

Hepatitis B or C can be transmitted through sexual intercourse or infected needles and can cause liver cancer.

Attitude can cause cancer and a poor outcome

No. Officially, attitude can't cause cancer or lead to a poor outcome; however, from my own experience I've found a positive attitude can dramatically increase your tolerance of treatment and your long-term success.

At the start of this book, I mentioned my brother and how he took the stairs to receive his diagnosis from the doctor and afterwards took the lift down. In his mind, he had just been given the official qualification to be sick and to act sick. Never mind the fact there was no difference in his health from going in to see the doctor and coming out; he was now entitled to play-it-up, to seek sympathy, and ultimately give up, which he did.

If you think you're at death's door, and you knock on death's door, eventually, it will open.

The good, the bad, and the ugly

Although there are various grades and stages for all cancers, I'd like to throw another three classifications into the mix. These (as far as I'm aware) are my own and are the result of observing and talking to various patients over the years.

One of the worst days in anyone's life is the day they discover they have cancer, but it can also be the day your life changes for the better. The first day for the rest of your life?

The good

A cancer diagnosis can never be considered good or lucky, but for those whose treatment is successful first time and for whom cancer never returns, it's a good result.

Depending on the treatment received, there may or may not be long term side-effects, but even if there are, it's a small price to pay to continue living.

On my journey through cancer, I've known a lot of people who have found themselves in remission after the first treatment and I have talked to a lot of them, both during and after treatment, and with very few exceptions they said cancer changed their lives for the better. When you consider the severity of a cancer diagnosis, you may think that's a strange thing to say. How can something so bad change your life for the better?

A cancer diagnosis focuses the mind. It makes you realise you're only here for a limited time. It makes you think about how you are living and have lived your life up to now—thoughts you would never have owned up to become foremost in your mind. You start to think how you should live the rest of your life as opposed to just living without thinking, which is what the gift of health allows you to do.

For me, cancer calmed me down (eventually), made me think, made me write this book in an effort to help others. It would never have been written had I not had cancer. I would have kept on chasing money and never taken the time to appreciate everyday things. Something as simple as a tree or a flower now puts a smile on my face, whereas pre-cancer, I had no interest and was unaware of the wonders around me.

A friend of mine had cancer that went into remission after treatment, and he has gone from being a bit of a twat to a cancer counsellor and he studies hard to be the best he can be. He's making a massive difference to other people going through the cancer experience, and, as he's been-there-done-that, they listen even more intently to what he has to say. He's had thank-you cards and letters about how he's changed/saved lives, which he would never have had if he had carried on in his pre-cancer ways. And no, he hasn't turned it into a business as he works with one of the major cancer charities. I met him several weeks before writing this, and he was going for even more training.

In his previous life, he was a scallywag, and that's putting it mildly. I suspect if he hadn't had cancer, he might well have died as a result of his activities, so cancer not only changed his life, but possibly saved it and enabled him to help others.

Due to the inactive time spent fighting cancer, it gives you time to reflect on your journey so far; mistakes and regrets you never realised you had pop into your mind, but now you have the time to learn the lessons necessary to avoid repetition; to live a more meaningful life. I'm not suggesting you'll become the best person on the planet, but you will be a better you.

The good classification is a great place to be, as lots of survivors can confirm.

The bad

I'm sure it won't come as a surprise to discover that the bad is when someone gets cancer and dies.

Unfortunately, there are still many people who don't make it, but thankfully, this number is reducing due to research, clinical trials, new drugs, and methods being refined and discovered all the time.

The side-effect is the death of the patient, but the short and long-term side-effects are present for those left behind.

As advised throughout this book, counselling is essential to help loved ones come to terms with the loss.

It doesn't seem to matter how much death is expected, it still comes as a surprise to everyone, and no matter how prepared they think they are, it's never enough.

Unanswered and unanswerable questions that mainly revolve around the word why, are ever-present, and it can have a devastating effect on those left behind if they fail to obtain closure, especially children.

Counsellors are specifically trained to help the families of people living with cancer, so although I hope this is a service you never have to use, it's useful to know it does exist, and making use of it should not be seen as a failure.

The bad classification is not a good conclusion, but it is always a possibility for anyone with a cancer diagnosis.

The ugly

Survival is the ultimate goal with any cancer diagnosis, both for you and your family/friends, and also your doctors, but sometimes success brings its own problems.

My ugly definition applies where the sufferer survives the initial and subsequent cancers, but is never cured or remission attained. Cancer moves from being just an illness to a state of being where it is ever-present but controlled with medicine, and this stage is known as chronic.

The dictionary defines it as—an illness persisting for a long time or constantly recurring. The term is often applied when the course of a disease lasts for more than three months and where the person is restricted in performing at least two activities of daily living such as eating, toileting, bathing and dressing, or requires considerable supervision to prevent injury or problems.

This is the stage I've been suspended in, on-and-off, since my original diagnosis, and I've had so many recurrences, I now refer to cancer as one of my hobbies. Some might say it's a silly way to look at a serious condition, but it's my way. I suspect it's a coping mechanism on my part as continually thinking about cancer and the ramifications would drive you nuts. It's got to the stage where if I don't have problems with it, I wonder what's wrong.

Irrespective of how you choose to look at it and deal with its implications, you now lead a curtailed lifestyle as you've been inconsiderate enough to allow yourself to get cancer yet again.

Inconsiderate is a weird word to use in the previous sentence and might seem incorrect, but having asked others, it seems to be how some of us think, and while we have no control whether it recurs, it feels like we bring it on ourselves, even though that isn't the case. In effect, we feel like we somehow failed.

For example, in 2016 I was feeling okay when a last-minute offer of a cruise presented itself, so I booked it only to find out a couple of weeks before I was due to go, they had found yet another tumour in my bladder. Of course, I didn't have insurance, as those of us who have had cancer over and over have little to no chance of obtaining travel insurance, and on the rare occasion it is offered, the cost is prohibitive.

The outcome of my diagnosis was the loss of the money paid for the cruise, but, if you consider a family in the same circumstances where holidays have been arranged from work, kids taken out of school, etc., and you have a significant stress event for the family as a whole, and, in addition, the decision has to be made as to whether or not everyone should stay behind or only the patient. If everyone stays, there is resentment from those deprived, and if they go, there is resentment from the patient and guilt for everyone else. It's an unwinnable stress bomb that is relevant to all aspects of living with cancer and caring for a cancer patient.

With the ugly cancer, it is important to consider the point of view of both the sufferer and the carer/family, as all parties are affected.

From the long-term carer's point of view, they may feel you're holding them back from living a full and normal life, and from your point of view, they're healthy, and you're jealous; and yes, jealous is the right word. It's not a planned perception on your part, but you've been dealt a lousy hand and they haven't.

Over time, there can be a steady build-up of resentment towards anyone who isn't suffering.

Sufferers can often be stubborn, and depression frequently enters into the equation both for the sufferer and long-term carer.

The loss of control the patient feels can drive them crazy, and I'm not necessarily talking mobility issues; more the fact their bodies have developed a disease that has the potential to kill and they have no control over it.

The inability to do things they were physically/mentally capable of before the disease is frustrating and serves to increase the stress on the patient.

Where there is more than one carer, it is usual for one to be more sympathetic than the other, which can mean the sufferer tends to prefer the sympathetic one over the one that will encourage them to do something they don't feel like doing, even though it's in their best interest.

When I had Stem Cell Treatment, it was very stressful, and my mental state was nowhere near where it usually would have been. I remember calling my wife several times one day and could never get a reply. As frustration turned to anger, I called her work and left a message to say I was being taken to a hospice (A home for the terminally ill) and not to bother calling back.

Friends who later became aware of this immediately dismissed it as a momentary blip due to the treatment, and I even excused myself with the same excuse, but consider how this message was received by my wife.

Patients don't usually do it with any intention to hurt, but more to ensure the recipient is paying enough attention, and although it's understandable, it's avoidable with a) the knowledge it can/will happen and b) the acceptance, expectation, and plan on how to deal with it when it arrives.

Looking back, it was a horrific thing to do, but at the time, there was no thought given to any potential shock at receiving the news

Conventional Cancer Treatments

Sometimes referred to as the 'cut, poison and burn' method by alternative therapy practitioners that don't recommend it; however, this is what worked for me and countless others I have met on my journey.

Surgery (cut)

Surgery can be used to diagnose cancer (such as removal of a lymph node) and remove some, or all, of a cancer tumour, including healthy tissue from surrounding areas called the margin, which is taken away in an attempt to improve the chances that all the cancer has been removed. Irrespective of the success of the surgery, it is usual to use adjuvant therapy (A belt-and-braces approach to remove any remaining cancer cells that may have been missed during surgery) to suppress secondary tumour formation (usually chemotherapy or radiation).

Diagnostic Surgery (cut)

Used to make a definitive diagnosis by analysis of suspect tissue, the surgeon performs a biopsy.

Incisional Biopsy (cut)

The removal of a piece of the suspicious area for examination.

Excisional Biopsy (cut)

The removal of the entire suspicious area, such as a mole or lump.

Laparoscopic Surgery (cut)

Normally referred to as 'keyhole' surgery.

Three small incisions are used to access the area using a lighted tube with a camera, and the offending tissue removed.

When they removed my kidney, this was the method used. I was left with two very small scars and one slightly larger which was used to remove the kidney.

Laser Surgery (burn)

A narrow beam of high-intensity light is used to remove cancerous tissue.

During my bladder cancer treatment, a laser was used to burn off the cancerous tissue prior to chemotherapy.

Ablation (burn)

Ablation is used if you have had previous surgery or if you're not considered strong enough to endure initial surgery. It is performed using a fine needle which is guided by an ultrasound or CT scanner, and inserted directly into the tumour and then heated with the aim of burning the cancer cells. Treatment takes around 30-60 minutes and you will be given a local anaesthetic to numb the skin. The side effects are usually mild and include pain in the area of the insertion which may last for 5-7 days, with the possibility of a fever, feeling unwell and tired. The side effects are due to the body eliminating the cells that have been burnt and it is recommended to rest and drink plenty of water.

Cryosurgery (burn)

Liquid nitrogen is used to freeze and kill abnormal cells.

Mohs Micrographic Surgery (Microscopically Controlled Surgery)

Normally used by a dermatologist who shaves off a skin cancer, one layer at a time, until all the cells appear normal when viewed under a microscope.

Chemotherapy (poison)

Chemotherapy is basically a variety of chemicals that have been proven to have success with various cancers. They are injected into the bloodstream in an attempt to kill all the cancer cells and stop them reproducing.

Unfortunately, they also kill normal cells which result in sickness, weakness, hair loss, etc.

It is an inexact science as no two people present with the same symptoms or stage of progression, but experience and research has provided us with details, records, and statistics showing how successful treatment is likely to be.

Essentially, it is the treatment that worked for me.

Hormonal Therapy (poison)

Hormonal therapy involves the manipulation of the endocrine system through the use of specific hormones, particularly steroid hormones, or drugs which inhibit the production or activity of such hormones (hormone antagonists).

The endocrine system is a network of glands (pancreas, hypothalamus and adrenal glands, pineal gland, pituitary gland, ovaries, testes, thyroid gland, and parathyroid gland) that produce and secrete hormones to organs and tissue.

The best-known example of hormonal therapy is the use of the selective estrogen-response modulator Tamoxifen for the treatment of breast cancer.

Cancer Immunotherapy (poison)

This is the use of the immune system to beat cancer by causing the rogue cells to commit cellular suicide or apoptosis. For example, Rituxan is drawn to a cell-surface marker on B cells called CD20. During my first lymphoma treatment this was just being introduced and I was given it in addition to CHOP. It is now a recognised therapy that produces results.

In my treatment of bladder cancer, I also have experience of immunotherapy in the form of BCG (Bacillus Calmette-Guerin) treatment, and it is very effective.

Radiation Therapy or Radiotherapy (burn)

Radiation therapy uses high-energy radiation in an attempt to shrink tumours and kill cancer cells.

It is normally prescribed by a radiation oncologist with intent to either cure the tumour or prevent growth of other cancer cells after a tumour has been removed.

Notes

Although I have indicated whether the procedures fall into the cut, poison, or burn categories, it is for clarification purposes only, and as shown, I have had many of the procedures throughout my treatment—none of which I would even consider refusing if they were ever necessary again.

"You can be a victim of cancer, or a survivor of cancer. It's a mindset." – Dave Pelzer

Mental Issues

The first thing that will have a significant impact immediately after diagnosis is your mental state. This happens before treatment has started, and even if the condition was expected, the fact it has now been confirmed will have the brain searching through all your life experiences trying to find a way to deal with it.

Your mind will be all over the place and you won't be able to concentrate. Sleep patterns may be affected. You will find yourself constantly thinking of the cancer, and the treatment, and your funeral; last thing at night before you go to bed, during the night, first thing in the morning and throughout the day. It takes over your life, and it is at this stage most people will pay a visit to their friendly local doctor, who—although trained to deal with cancer patients—isn't going to be a great deal of help.

Depending on your doctor, it is usual with a diagnosis of cancer for the patient to be prescribed anti-depressants. This is usually as a result of either a personal request, due to the mind becoming muddled and an inability to concentrate or think of anything for any period of time without an overwhelming sense of foreboding and panic, or a recommendation from a friend/relative who has your best interests in mind. The wakeup for me came when I did a course on psychology with the Open University and it explained the differences between internal and external problems (nature vs nurture) that can lead to depression.

Keeping it at its most simple; depression can be brought on gradually by pressures at work or relationship problems or any number of other issues, and these are known as external triggers. It's not a chemical imbalance in the brain which would be an internal issue, and the new way of trying to solve this type of problem is through analysis into what is causing the problem in the first place (cancer, treatment, potential death), gaining an understanding of why your mind is not processing the information, and suggesting ways to combat it, rather than popping a few pills.

It's easy for most people to determine if a another is depressed as it displays physically, with slumped shoulders, lack of movement, withdrawn attitude, etc., and one of the quickest ways to improve mood is movement. Movement is improvement, motion is lotion; exercise releases dopamine (the feel-good hormone), and it can be as simple as a walk around the garden to get a little lift. Is it a quick fix? No, but, little and often has rewards. Again… you have to participate in your own cure; you have to do things you never considered before and accept that although they may not bring immediate results, the cumulative effect is what we're after.

Sometimes, the best way to reset is to simply let it out, which can be done with a relative or friend, or even somewhere quiet where you can cry, scream, or shout. Everyone has their own coping mechanism, but all too often, expectations of what others may think restricts action. Give yourself a chance and stop worrying about how others might view your behaviour. If you do bottle it up, you're only storing it until such times as it explodes, which is when family and friends will be on the receiving end. The phrase, 'we hurt the ones we love' is there for a reason, so whatever you do, avoid at all costs.

At their best, the pills on the market can take weeks to have any real effect anyway, so it's not something that should be prescribed for cancer patients in an effort to sort out something which is clearly an external problem. The main concern is you have been given a life-changing diagnosis and your brain is trying to deal with it to the detriment of all else. The best advice I can give is to seek professional help by talking to your consultant or one of the counsellors from the major cancer charities.

"What?" I hear you ask. "Like a psychiatrist or shrink?"

Yes. There. I've said it, and I know it's not what you want to hear, and some of you will be stoic and think it's a failure to even consider asking for help, but just think of it this way. When you have car trouble you take it to a garage. If it's mechanical, a mechanic fixes it, but if it's electrical, then an electrician fixes it, or if it's had the paintwork damaged, a painter fixes it, or if it's been in an accident, a bodyworker fixes it. Your body is just like a car. When you break an arm, you go to casualty/emergency and they put it in plaster, when you have cancer you see an oncologist or haematologist, but when your brain is overloaded and muddled with thoughts of cancer, you need to see someone to help you process the information.

It's not a failure. It's common sense. It's practical. It's using the facilities available to you to fight cancer in the best way possible.

From my experience, you will see a psychologist and not a psychiatrist. The difference is a psychologist won't prescribe you with medication but will help you work through your understanding of what your body is going through and suggest methods to deal with everything.

Think about it. It makes a lot more sense and it's going to have a positive effect on your mind after the first consultation. Understanding the why, and how to deal with it, makes life a lot easier.

You can also get immediate help from any of the major cancer charities as they all have trained counsellors who have experience with lots of other patients and can work wonders with your worries.

Lots of people see asking for help as some sort of failure, and this is particularly true once you pass a certain age, but, get over yourself. This has hit you and there is help available. It's a no-brainer to take advantage of it.

All of the above was true for me and a lot of other people I met on the cancer journey; however, as each of us are different, I recommend that if depression rears its ugly head, you seek help from either a medical professional (preferably) or ask someone from one of the major cancer charities to help.

Do not start using St John's-wort, which is a herbal remedy recommended for depression by practitioners of herbal/alternative medicine. It compromises the tumour fighting abilities of chemotherapy and can have adverse side effects.

The best advice is not to use any supplements or therapies unless specifically recommended by a real doctor. Later in this book you will find out about some doctors who have either bought bogus qualifications off the internet or just haven't bothered with any form of training and simply use the honorific without any foundation.

The other major impact which is usually never explained or expected is the way your diagnosis will affect your closest relatives. Your spouse, your children, your parents, your relatives, your workmates, etc.

"But I'm the one with cancer," I hear you say. Yes, but if you put yourself in someone else's shoes, you'll start to understand. They start off asking themselves if they will lose their loved one and move on to how quick it all was, and how could it happen to them. How are they going to deal with the death? Yes, they too will jump to conclusions.

The five stages of grief. (DABDA)

Cancer is a roller coaster of emotions. From the day you receive the initial diagnosis, to the last day of treatment and beyond, your mind will play tricks on you, and it helps if you not only know what to expect once your emotions and feelings go on a rampage, but how to accept and deal with them as they appear.

The main problem with these emotions is the simple fact that nobody tells you about them. You initially get hit with the denial stage and can go straight to depression, which isn't in any way helpful in your fight.

You might have noticed the acronym DABDA above. It stands for Denial, Anger, Bargaining, Depression, and Acceptance.

In 1969 a Swiss-American psychiatrist called Elisabeth Kübler-Ross published her book, 'On Death and Dying', which introduced her theory on the five stages of grief, and they are very relevant to a cancer diagnosis.

Although widely accepted as an international model, it is important to understand that everyone will have a different experience at each of the levels. Some people might not experience some of the stages at all, while some might go through them in sequence or out of sequence or revisit them. There is no right or wrong.

The stages are listed in the usual order they appear and are a guide of what to expect, but in reality, you can expect everything and anything hitting you at any one time.

The main thing to remember is this isn't unusual. It's a process the mind uses to cope, so don't feel guilty.

Denial

If you've been expecting a cancer diagnosis due to ill health or family history, this stage may either affect you less, or not at all, but if you've been of the opinion you were healthy and suddenly been diagnosed, then it's probably going to pay you a visit.

In this stage the mind denies the diagnosis altogether, refusing to accept it as fact.

Phrases such as: 'Not me, I'm healthy,' or 'Nothing will happen, I'll cure it myself,' or 'They've made a mistake,' may play through your mind over and over. It's not something you can control unless you know the process, but even then, the mind tends to do its own thing.

Denial is the way the mind chooses to deal with the diagnosis; it helps us to cope in the short term. It is nature's way of deciding how much we can handle. At this stage, you already know what you are facing is a reality, but the denial stage can help to pace the mind and give it time to absorb the situation.

You may experience feelings of numbness and wondering if or why you should go on, but ultimately it will pass.

How long does it last? There is no answer I can give as it depends on a lot of things such as life experience, intelligence, beliefs, demeanour, etc., but the very fact you are now aware of its existence as a normal process should help you get through it much easier.

On my journey, I didn't experience the denial stage as the diagnosis was not only expected but welcomed, due to problems in the previous two years.

Anger

Once the denial stage is concluding, your thoughts might turn to anger as to why you have been chosen to face this disease. Phrases such as, 'This is unfair,' or 'Why me?' or 'What have I done to deserve this?' might take over in your mind, and the realisation that, 'Yes. I do have cancer,' can push you over the edge.

Anger is dangerous as it has no limits. It can manifest in screaming, shouting, breaking things, using phrases to specifically hurt those around you, and sadly, physical violence in some cases. Once the fog descends, even the most timid person can start to throw their weight around, and the people on the receiving end are usually those closest; spouse, father, mother, children, siblings, friends, and colleagues will all suffer at this stage, and while it is you accept this is a normal and necessary stage to go through, it is also a stage that has to be managed.

Sometimes, anger can make you look for a scapegoat, and it is also normal to blame the doctors for not diagnosing it soon enough or even for diagnosing it in the first place. You will blame anyone and everyone, and even though your rational mind tells you it's irrational, it's extremely hard to get control.

It's a theme throughout this book that there is help available and being stoic and not asking for it is a recipe for disaster.

Accept that you will feel angry. The more you accept it, the quicker you can pass through this stage.

Be aware it can creep up on you and take over if someone says something you don't agree with, or the kettle is filled with too much or too little water, or the batteries in the remote are flat.

It's easier said than done, but, when you lose control, try to regain it by going somewhere quiet and simply thinking about the big picture. If you throw the remote at the TV, you're going to have to replace the telly, which puts even more stress on you, which makes you angry all over again. Take a step back and think, but don't beat yourself up. The fact you've taken control and realised the problem exists is a massive achievement in itself, so work from that point on and give yourself a pat on the back.

If you do lose your temper, fix it. Apologise and move on. Accept it's not your fault and forgive yourself.

Again, for me, this stage wasn't one I experienced with the initial diagnosis as I've always had a pragmatic approach to life and know things don't necessarily happen for a reason. When something unexpected happens, there's not much you can do about it, other than deal with it as best you can.

I did have bouts of anger during treatment later (see: Roid rage) which were unrelated to the diagnosis, and yes, I broke things and at one stage my daughter was making a lot of noise and after repeatedly telling her to keep it down, I lost it. As parents, we weren't into hitting the kids, but I punched her on the arm; only once, but once is one time too many. I think she was shocked more than anything else and there was no bruise the next day, but in my diary I wrote, 'I was a complete bastard tonight, I hit my girl.' I didn't need to write anything else as I knew I'd never forget it. Yes, I regretted it immediately and tried my hardest to make up for what I did, but you can't. Irrespective of forgiveness and understanding, you'll never forgive yourself.

Please pay attention to this particular section as it can overwhelm you without warning and lead to disastrous results.

Bargaining

You've denied you have it, you've got angry about it, and now at stage three, you will appeal to whatever deity you believe in to give you a break.

Could it be a complete cure, or lesser diagnosis, or at least a postponement is possible?

Irrespective of your beliefs, most people like to think there is some higher power managing everything, and so bargaining comes into play; even with yourself.

'If I do (whatever sacrifice you're prepared to make), can I survive?'

'I'll never smoke/drink/do drugs again, so make it go away.'

'I'll jog every day and eat healthily and it'll go away.'

'If only . . . What if . . . I'll change . . .'

None of them work. No effect whatsoever. Nada. Zilch.

It is also usual to offer to stop things that we have always known to be wrong, such as smoking, and you need to be careful not to start blaming yourself. You can't go back in time and undo anything. What is done is done. Accept it and move on; you've more important things to be concentrating on.

Although this book is specifically targeted at cancer sufferers, the process of grief applies to everyone involved from the date of diagnosis and includes close family members worrying on your behalf.

A horrible example of extreme bargaining is: 'Please, God, take my wife/brother/father instead of me', which is outrageous, but does happen. The mind is just too mixed up to think rationally and things you would never have previously considered raise their ugly head.

I was guilty of bargaining, and frequently prayed to a God I never believed in with various deals I was prepared to do if only…

For some reason, He never replied, or maybe He did and that's why I'm still here. Who knows?

Depression

It is essential to realise that depression can creep up on you from the minute you are diagnosed, during treatment, and after treatment, and it's not just you; members of your family can be affected as well.

The feeling of having to relinquish control over your life and put it in the hands of doctors, and being powerless, can overcome you with feelings that can make it a struggle just to get out of bed in the morning.

'I give up.'

'Nothing matters anymore.'

'It's not going to work.'

'I'm dying and there's nothing I can do about it.'

All of the above and more will invade your thoughts, but it is important to understand this is not a mental illness. It is a normal and natural response to external pressures that have suddenly been exposed in one ugly package.

When we're under pressure, the brain will search frantically for a solution and can simply overload your rational thought process. If someone close to you was diagnosed, the stages of grief would be much less, and you would be in a position to give helpful advice due to the fact you're not the one under the most pressure, so you have to include that in the equation and think it through.

Depression—if left to its own devices—can ultimately drive people to suicide, so talking things through (honestly) with a professional can have immense benefits. Don't be afraid to ask for help.

It can also be helpful to look at life with a 'glass-half-full' attitude. Think about it. You're not dead. Someone, somewhere, is worse off than you. Someone with the same diagnosis has already beat it.

I'm repeating myself, but again, when you realise you're going through this stage, you need to accept it as natural and forgive yourself.

For me, this stage was the worst. Later in the book I will tell you about my suicide attempt, but for now, it's enough to say it snared me. It manifested itself in anger against the world, and I said a lot of things I now regret. It's one of the problems doctors frequently encounter with cancer patients and the usual remedy is to 'pop a pill' to cure it, but as I said before, depression, in this case, usually isn't caused by internal mechanisms going wrong, rather it is a reaction to the diagnosis.

One of the other problems with a diagnosis of depression is that it's like a qualification for some. People do or say something wrong, then excuse it with, "Oh, not my fault. I'm depressed." It's like the doctor has given you a get-out-of-jail-free card.

If a doctor says you have depression, it must be correct, but in the majority of cases, people say how they feel; "I think I'm depressed, Doc," and the doctor says, "Yes, it does sound like you're depressed," and you eagerly agree because you want something to lift your mood—you want a quick fix.

You get the pills, and because they're for depression, it follows you have depression, so you better act like you think a depressed person would act, and behave like you think a depressed person would behave.

Newsflash, you probably aren't depressed. Your mind is struggling to process your diagnosis and the future and has never been under so much pressure, but that's not depression, it's pressure, and the good news is it can be dealt with, and the even better news is that you are probably the best person to do it.

Before you visit a doctor, figure out in your mind why you need the appointment in the first place. Take a quiet 10 or 15 minutes, or an hour, or a day, or go for a walk and ask yourself, "Why am I feeling like I'm feeling?"

The obvious answer is cancer, but we're looking for the not-so-obvious answers.

Write everything down you can think of, and it doesn't matter how silly or trivial you think it is; write it down.

I've got cancer.

I'm dying.

My mum/dad/brother/sister/neighbour/friend/work colleague/pet died of cancer, so I'll die too.

I can't work/they need me at work.

We're broke.

This will finish my relationship/marriage.

Etc., etc.

Then take each answer and give it five minutes of intense analysis.

What is the worst that can happen?

What is the best that can happen?

Why would the worst happen?

Why would the best happen?

Am I overthinking this?

Does this really matter at this time?

Can I control it?

Can I delegate control to someone else?

Etc., etc.

Rationalise everything out on the page and in your mind, and you will find solutions and realise that some of the potential problems aren't problems at all.

The mind can torment, but if you already have the answers, it's a lot easier to deal with, and no amount of pills can give the answers you can.

A good exercise is to imagine yourself in the future having beaten cancer and looking at everything you thought were problems. Would you still agree with yourself that they were problems, or wonder why you even bothered writing them in the first place?

It also helps to realise that other people have been in your position too. Some have dealt with it well, and, of course, some have dealt with it poorly.

How did those who dealt with it well do it?

How did those who dealt with it poorly do it?

Yes, I realise you don't know precisely what each example did, but you have an incredible brain that can easily throw scenarios at you, and you simply modify the scenarios to suit you. We all have an imagination, so don't self-limit because you believe you can't come up with answers. If I gave you the answers, they would be my answers, relevant to my circumstances, so not much use. Do it for you—you're the only one who can.

"*Once you accept you're not as smart as you thought you were and realise you're a lot smarter than you thought you were, things change.*" ~ Lawrence Wray

Nothing is guaranteed.

Survival is not guaranteed, which means that death isn't guaranteed either.

If it's all a bit too much, that's understandable, but it's really very simple to get it sorted; just ask for help.

Don't ask for antidepressants, and don't use the word depressed.

Don't say, "I need to talk to somebody because I'm depressed," because a) you probably aren't, and b) you're not qualified to make that decision. But what you can say is, "I'm really worried and confused, and I think that if I discussed some of my problems with someone who could give me good advice and point me in the right direction, it will help."

The first step is a willingness to accept that you have a problem, the realisation that other people have probably had the same problem, and the understanding there is always a way to improve things. (Which doesn't necessarily mean an ideal solution, but your health is the priority, so be reasonable.)

Too many people want to pop a pill for anything and everything that ails them, and it doesn't matter what it is. Life doesn't work like that.

Give yourself a lot more credit for having more intelligence than you think you have; you have a great brain that can sort out all manner of things, but people self-limit for various reasons that aren't relevant. My brain doesn't know what to do. I'm not smart. I wasn't good at school. I didn't finish school. I'm dumb. I'm not good at my job. Etc.

None of these reasons are valid for anyone. Trust yourself. You've got this far, so you must be doing something right.

The best advice I can give is to plan for it and expect it, but seek advice from professionals before you experience it and ask for help.

Acceptance

Now we're getting somewhere.

If you have achieved this status, give yourself a pat on the back.

You're aware you have problems and you can't bargain your way out of them, you may still occasionally face depression or get angry, but you know what to do.

You now have a new reality that will, hopefully, be temporary.

'Such is life.'

'Where do I go from here?'

'What next?'

And the ultimate one: 'I'm ready for the future. Bring it on.'

Some people say they can't stop thinking of their funeral, but I never really gave it much thought. I've always been a dreamer and so I kept looking to the future as mine. My future, my path, my decision to make.

Acceptance isn't defined as being 'all right' or 'okay' with the situation you find yourself in, but the fact you have now accepted everything as the new normal. Your mortality or inevitable future is okay with you. It was never your fault, just one of those things.

Life will change and problems will arise as a result, but you can take whatever life throws at you.

You (probably) won't be able to jog your usual six miles, but you can read, or play table tennis, or snooker/pool, or knit, or whatever calms and keeps you distracted. Do little and build it up slowly.

Replace what you can't do with something you can. Distract yourself and get on with it.

As I accepted the diagnosis from the start and was eager to get started beating it, I (more or less) went to this stage straight away.

Treatment

Once treatment starts, the chemotherapy can play a huge part in causing confusion, and irrespective of the order shown above, you can find yourself jumping in and out of stages throughout your journey, so accept it as a possibility, be strong but ask for help when you need it. Don't wait. Don't think you're stronger. Get any help you need the second you realise it might be a good idea.

More Stages?

If you search the internet, you will find sites that contradict this theory of five stages and some go up to as many as thirteen, but in reality, everything you ever need to know is covered in the five we've looked at, and if you spend your time looking to find more, you're only adding to your problems.

You might find it helpful to refer to this section as and when you may be experiencing problems. If you find that even after understanding the stages, things are still getting you down, don't worry, it's natural, but it is at this time you will need to seek help.

Seeking help is sometimes easier said than done, as human nature sees needing help as a failure and something that should be avoided, but what have you got to lose by trying? My sincere advice is to overcome your reluctance and give it a go. At the very worst, it might take time to help, but having been there myself and been reluctant, it's an eye-opening experience that definitely does help.

"*You get one chance to get it right, so come out swinging and fight as you've never fought before.*" ~ Lawrence Wray

It's your funeral

Need a dose of motivation?

Sit down, close your eyes, relax, take a couple of deep breaths, and imagine watching your funeral in your mind.

Watch your loved ones gather around and talk about you, like you aren't even there (which, of course, you aren't).

See the shiny coffin with the fancy handles, and the easel with the blown-up photograph of you smiling blissfully, before your death.

The flowers look lovely too, only in the afterlife you can't smell them; still, nice touch.

Your closest relatives are heartbroken and inconsolable, and you spend a couple of minutes sympathising and regretting.

Then you float up over the mourners and listen to the lovely things they are saying about you, then, as you glide over some more mourners you overhear a conversation where somebody says, 'He/She just gave up.' 'There was nothing more we could do.' 'He/She just stopped fighting.' Now, the question is, how would that make you feel if you were looking down and heard that?

Would you want that second chance to fight?

Would you do things differently?

Would '*you*' go into battle for '*you*', given another chance?

I think you can see where I'm coming from, but here's the thing, you have that chance now. Now is the time to give it your all. When it's too late… it's too late.

When would 'now' be a good time to give 100%.

There are no second chances in this fight.

You win, or you die.

My Story

It's hard to say exactly when my cancer story started. I was seventeen when my mum died of cancer, but this was a fact I only found out about some thirty years later. Growing up in Northern Ireland, every health issue a woman had was simply put down to 'women's problems' and left at that. It might have been nothing more than a toothache, but this catch-all phrase meant no further questions would be answered, so it was best to just accept it and move on. I suppose had I been aware, I might have considered the possibility cancer would eventually pay me a visit, but ignorance was bliss.

I married when I was twenty-six, had my daughter precisely one week before my thirtieth birthday and a son just over three years later. Everything was on track and I was following the expected route as best I could, but things were always up and down as I had been self-employed since I was twenty, so sometimes we were well off, and sometimes not. When times were good, we had frequent holidays and spent like it would never end, and when times were bad, not so much.

Other than the occasional cut or bruise, I was in good health. I jogged six miles, three times a week, did weight training and mountain biking, and at that time I didn't drink much. Sore throats and inflamed tonsils were my thing, and eventually, it was decided they (my tonsils) should be removed, so on 29th May 1999, I attended a hospital to have them taken out, which was my first time being admitted to a hospital.

I've always had a problem with weight as I love food; a side-effect of having too much income at the time (whatever happened to that?), hence the need for all the exercise, so in 2000, I and a mate walked, jogged, ran or mountain biked up the Cave Hill every lunchtime. The Cave Hill overlooks Belfast and is 370m/1213ft above sea level and has great views at the top, and we were up so frequently that we not only found lots of alternative ways to reach the top but made some new paths for others to use. If we walked, we wore backpacks with two stone in each one, and if we jogged, we reduced it to one stone.

We were both the same age, both working for ourselves in similar businesses and both overweight but fit, with me being the fittest of the two. Every day we would set a timer and try to beat the previous record, and usually, we did, only things started to change when I found it increasingly difficult to keep up with him. So I guess my cancer story probably started then, which was around late 2000.

I went to a doctor who did blood tests and concluded there was nothing to worry about and maybe it was just a bug (Maybe? A bug? Ya think?). I would strongly advise anyone to always get a second opinion if they feel the diagnosis isn't accurate as I really felt the lack of energy wasn't down to any bug. Doctors are just like the rest of us and can have an off day due to any number of things. We're all human.

October 2000-April 2002

The decrease in fitness was quickly followed with a rash/itch on the inside of my right leg. I again went to the doctor, who prescribed cortisone cream. This seemed to do the trick initially, but the rash/itch came back again within days, so I stopped using the cream and was prescribed an antibiotic instead. This continued on-and-off for at least a year, and even though some mornings I woke up with my nails black with skin and blood—from scratching through the night—it was never considered life-threatening. I suppose, on reflection, it was no big deal, and definitely not an immediate sign of cancer; but herein lies the problem, it is an early indicator of Lymphoma.

I developed a slight cough after that; a tickly one. When I was trying to carry on a conversation, I frequently had to stop several times. I hoped it would clear up quickly, but it didn't. I would cough my way through telephone conversations, and cough at the table, and cough at night. I visited the surgery and was told it was simply a virus that was going around and it would sort itself in time. I'm getting ahead of myself here, but the first time I was prescribed Prednisolone (Steroids), both the cough and itch vanished overnight, never to be seen or heard of again.

After that, my sleep patterns became erratic as my back was extremely sore and nothing would take the pain away (I was always on painkillers).

I started sweating in the night, and this escalated to the point where I was taking a yellow bucket (that I bought specially for the job) to bed to hold the wet t-shirts. Some nights I slept on a bath towel to absorb the moisture, but inevitably, the sheets were changed at least once. At the end, it was possible to wring the t-shirts out. I again visited a doctor. He looked at me and told me I was overweight and advised me to stop eating so much. He didn't even examine me. I would point out that at this stage I had lost around three stone from a starting weight of over seventeen stone (238 pounds/107.95kg).

Disturbed sleep continued and progressed from a bad back and sweats to pains in the chest which forced me to lie in a face-down position with my arms under me to support my body weight, and again, with hindsight, I should have sought a second opinion.

The next adventure was rigors. I didn't know what they were called until I eventually went into hospital to start treatment, but basically, I was lying in bed freezing. Just the opposite of what I'd been used to. Two quilts and a hairdryer blowing constantly were required to get me warm, but once I was heated up, I immediately started sweating again. I actually chipped one of my front teeth from chattering. Another visit to the surgery and blood tests were authorised to get to the bottom of it.

I started to drink to help me get to sleep. I once knocked back four tins of beer, a bottle of wine, and a bottle of Jack Daniels between lunchtime and bedtime. Crazy or what? But I never got a hangover. The drink simply helped me sleep. I asked another doctor and he advised me to cut down but didn't investigate the 'why I was doing it' bit and advised that I was self-medicating and not to worry.

Habits like that can kill you, or forever wreck your liver. I was never a heavy drinker before and my intake now has reduced substantially, and anyway, I could never have afforded (financially or physically) to continue putting it away like that.

The next symptom—a good one this time, but obviously not for everyone—was weight loss. I couldn't eat. Friends who had been out for meals with me knew I could shift a plateful of food faster than anyone, and if you weren't careful at the table, I'd have a go at clearing yours as well. But here I was now, picking at my food, and sometimes not eating at all. For my Christmas Dinner 2001, I ate virtually nothing (which didn't go down well) and had lost just over five stone. I was ecstatic, but it wasn't good as I was very weak and tired all the time. People were always commenting on my weight loss, and after I had been diagnosed, I told them I was on the 'Big C' diet. I had a black t-shirt printed with the words, 'I lost 5 stone on the Big C diet.' I wore it in a shopping centre once and people actually stopped me and asked where they could get more details as they assumed it was like the Atkins diet which was popular around that time. Oh, how we laughed.

At this time, I owned a balloon business and, coincidently, the most memorable balloon release was for a cancer charity. I took my kids with me and we drove the forty-odd miles, but after the first ten, I had to stop for a sleep, then again, and again. Then while I was driving, the front tyre blew; I managed to keep control and pulled onto the hard-shoulder. I started off as a mechanic when I was sixteen, so changing a tyre wasn't a problem, but the boot was filled with gas tanks for the balloons, so I took them out and stood them behind the car, then got on with changing the wheel. I had nearly finished when I heard sirens, I looked up and two police cars were approaching, then they abruptly stopped. The doors opened and the cops jumped out, guns drawn. Seriously? Turns out that having what looked like missiles sitting on the ground (gas tanks) had prompted a member of the public to make a call. I showed them the tanks, explained what had happened and managed to have the police escort me to the venue. Yeah, there was a time when Northern Ireland was like that.

Before I was eventually diagnosed, I visited the surgery every Friday for ten weeks, and each week they took blood, had it analysed, but discovered nothing worth further investigation.

Thankfully, things have changed dramatically, and doctors are now more aware of the signs of cancer, but back when I was having problems, they weren't known about by local GPs as they are now. As with everything in life, it takes time to educate everyone (including professionals) about potential problems. There was a specific test that could have been carried out on the blood which would have analysed the LDH levels (Lactate Dehydrogenase—no I can't pronounce it either) that are used to detect the death rate in growing tumours as they produce LDH as a waste product and would have flagged the problem immediately, but as cancer was never considered, the test was never carried out.

Again, and I can't stress it strongly enough; always ask for a second opinion if you feel you aren't getting anywhere.

Things came to a head when I couldn't work and couldn't stay awake during the day. I arranged for an appointment with my own doctor this time (not a partner at the practice), and he referred me for tests at Whiteabbey Hospital. Previously his colleagues had arranged for tests for everything from hiccups, kidney stones, and thyroid problems, to pregnancy, so I couldn't wait to see what was in store for me now. My doctor didn't say I had cancer, but the symptoms all together were worrying, so he sent me for an ultrasound scan (the ultrasound scan is where they put jelly on your belly and look at your insides on a monitor), to be followed by an endoscopy test (which is where you swallow a small camera) some days later.

I knew something was seriously wrong and asked numerous times if it could be cancer, but was always assured it wasn't and there was nothing to worry about; they'd get to the bottom of it (eventually). But… of course, it was cancer.

I had the ultrasound done and was getting ready to leave when the radiologist asked me to wait. She left the room and came back with another doctor and he repeated the test. This guy was old and had gold half-moon glasses and looked like he knew what he was doing, so I trusted him from the start, and yes, maybe this was a flawed judgement, but that's just me. I asked him what was wrong as I was sure this wasn't a normal occurrence. He said he couldn't tell me, but after I hassled, pleaded and begged, he did say the lymph nodes were enlarged which was worrying and would need further investigation. I immediately asked him about cancer, but he wouldn't discuss it further. In my mind, and after researching it on the internet afterwards, I knew it was a strong indicator of cancer.

Ultrasound Scan

Sometimes referred to as a 'sonogram', an ultrasound scan uses high-frequency sound waves to create an image of the inside of your body.

There is no radiation involved, so it's completely safe.

A (freezing cold) lubricating gel is spread over the area to be scanned so there is continuous contact between the probe and skin.

The probe emits sound waves that bounce off different parts of the internal organs to create 'echoes' that are picked up and turned into an image on the screen.

Pain rating is 0/10. Nothing to worry about, except drying off the gel afterwards. It's sticky.

Problems afterwards? None.

You're putting what down my throat?

Tuesday 16th April 2002

Before I was diagnosed correctly, I needed to have an endoscopy test. It involves the patient swallowing a long tube with a tiny camera at the end to inspect the throat, oesophagus, stomach, and the beginning of the small intestine.

Was I panicking? Yes.

I could use a lot of very inappropriate language to describe my reservations about this test, but let's just say I was worried.

Down my throat?

Awake?

Asleep?

Would I choke?

Would I die?

Would it hurt?

Would I need stitches?

Would it work?

What would it find?

On and on it went.

My wife was with me and we were sitting in the waiting room, the sweat dripping off my forehead and my hands clammy and shaking.

The nurse came with the paperwork and I held her hostage until she explained every aspect of the procedure and answered all my questions. (I have always found I crave information about everything)

I was offered a general anaesthetic or simply having the back of my throat frozen. I choose the latter option as it meant I could leave immediately afterwards.

You haven't read enough of this book yet to conclude I'm very open to all sorts of ideas. Anything and everything that can potentially help is on my radar. In business, I consumed self-help books and books on positive mental attitude, so I found myself using some of the suggestions.

I told my wife I was going to sort things out in my mind and wouldn't be talking until they came for me. I calmed myself, closed my eyes, relaxed back into the chair, and visualised the whole thing from start to finish.

The visualisation process

I watched me opening the door.

Walking into the room and lying on the bed.

Opening my mouth.

The doctor squirting something down the back of my throat to freeze it.

The long intimidating tube being picked up and dangled over me.

Looking at it and thinking it wasn't so big.

Leaning my head back.

The doctor putting it in my mouth and me being amazed at how easily I swallowed it, without any gagging or discomfort.

Me, breathing very deeply as the nurse recommended.

Me, feeling absolutely no pain and thinking how easy it was.

The doctor eventually pulling the tube out.

The doctor congratulating me on being the best patient he ever had.

At the end of ten minutes, I was looking forward to it, and when the nurse did call me, I nearly sprinted into the room.

The outcome? Okay, he didn't congratulate me, and I was lying on my side instead of on my back, but I had no problems. It went just as I'd visualised it would, and I would do it again without hesitation.

The doctor who carried it out was another I liked from the off. I don't like wishy-washy-maybe doctors who don't say what they think, but even before he did the procedure, he said it was probably a waste of time after the results of the ultrasound. I asked him what he thought it could be, and he simply said, "Lymphoma."

He was a very 'straight to the point' type of doctor, which I prefer. He told me he thought it was lymphoma and that was good enough for me. That was the first time I had a diagnosis by a doctor, even though it was an unofficial opinion.

I went home and used the internet to find out about the various types of lymphoma and found that Non-Hodgkin Lymphoma was spot on for me, thank you very much. He was right on the mark as all the classic symptoms were present.

The point I am making is that instead of the dread I expected to feel and had been feeling before arriving at the hospital, I must have been his most enthusiastic patient. I had accepted it was definitely going to happen; I needed it and had no choice, so by simply playing out the whole thing in my head and seeing a positive outcome, I had conditioned myself to expect a positive result. No pain, no gagging, no problems—well, other than the fact he confirmed I had cancer, which I was expecting anyway.

This was the start of a new period in my life where I took control.

I remember talking to my consultant about pre-conceived ideas just before the cancer treatment started, and she explained that most people have an expectation of what chemotherapy entails.

Mostly it's about sickness and hair loss, as that's what most people associate with treatment. Some people are more afraid of the chemo than the actual cancer, and especially potential hair loss. You go in looking reasonably normal, then the nurses inject you with some vile liquid that makes you projectile vomit, weak, even sicker than when you just had the cancer, and your hair falls out. Who would want that?

Hair loss is not an inevitable side effect of chemo, and you might not lose it as it depends on the chemotherapy you will receive, but your chemo nurse will be able to advise you; however, if you're on one of the drugs where it is an expected side effect, it's unusual if it doesn't fall out.

I knew it would be an unbearable process if I allowed myself to think that way, so instead, I thought about going into a futuristic world where they injected you with chemotherapy that not only cured the cancer but made you feel good. I took the long view that in this world, not only would the cancer be cured, but afterwards, while others were suffering, I would feel brilliant, sort of bionic. That visualisation changed my mindset from that of every other patient. I looked forward to my appointments because I knew they would cure me and make me better than I had ever felt.

It's all about how you look at it.

I remember when I was a kid, my parents made me do piano lessons and the inevitable exams. I hated exams and was always nervous, until one day when my mum couldn't take me, my piano teacher took me instead. In the waiting room, she asked me if I was nervous and I answered, "yes." She told me it was my chance to show off just how good I was (I wasn't) and how it would be an exciting adventure. She said I wasn't nervous; I was excited as inside I knew I was prepared. She explained how good I would feel if I was the best pupil of the day and passed everything with flying colours. When they called my name, I trotted off immediately and had no fear of the examiner. I passed with distinction.

What I'm trying to get across is how the mind can sabotage you before you even start. A positive mindset isn't magic, it's simply allowing yourself to be open to new ideas without the normal baggage.

Had I maintained my negative mindset, my experience wouldn't have been anywhere near as good. I would probably have choked and gagged as the camera went down, I might have panicked halfway through and tried to pull it out, but no, none of that happened as I had conditioned myself to know that wasn't going to happen, it was going to be a good experience.

Endoscopy

An endoscope is a flexible tube with a camera and light at the end that is used to look at the inside of your body.

If you are worried about the procedure, ask the doctor to show you the tube and explain what will happen next.

Although they use different names for the scopes, the same procedure can be used to look down your throat, up your anus, into the bladder, or into your abdomen—by use of an incision—in keyhole surgery. They also have the ability to remove small samples of tissue for analysis, which is known as a biopsy.

I've had all four performed and never had any problems or pain.

The time taken can vary between fifteen minutes to an hour, but the thing to remember is that once it's in, there is no feeling from inside the body and no pain. During the procedure, they will encourage you to breathe deeply, and I recommend you take this advice seriously as it not only makes it easier but relaxes you and takes your mind off the camera.

You may be wondering at this stage the relevance of the endoscopy test, and although it isn't standard procedure for a lot of cancers and turned out to be irrelevant to my diagnosis, I have included it to illustrate how the mind can be manipulated to view a procedure with enthusiasm and positivity, rather than trepidation and worry.

The result of the examination will be the same irrespective of your attitude, but your experience before, during, and afterwards, can all be modified in your favour by simply concentrating and conditioning your mind prior to even entering the room.

Pain rating is only ½/10. (if even) Nothing to worry about.

Problems afterwards? Yes, but not what you think. Think of a tune, and you will be able to play it with your bum all the way home. Yes, they have to inflate you when they put the scope down, and it has to come out somewhere, so wind the windows down.

Tuesday, 23rd April 2002 (7 days later)

The following Tuesday I had my first CT/CAT Scan at Antrim Hospital. They gave me barium to drink, which, contrary to popular belief is not that bad. Barium sulfate is a contrast agent that coats the inside of your throat, stomach and intestines, which gives a clearer CT Scan.

I drank it, waited for around an hour, and then went in and had the scan done. Nothing to it.

One thing to watch out for is the dye they sometimes inject before the scan starts; it gives you an intense feeling that you want to urinate or just have, but don't worry, you won't.

Once the machine starts the scan, it's loud, but if you can, just close your eyes and go to your 'happy place' and it will be over before you know it. The way I did it was to take five deep breaths, then get on a chair lift (in my mind), and at the top I stand and ski off perfectly down the most fantastic slope imaginable, all with perfect parallel skis, then, when the noise starts in the CT scanner,

I imagined it was a piste basher/Snow Groomer driving alongside me. It might sound a bit weird, but it's your mind, and that's a place where anything is possible, in fact, the more outrageous the better, so not only did I ski down the slopes—I skied up them as well. When I went over a bump, I was airborne for minutes. Done well, it's a place you won't want to leave, and the noise of the scanner is absorbed and translated into something else in your experience.

The distraction wasn't planned, but when they told me I had to lie still for half-an-hour, I knew I had to do something and skiing just appeared. Everyone has something they like doing, so design your own 'happy place' before you go and just relax. It's a worthwhile exercise as you will find yourself using it over and over, and the more you do it, the easier and more enjoyable it will get.

Sometimes they will ask you to inhale and hold your breath, but the instructions are clear and easy to comply with.

The only bad part of the scan was waiting for the results.

CT Scan

A computerised tomography scan, to give it its proper name, or CT/CAT scan. It uses X-rays to create detailed images of the inside of the body which include organs, blood vessels and bones.

It can be used to diagnose conditions such as cancer, strokes, blood flow problems, and injuries.

With cancer patients they are used frequently to check the size of tumours before, during, and after treatment.

Scans are quick, painless and generally safe; however, there is a small risk of allergic reaction to the contrast dye, and you will be exposed to a small amount of X-ray radiation which is the equivalent of between a few months and a few years (depending on the time taken in the scanner) of exposure to natural radiation from the environment.

When you receive confirmation of your appointment, it usually includes details of everything, including any fasting requirements.

If you already have any conditions or are pregnant or on any medications, it is essential you let them know before the scan is carried out.

You may be given a drink or injected with a die called a contrast to help improve the quality of the images.

The scanner is an intimidating piece of equipment, and you will be passed through a tunnel, so if you have issues with claustrophobia or are just worried, they can give you medication to help you relax, but really, it's easy.

Once they start the scan, it is noisy, so don't be alarmed. You may be offered earplugs or headphones, but if not, it's not a problem.

After it's finished, you usually get tea/coffee and biscuits and will be asked to wait for around an hour to make sure you don't have a reaction to the dye.

You can ask for the results, but the answer is usually that they have to wait until a consultant reviews them, so don't worry as there is nothing you can do until you get your next appointment.

Pain rating is only ½/10. (and that's only if they have to inject you with the dye) Nothing to worry about.

Problems afterwards? None.

Friday 26th April 2002 (3 days later)

I went with my wife to see Dr Rodgers again, and he brought us in, sat us down, and broke the bad news officially. He had received the CT Scan results and had major concerns about my swollen spleen, liver, heart, and lymph nodes. He predicted chemo would start within a week at Antrim Hospital.

I didn't react badly; in fact, I didn't react at all as it was the news I had been expecting. I knew that now we could start to do something to put things right. He obviously hadn't expected this reaction and advised me he had a nurse arranged to meet me after the consultation. I assumed (in my naivety) that this was to immediately start treatment, but she just wanted to calm me down, give me a cup of sweet tea and talk things through. I didn't need her, although I appreciated the thought. I just left and went home, glad it was confirmed.

"Either cancer will end up in a coffin or I will... and it ain't gonna be me." ~ Lawrence Wray

Relatives, friends, loved ones.

We're early in the process at this stage and you might (or might not) have noticed I mention my wife was with me during visits, but I don't deal with her in any way. It's as if her thoughts and feelings are irrelevant; after all, it was me that was sick. But the relationship between the patient and the family is a very relevant and important part of the process.

This is mistake number one. Nobody tells you anything about this at the hospital as it's their job to treat the person who is sick, and only them.

When a life-threatening illness visits; it not only affects the sufferer, but the immediate family as well. The phrase, *When someone gets cancer, the whole family get it as well*, is relevant.

You're caught up in thoughts of treatment and ultimately death, so it's not surprising that family are looked on as 'having to be there for you' as you would be for them. But it's not that simple.

I have mentioned I had symptoms for two years before diagnosis and abused alcohol, which I had never done before. I had lost a lot of weight and there were days I didn't eat anything, which meant I was happy losing weight; but throw in a bottle of Jack Daniels on an empty stomach and the results aren't surprising, yet, I carried on, oblivious.

There were nights when I drank and simply went to bed, woke up the next morning and carried on, but there were nights when I passed out on the floor and couldn't be moved, or I was sick in the bathroom, and on one occasion, I was sick on the living room floor.

When we were going together (dating), way back in the day, my wife was a care worker in a home for the elderly, and she frequently told me about how someone had died that day or had an accident; and I remember the night when I was sick on the floor and told her to, "Clean it up, it's your job." Boy, was I an asshole, or what?

At the time, I was severely inebriated, and as with alcoholics, it's not unusual to wake up the next morning and remember nothing of the night before, but eventually, memories start to materialise and, of course, you are reminded by the person you offended. I'm not going to make excuses here, but there is nothing more confusing than someone telling you about something you've done you have no recollection of. Add to that the fact she had her own job, our kids to look after, my cancer diagnosis, and you have a recipe for disaster.

As a sufferer, you have to have empathy with your partner, friends and relatives, but this is usually only learnt much later as happened with me. It's not something that comes naturally, but forewarned and all that.

Take the time now to sit back and think about how you would cope if the situation was reversed and you were the carer. How would you juggle work, school runs, shopping, hospital visits, all while worrying about whether or not your partner will survive and how the finances are going to be impacted? Your care is in the hands of the doctors, which is as it should be, but for the others in your life, there is (usually) little or no help offered, and although there is help available, most people see it as a failure to ask for it, which is just silly. Why would you not take advantage of any and all help available? You, as the sufferer can ask your consultant/chemo nurse for more information on behalf of your carers and family. Get the wheels moving and make it easier for all concerned.

My son was eight years old and my daughter was eleven years old at this stage, so you can imagine what my kids were going through, yet I never sat down with them and talked it through, though I now know my wife did.

The problem is that irrespective of how mentally strong you think you are, you are so wrapped up in yourself and your predicament that your mind has probably never had to deal with so much at one time—and especially when you throw in mortality and the ever-present thoughts of death.

Mental processes you do every day without thought become more challenging, not because they are, but because your mind is otherwise occupied.

Temper changes, tantrums, and opinions like, ‘you don’t understand what I’m going through,’ while accurate in the context of the sufferer’s mind, don’t help. Not only do you have to figure out how you’re going to tackle the treatment, but you need to put yourself in the position of others and meet them half-way.

Nobody will prepare you for this, and nobody can. I’ve given you a very limited picture about some of the problems, but it’s something you’re going to have to sit down and really think about when you’re on your own. Imagine for a second how you would cope if it wasn’t you, but someone close to you.

Saying, “I’m sick,” or “get me this,” or “get me that,” or “don’t you love me?” etc., are things you as a person wouldn’t normally say, but you have to accept that going through diagnosis and treatment, you won’t be the ‘normal’ you. You won’t plan on saying any of them and, inevitably, you will play the ‘cancer card’ at some point. On the other hand, the people you’re going to be saying these things to need to know what’s happening, why you’ve changed, and ultimately, how to cope with the comments.

Coping with the comments means them realising it’s not the ‘normal’ you, and in that instance, reminding you of that fact. You—as the sufferer—need to realise what is happening when you’re reminded of that fact, accepting it and modifying your behaviour appropriately. It's damned hard when you're in the middle of a tantrum, but now you know, you can plan for it.

It's hard for someone who has never had cancer to get their mind around it; someone who has always been in control to suddenly lose it for no real reason, then, when it happens, they've already committed to that course of action so feel compelled to reinforce it and… there's no easy way to say it, but they make it worse to validate their mindset, and even though they know they're doing it, they're helpless.

Once you have the diagnosis and treatment has started, the attitude towards you slowly changes from one of extreme sympathy to, 'just get on with it.' Yeah, human nature adapts quickly, but not for the patient.

Unlimited help and sympathy is always available at the start of treatment, but your illness becomes the norm and from the second treatment onward (unless there's a blip) you are gradually left to get on with things. You know what to expect as you've done it before and survived.

It's horrible, but as I say, human nature; but now you know about it so when it happens (and it will to some degree), you'll not take it personally, because if it was the other way around…

Of course, on the other side of the coin there are those who expect everyone on the planet to go out of their way for them as they have *cancer*, but don't forget you are not unique, and you (mostly) have the ability to do lots of things for yourself without relying on others too much. The more you do, the better you feel. You can abuse it and take advantage, but think about it; you're robbing yourself of the power you have, you're ultimately making yourself feel worse than you are, and that's not good.

The initial aim is to wrap the sufferer in a cloud of acceptance and ignore anything untoward with the explicit excuse that as they're sick, it's understandable. It is, but it's not the right way to go about it.

Resentment and frustration can build to a point where you or they eventually explode, so it's better for both parties to point out when something is unacceptable and explain the reason why, then something can be done about it before it becomes a problem.

You must appreciate how your condition affects others on a daily basis, both on a mental and physical level. The thoughts running through their minds vary from impending death to practical everyday matters, to financial implications; and all take their toll, and it's not unusual for depression to affect those around you during your illness.

It was only after I had finished treatment my wife confided she had seen a counsellor on a regular basis and taken advice on how to cope. It was a revelation to me as she hid it so well, and that's yet another problem, as your partner can no longer share things they normally would have done for fear of adding to your burden, and while that's understandable, it's also understandable their problems continue to grow.

The best advice I can give is to seek counselling for the family unit as a whole right from the start, and take advice on what everyone can expect and how to avoid confrontation and a build-up of worries. It's an ongoing process and problems will arise that no one can predict, but help is available. The hospital can help, and the various cancer charities all have professionals that can give advice. You might also consider joining a group where other sufferers and survivors meet up to discuss their circumstances and offer advice. Facebook has some excellent groups where others share their experiences and I have listed some of the ones I am in later in the book under Facebook Support Groups.

Please don't do it alone as I tried to do. Be strong, but listen to others and seek advice.

What do I tell my kids?

There is no one answer that fits all. It depends on your kids. It depends on your relationship with the kids. It depends on the diagnosis. It depends on their age. It depends on their maturity. It depends...

I wouldn't recommend you come straight out with it and say, "Mum/Dad has cancer and will be dead in six months. Bummer. Let's move on."

You can't do that.

At the same time, you must be careful not to make a promise you may not be able to keep. Each case is different. Again, as I've said many times in this book, seek advice. Experts can advise on this type of thing as they've experienced similar cases many times.

It may be an idea to bring your children with you to treatment and involve them in the process, but that may not be an option.

Initially—until you know what you're dealing with—I would say nothing.

The one big warning I have to give is if a doctor gives you an estimated date of demise, do not tell your children because—as has been proven repeatedly with me—it's not guaranteed. It's just a guess.

The other big plus is the fact that you have your kids to fight for, and it's a big motivator when you want to see your kids graduate, get married, or become what you know they can become. It's a free motivational force to get you through the worst times.

Monday 29th April 2002 (3 days later)

My first of many visits to Fern House at Antrim Hospital was on the Monday following the diagnosis, which was the service I had hoped for. Get on with it as quickly as possible.

My wife went with me, and it was an intimidating experience. We went into the waiting room, and guess what? Everyone there was sick. This was a complete surprise to me; I think I expected to see healthy, happy smiling people.

Blood samples were taken and analysed straight away, and then we met a consultant for a brief talk about possible treatments, and then Dr Kyle, who again confirmed I had lymphoma.

I think it's very important to both like your consultant and have confidence in him/her. (I wrestled with putting 'like' before 'confidence', but I decided that's my preference)

I liked my doctor from the first time I met her. She was straight to the point, professional, and answered all my questions without hesitation or reservation.

I was sent home with an inpatient appointment for the next day in the main hospital.

Tuesday 30th April 2002

I was given a bed and started to learn the nurse's names. Some bloods were taken, and a cannula fitted, but for the first day in hospital, that was it.

Cannula

A thin tube that is inserted into a vein and taped into place to administer medication. It can usually be used for up to forty-eight hours. Easily attaches to a drip or syringe.

Pain rating is 1/10. You will feel a sharp prick as it goes in, but other than that, it's easy. Once in, you won't feel anything.

Problems afterwards? None.

Distraction Techniques

Unfortunately, the journey through cancer treatment has many unpleasant procedures, like getting blood taken, or having a cannula inserted, or boring procedures like a scan; so when something is about to happen that you're not looking forward to, distraction techniques are a great way to make the process easier. For example, when I am getting a C.T. scan, I simply go skiing. I see myself stepping onto a chairlift, going up the mountain, looking down at other skiers, and I ski onto a perfect piste; I can even smell the snow. The turns (in my head) are perfect—real life, a different thing—but in my head they're perfect, and I can spend 20, 30, 40+ minutes in a scanner doing nothing more than having the ski run of my life. I do jumps and 360s and back-flips, and I can even ski uphill, and the more complicated the ski run, the less time the brain has to concentrate on reality.

Anyone who practises meditation can easily do this, but it's not hard to do it well the first time.

Long boring procedures are ideal for this method.

The last scan I had (17th August 2021), the radiographer had to shake me at the end of the scan to tell me it was over. I told her where I'd been and she thought I was nuts, but... I was so engrossed in the process I didn't even know the scan was finished and I was back outside the scanner.

For procedures with a little pain, something as simple as pushing your thumbnail into your forefinger can take your mind off an injection. You know how hard you can push your nail into the flesh, so you know the level of pain you can take, and when you have it at maximum, the brain is tricked.

Motivational speakers frequently say to their audience, "I want you to put your right hand in the air as high as you possibly can," and everyone instantly raises their hand; then the speaker says, "Higher," and almost everyone raises their hand even higher.

The initial instruction was, "…as high as you possibly can," which means that virtually everyone ignored the request and didn't go as high as they could, so, my advice to you is to pick a distraction technique (more than one at the same time is okay) and before anything happens, you use the technique, but… no half measures. Do it as hard as it's possible for you to do it. If you're making a fist, you need to see nail marks in your palms when you relax.

Do it half-hearted and the brain has spare capacity to concentrate on two things at once, so you'll feel uncomfortable until you tense further, which begs the question, why didn't you do that in the first place?

People frequently kick their legs out when getting an injection, and, to a certain extent, it helps with the initial nip, but again, if you prepare your brain and use your technique 100%, the focus isn't on what's going to potentially happen, but what you've already initiated.

Suggestions and process for cannula/injection, etc

First things first, find out what is about to happen.

Find out how long it's going to take.

Pick your technique/s.

Relax. Ask for time if you need it.

Prepare your brain and visualise your outcome

All the above sounds like it's going to take a while, but in reality, it's maybe only a minute.

Make a fist.

Tense your legs.

Push your thumbnail into your finger.

Pinch the inside of your thigh.

Pull your hair.

Bite your tongue/cheek (but don't draw blood).

Clench your teeth till your jaw hurts.

Close your eyes tight.

Tense your stomach.

Push your knees together using your legs only.

Curl your toes.

Press your feet hard to the ground.

Tense your leg muscles.

Pinch your earlobe

Push your feet together using feet and legs.

…or come up with one of your own.

With any distraction technique, you should always initiate it before you need to, so if you're getting an injection, you should be nipping your earlobe—or whatever method you choose—before the needle is anywhere near your skin.

I normally prepare with my eyes closed and on a couple of occasions I've told the nurse I was ready, only to be told it was already done. That's how good these techniques can be, and they're really, really simple. There's nobody on the planet that can't do these.

For longer procedures (which in fairness are usually just uncomfortable and not really painful) there are an unlimited number of techniques available, but something as simple as multiplication in your head can work well.

13 times 13.

What day and date will it be 23 days from today?

What day will your next birthday be on?

Count backwards from ninety-nine in threes or count forwards in sevens starting at four.

Pick something you know is going to be complicated or immersive (like skiing, deep sea diving, motor racing, flying like superman, jumping out of a plane) and run with it. Anything that takes over your brain to do something else distracts.

Recite the alphabet, but don't do a, b, c, d, etc., but do it every other letter a, c, e, etc.

Do the alphabet backwards z, y, x, w, v, etc.

Think of a word and spell it backwards in your head (makes of cars, colours, numbers).

Basically, any mental exercise that distracts works, and as I say, anybody can do it. In addition, the nurses want to have an easy time too. They want to be able to get your vein or carry out the procedure, and if you're relaxed, it makes it easier.

Breathing also plays a big part. I sometimes use the seven-eleven technique. Breathe in for a count of seven and exhale for eleven. Nice, big, deep relaxed belly breaths.

Don't allow yourself to be rushed (but don't take the piss either) into a procedure you're not prepared for. Just say to the nurse, "listen, I am too tense, can I get myself relaxed?" Believe me, they want you relaxed as much as you do, so a minute to have an easy procedure versus having multiple attempts as you're too tense is preferable for both parties.

Whichever technique/s you choose, close your eyes while you're doing it and hopefully—as has happened with me—the procedure will be over and you won't have felt a thing.

Again, it's worth repeating that anything you do needs to be 100% commitment before anything happens.

Fuck, fuck, fuckety-fuck

Stick a needle in me and (you're going to find this hard to believe) sometimes I swear. In fact, lots of people do and the nurses are used to it. Now, for clarification, I'm not suggesting you shout out at the top of your voice, but a short sharp (insert preferred word here) between clenched teeth does work wonders to reduce the impact of pain.

In fairness, swearing is not as effective as the distraction techniques mentioned above as they are 'preparation for' whereas swearing is a 'reaction to'; but it still works.

If you're using the distraction techniques properly with 100% commitment, you shouldn't feel anything, but if you're at 98% and something nips, feel free to throw out a choice swear word or two to help.

As a reaction to pain, swearing works wonders as anybody who has ever hit their finger with a hammer can confirm, but it's not just a reaction; it has now been proven to reduce pain.

Sixty-seven undergraduate students were enlisted at Keele University in England in a study approved by the Keele University School of Psychology Research Ethics Committee, to establish whether or not swearing makes a difference in response to pain.

Students were tested twice with one group allowed to swear and the other not; then they were switched around.

One group was allowed to swear using a word of their choosing (fuck, shit, wanker, etc), and the other group had to use a neutral word to describe a table (flat, useful, wooden, sturdy, etc).

The participants were connected to heart rate monitors and a galvanic monitor (which measures stress, anxiety, and fear).

When the participants were swearing, their heart rates went up, and the level of pain experienced went down, which meant that those who swore were able to keep their hands in the water nearly 50% longer than those who didn't

The results were:

Male volunteers could tolerate the ice water for an average of 117 seconds without swearing, which jumped to 195 seconds when swearing was allowed. (+78 seconds)

The figures for the female volunteers started at 106 seconds and jumped to 174 seconds when allowed to swear. (+68 seconds)

I think you'll agree; there is a substantial difference between gosh-diddly-darn-it and fuck.

Interestingly, the swear words used had an effect on the level of pain and time the volunteers could tolerate. If they used the word bum, it was a much-reduced time than those who used the word fuck. Those who use the word, motherfucker, were able to beat those who use fuck on its own, and those who used cunt (which I know will offend a lot of people, and I apologise), we're able to beat those who used motherfucker or fuck.

The more swear words used, the stronger the swearing, and the more aggression used while they were saying them, the more their brain could tolerate the pain.

Another interesting discovery was that people who don't usually swear get even greater pain relief as a result.

Even with reduced intensity swear words, volunteers were able to keep their hands submerged longer than those who didn't swear.

So, if you accidentally close your finger in a cupboard door and say, shucks, or darn it, you're going to feel a lot more pain than if you let out a shit, or fuck, or motherfucker, or... whatever you choose.

In addition—for those of you who may be thinking tut, tut, swearing is a ridiculous thing to do and shows a lack of vocabulary—a 2015 study showed that people who were well educated were much better at coming up with swear words than those who were less educated.

Swearing is also a sign of creativity as it originates in the right side of the brain, which is acknowledged to be the creative side.

It's also a safer way to display aggression; rather than rushing across a room and punching somebody in the face, you simply tell them to fuck off and that's it finished without the need to visit casualty/ER

So, all in all, swearing is good.

Doctors and Nurses

I don't think anyone decides to work in the medical profession for the remuneration, as the pay isn't that good compared to the amount of mental stress they have to work under, instead, it's mostly a profession of choice based on the desire to make a difference by helping people and producing a good outcome. I've been through the system over the last nineteen years and have never met anyone who was there just for a pay-check at the end of the week.

They have—without exception—always been on my side, fighting on my behalf with the aim of achieving a cure. So, with that in mind, if the medical professionals are fighting on your behalf to cure you, then the only weak link in the process is you. What are you doing to get better? It's essential that if they tell you to stop smoking, stop drinking, drink plenty, eat healthy food and exercise, you do exactly that.

I think it's relevant at this point to realise you've now delegated your life and wellbeing to the medical profession, so do everything they advise and do it with enthusiasm.

This is where everything changes. You have the choice of working with these people, or treating them as if they work for you—which is in effect what they do—but the word empathy springs to mind, and that's why I immediately started learning the doctor's and nurse's names.

If you, or I, were working in a hospital and had a patient who was always complaining and always ringing the alarm asking to have water poured, or pillows plumped, or tuck them up in bed, or scratch their leg, or stupid things they can easily do for themselves, then irrespective of the professional requirements, it's human nature to get pissed-off with people, no matter how sick they are.

You can be sick and be decent, or you can be a pain in the ass. Guess which one gets you the best attention.

The old story of the boy who cried wolf is relevant. If you never ring your buzzer, the one time you do ring it, everyone comes running because they know you don't abuse it, and if it's ringing, something is definitely wrong.

You have a team behind you, and you won't realise how good they actually are until you come out the other side and think back. During treatment, they look after you, and some people translate that care into thinking they're in a hotel, and that's the wrong attitude. They are people doing a job, and yes, they can do it well, or like the rest of us, they can have an off-day. Get them on your side and *good* doesn't come close to what they can achieve. Work with them, and work together, and the result will be magnificent.

I don't know everything that works; but here are a few ideas I have used, which seems to have built a good relationship almost immediately.

When calling for a nurse, initially use the little button beside your bed if it's urgent or wait until you see one and give them a wave. Do not yell out, "Nurse, Nurse," as if calling for a lost child.

Don’t forget, priorities in a hospital can be critical, and just because a nurse or doctor can’t immediately come to your bedside, doesn’t mean they’ve forgotten about you. They could be attending to an emergency, and even if it appears they are simply having a conversation and ignoring you, they could be discussing something important relating to another patient’s care. If you think about it, the next time the emergency could be you, so would you want them to be running off to fill somebody’s water jug or plumping pillows?

Do not dare click your fingers at them for attention. A waiter in a restaurant would be offended if you attracted their attention like this, and you will need the nurse at some stage, so it’s not an option.

When a nurse or doctor is talking to you, they usually have the advantage of your name being shown above the bed, so they don’t have to remember it, and I think it lends a nice touch to the conversation, so I always try to find out the first names of everyone I come into contact with and use it every time I address them, that way it’s more personal.

Don’t waste their time asking them to pull your bedclothes up for you, or plumping your pillows, unless you’re at death’s door, or really can’t do it for yourself. They have better things to be doing.

Don’t continually ask, “when can I go home?” It’s simple to answer, and I’ll answer it for you now without even knowing your medical history; you can go home when the doctor tells you; not before. Nurses don’t make these decisions. As you probably know, there is usually a shortage of beds, and the doctors are continually looking to free beds for other patients, but although you might feel well enough to leave, you could catch an infection or encounter other problems once you go, which would not only mean another stay in hospital, but potentially, a longer stay, simply because of impatience. The doctors are the experts and they will discharge you only when you are healthy enough to do so.

By way of illustrating some of the problems nurses have to deal with; I can remember lying in bed hooked up to drips, and in the bed opposite there was a woman who was continually moaning and grunting. She didn't seem in pain and waved to the rest of us indicating everything was okay, but the groaning continued. I didn't pay an awful lot of attention after that, but I did notice when the noise suddenly stopped. I looked across and she was pressing the button for the nurse to come and help. When the nurse arrived the woman said, "I've had an accident," and pointed below the bed clothes, then she said, "It's bad. A lot came out."

I'm not gonna beat about the bush, but my thoughts were: You bitch. It took you twenty minutes to make the mess, but this morning you were able to get up and go to the newsagents to buy a paper, but you're too bloody lazy to get up and go to the toilet?

I and other patients told the nurses what had happened, but typical of all nurses, they simply shrugged and said, "It's all part of the job."

But it's not. It shouldn't be.

Treat the staff like you would like to be treated and you can't go wrong.

I don't like that doctor

All the medical professionals I've ever met were amazing, and that's a fact. They all did their best; however, two doctors stood out because they were what some people would call ignorant, or even arrogant.

It would be fair to say their bedside manner sucked.

There were times when they barked at some of the other doctors if expectations weren't met, and when they came in, if you hadn't done what they asked you to do, you should realise they never asked in the first place; asking was for mortals—a demand had been issued, not a request.

They were two of my favourite doctors because they didn't waffle.

They said, "This is what you've got. This is how I'm going to treat it. This is the best treatment for you. End of."

Some patients said, "I've asked for them not to treat me because they're ignorant."

The fact was, their attitude and demeanour sucked; of that, there was no question, but these two gave me so much confidence in their ability, I insisted they look after me.

The nurses dreaded a visit from either, but they all said the same thing, "They're the best at what they do."

There was no, 'that might work', or 'we could try that', or 'maybe'...

They were methodical; they didn't make an instant decision, they read all the notes, checked everything, and then said, "You need ABC." If somebody else suggested XYZ, they were shot down in flames with an explanation why they were wrong.

Yet some people refused to have them treat them because they didn't like their attitude.

Ladies and gentlemen, if they are the person best qualified to get you to the other side, bedside manner is irrelevant. They are not there to be your friend; they are there to save your life.

They don't have time to stand and hold a conversation about how the weather is, or how your local football team is doing or the state of the world. Nope, they're too busy working miracles every day.

The most relevant question I can ask is, do you want a nice doctor, or do you want the best doctor?

If you prefer the nice one, you need help.

Do they ever make mistakes? Yes, but every doctor makes mistakes; however, these guys make mistakes a lot less frequently. They study hard. They work hard. That's why they're the best.

They take cases others have given up on, and when death comes calling, they step up and say, "Not on my watch."

That's the kind of doctor I want on my team.

A doctor who makes decisions based on asking 20 people and getting 20 different suggestions and then picking one out of a hat isn't for me.

In fairness, that's an over-exaggeration, but it gets the point across.

You want somebody that has experience; has seen what you've got and been successful many times before.

I go back to a boxing analogy; if a boxer goes to his corner and the trainer hits them a smack across the face and says, "Waken up. You could beat this sucker with one hand tied behind your back any day of the week. Now get out there and finish it, or I'm out." What is the boxer going to do?

The trainer is crude, or ignorant, or arrogant, but it works.

With cancer, whatever works is what you need.

Dr Bishop is the Director of Hematopietic Stem Cell Transplantation Programe at The University of Chicago Medicine, and says that his approach to treatment is that aggressive is best and that is what he recommends. He views treatment as a war with the ultimate goal of a cure. He often recommends treatments that are associated with an increased risk of death but offer a higher chance of cure, but he also presents treatment options that are less toxic, but that offer a lesser chance of cure. He says that as long as the patients are aware of the potential risks and benefits of both treatment options, he is comfortable with providing the aggressive treatment if that is what they decide.

For me, this would be my choice every time. Throw everything at it, including the kitchen sink.

Specialist terms you may encounter on your journey

Anesthesiologist

A doctor who specialises in giving drugs or other agents (gas, epidural, etc) that cause a total loss of feeling or relieve pain, most often during surgery.

Colostomy

A surgical operation in which the colon is shortened to remove a damaged part and the cut end diverted to an opening in the abdominal wall to evacuate faecal (poo) waste.

Cystectomy

A cystectomy is the surgical removal of the bladder.

Dietitian or Nutritionist

An expert in the area of nutrition, food, and diet who can advise on how to eat healthy.

Dosimetrist

A person who calculates and plans the correct radiation dose (amount, rate, spread) for cancer treatment.

Endocrinologist

A doctor who specialises in the glands of the endocrine system, such as the thyroid, pituitary, pancreas, pineal, and adrenal glands.

Enterostomal Therapist

A person (usually a nurse) who has been trained in enterostomal therapy to teach people how to care for ostomies. (surgically created openings such as a colostomy bag for the collection of poo, or urostomy bag for the collection of pee)

Gastroenterologist

A doctor who specialises in diseases of the digestive (gastrointestinal or GI) tract.

Genetic Counselor

A trained health professional who helps people decide whether to have genetic testing done and understand the risk of a genetic disorder within a family.

Gynecologic Oncologist

A doctor who specialises in cancers of the female sex (reproductive) organs.

Gynecologist

A doctor who specialises in female health issues, including sexual and reproductive function and the diseases of their reproductive organs, except diseases of the breast that require surgery.

Hematologist

A medical practitioner who specialises in diseases of the blood and blood-forming organs.

Blood cancers such as Non-Hodgkin Lymphoma, Leukaemia, etc., where there is no specific tumour to remove/treat.

Treatment is usually by chemotherapy.

Nephrologist

A doctor who specialises in kidney diseases.

Neurosurgeon

A doctor who specialises in operations to treat problems involving the brain, spinal cord, or nerves.

Occupational Therapist

A therapist who works with people who have impairments or limitations to help them develop, recover, and improve the skills needed for daily living and working. They use specialised activities as an aid to recuperation from physical or mental illness.

CANCEROLOGY

Oncologist

A medical practitioner qualified to diagnose and treat cancer and specifically tumours.

Basically, someone who can treat you if there is a mass of tissue caused by abnormal growth, whether benign (not harmful in effect) or malignant (can spread to other parts of the body with ill effect). Treatment can be surgical or a combination of surgery, chemotherapy and radiotherapy, depending on the specifics.

Ophthalmologist

A doctor who specialises in eye diseases.

Orthopedic Surgeon

A surgeon who specialises in diseases and injuries of the muscles, joint, and bones.

Otolaryngologist

A doctor who specialises in diseases and injuries of the ear, nose, and throat. Also called an ENT doctor (Ears, Nose, and Throat).

Palliative Care Specialists

A team of doctors, nurses, and pharmacists who help keep a person comfortable by managing symptoms, such as pain, nausea, or fatigue. They are not trying to cure the disease, but help the person have the best possible quality of life. They can help at any stage of cancer, from diagnosis to the end of life.

Palliative care doesn't translate as *the end*, as I was given it and survived.

Pathologist

Someone who specialises in diagnosing and classifying diseases by lab tests and by looking at tissue and cells under a microscope. A pathologist determines whether a tumour is cancer, the cell type (where it started) and grade (how fast it is likely to progress).

Paediatric Oncologist

A doctor who specialises in caring for children and teens with cancer.

Paediatrician

A doctor who specialises in caring for children and teens.

Physical Therapist (PT)

A person who helps examine, test, and treat physical problems, and uses exercises, heat, cold, and other methods to restore or maintain the body's strength, mobility, and function.

Phlebotomist

Someone who specialises in drawing blood for analysis.

Now this person is your friend, as chemotherapy damages your veins and makes it hard to draw blood. I had occasions where someone tried, and after four or five unsuccessful attempts had to either call a doctor or a phlebotomist.

There are no guarantees, but they are so used to dealing with this problem that phlebotomists are usually better than doctors, so when you meet yours, make them your new best friend.

Psychiatrist

A medical doctor specialising in the causes, treatment, and prevention of mental, emotional, and behavioural disorders. Psychiatrists provide counselling and can also prescribe medicines or other treatments.

Psychologist

A specialist who assesses a person's mental and emotional status and provides testing and counselling services.

Pulmonologist

A doctor who has specialised experience and knowledge in the diagnosis and treatment of lung (pulmonary) conditions and diseases.

Radiation oncologist

A doctor who specialises in using radiation to treat cancer.

Radiologist

A person who uses X-rays or other high-energy radiation to take detailed pictures of the inside of the body.

This includes Ultra-sound (even though it doesn't use x-rays), CT, MRI, and PET scanners.

Respiratory Therapist

A person who works with people who have breathing problems. This can include breathing treatments and managing patients on ventilators (breathing machines).

Sex Therapist

Someone who specialises in sexual changes (for example, after treatment for cancer). It's common for a sex therapist to work with both partners, rather than just one person.

Social Worker

A person that can help in dealing with social, emotional, and environmental problems that may come with illness or disability. They can help people find community resources and support services, and provide counselling and guidance to help with issues such as home modifications, nursing home placement, and emotional distress.

Speech Therapist

Someone that can help with speech and swallowing problems.

Surgeon

A doctor who treats diseases by cutting or removing parts of the body. (Surgeons'—depending on qualifications—are normally referred to as Mr or Miss instead of doctor)

Surgical Oncologist

A doctor who specialises in using surgery to treat cancer.

Thoracic Surgeon

A doctor who operates on organs and muscles in the chest (lungs, ribs, breastbone, diaphragm). Thoracic refers to the thorax or chest.

Urologist

A doctor who specialises in treating problems in the urinary tract in men and women (Bladder cancer).

Urostomy

An opening in the belly made during surgery to permanently or temporally re-direct urine.

Thank God. Without Him, I would be dead.

Imagine being a nurse or doctor who sat with a patient one night because they felt sorry for them. They talked, and consoled, and encouraged, and explained, and they got things back on track.

They left that morning thinking, ‘Wow, I really made a difference. That patient’s attitude has changed from negative to positive, and not only do they understand better, they are now enthusiastic to get on with it.’

The nurse or doctor is on a high because they made a difference, they did their job well, and some people will say, “So what? That’s their job,” but we all know you can do your job or you can live your job. Medical professionals tend to live their job, sometimes to the detriment of their lives outside. They don’t do the bare minimum to get the day in; they immerse themselves in providing the best care for their patients.

Now, imagine them seeing a post on social media from that person they helped that night that reads, ‘Thank, God. Without Him, I would be dead. He sat beside me on my darkest nights, the ones where I couldn't cope, and He held my hand and reassured me things would be okay.'

Really?

Not the doctor or nurse but an invisible being.

Some will say perhaps it was God acting through the doctor or nurse.

Seriously?

No, that was the goodness of the nurse or doctor when they empathised with a patient—nothing to do with a God instructing them to do A, B, or C.

Credit where credit is due; when somebody sits with you throughout the night and does the job and pushes their limits to get you to push yours, why the hell would you thank God? Thank the person who did the job.

Okay, so it was a rant (I tend to have the odd one, so forgive me), but… put yourself in the shoes of the doctor or nurse the next time someone needs their help throughout the night; are you going to want a repeat of the last time where God got the credit? Would you have a slight hesitation? Would it even cross your mind?

If you're being completely honest, you might have a hesitation and it would definitely cross your mind.

Credit where credit is due.

The power of God, or the Gods, or…

This next section is my personal belief and is not intended to offend, but after spending so much time in hospital thinking and studying various religions, I arrived at the conclusion there is no supreme being looking after humanity. But… I do recommend you read the next section and understand it's done with good intentions.

If it does offend, I pre-apologise. It was not my intent, but it is honest.

God's got it easy.

You have cancer, so you pray to the Almighty to survive, but if you die, people will say that God wanted you by His side, and if you survive, they'll say God is good.

God's got a great gig going; He can't lose. It doesn't matter how it turns out; live or die, God's a great guy.

People seem to conveniently forget that He is the one who let you get cancer in the first place.

But of course, He doesn't exist. So, it's all BS.

Prayers can be dangerous.

Some people have a whole church congregation saying special prayers for that one person with cancer, and it can be dangerous. I bet you're wondering just how prayers and danger could be connected.

Let's face it, praying for a good outcome is one of the nicest things anyone can do for a friend. It's happened to me, and I have appreciated it many times, but for some, the trust in the power of the Almighty translates into a firm belief, 'As everybody's praying for me, and there is such a power in that, how can I lose?' And so they don't fight as hard as they would if they didn't have the backup of a church congregation praying for them. Call it faith or call it belief; it can be dangerous because if God's got your back, how can it not turn out right?

You are your own God. You have your own power. Only you can fight your cancer, and as I said earlier, you can't delegate the fight to somebody else, and that includes supreme beings with beards in the sky.

God? He hasn't got your back, because He doesn't exist. But I tell you who does have your back—your medical team, the nurses, doctors, consultants, surgeons, etc. They do have your back, so if you're going to have faith in anything, have faith in yourself and your team.

Right at the start of the book, you read the joke about the guy saying over and over, "My God will save me," and he drowned. If that isn't a hint, I don't know what is.

"You gain strength, courage, and confidence by every experience in which you really stop to look fear in the face. You must do the thing which you think you cannot do." ~ Eleanor Roosevelt

Wednesday 1st May 2002

Things were eventually moving in the direction I wanted, and I had my appointments for both a lymph node biopsy and a lumbar puncture.

I was wheeled away first thing in the morning to have the biopsy on a lymph node in my abdomen first (a very small operation), and apart from an injection to freeze the area there was no pain. I lay on the bed and went to my 'happy place', same as in the CT scanner.

Biopsy

To confirm if a tumour is malignant (cancer), a surgeon may remove part of it by either a needle biopsy (yes, using just a needle) or by a small operation. The sample is then examined by a histopathologist (a clever dude/dudette who analyses tissues) who can tell whether or not it is malignant and exactly what type of tumour it is.

When the sample is analysed, it can be determined if there are any abnormal cells such as cancer, and allocated a rating indicating the degree of inflammation or the aggressiveness of the disease, which also gives an indication of the overall prognosis (long term outlook).

Once the results are available, they can be used to determine the most appropriate treatment, based on previous findings from other sufferers.

Various types of biopsy are available and include:

A punch biopsy, where an instrument punches a small hole in the skin to obtain the sample.

A needle biopsy, where a hollow needle is inserted using X-ray, ultrasound, CT or MRI scan to locate the area.

An endoscopic biopsy, where an endoscope is used to remove tissue from inside the body.

An excision biopsy, where an incision is made to remove tissue.

A perioperative biopsy, where someone is undergoing an operation and tissue is removed for immediate analysis during the operation and before completion.

Most biopsies only require local anaesthetic, which means it's usually a day procedure; however, an overnight stay is usually required if the procedure is carried out under general anaesthetic.

Pain rating is only 1/10. Nothing to worry about.

Problems afterwards? None. (or so I thought)

Lumbar Puncture

I had been given lots of books on Non-Hodgkin Lymphoma to read by Bernie O'Neill—who was my allocated chemo nurse—who promised to look after me (a promise she kept), and I had read all about the lumbar puncture biopsy and was panicking by the time Dr Kyle came to take the sample in the afternoon, but all was well; she talked me through the procedure, gave me a sedative and told me to lie on my side, relax and pull my knees up to my chest.

The sedative (I found out later) was oramorph (morphine), and the area was numbed with an injection before the procedure.

A lumbar puncture is commonly known as a 'spinal tap' and is a procedure where a needle is inserted into the spinal canal to collect cerebrospinal fluid for testing.

I can remember having a sense of pressure around the area, but no pain.

As the needle went in, it was like a sharp nettle sting, and although it was a bit uncomfortable, it was easy.

Pain rating is only 1/10. Nothing to worry about.

Problems afterwards? Slight bruising, but no pain, although some patients experience headaches.

Thursday, 2nd May 2002

Another relaxing day reading books after having stuffed balloons through the night.

Balloons? I still had a balloon business in the real world and had to stuff little pieces of paper into each balloon that indicated if the ticket was a winner or loser. Once the balloons were inflated, they were given out to anyone who had bought a specific alcoholic drink, then they popped the balloon to find out if they had won a prize. The nurses thought this a welcome diversion if nothing was happening on the ward and helped me stuff 2000 balloons for the weekend.

Dr Kyle confirmed that after looking at the results from all the scans, the cancer was in my spleen, liver, heart and lymph nodes, and chemotherapy would start immediately (next day) and would last for six sessions, twenty-one days apart, and I would be in until Saturday. The chemotherapy regime I was to have was called CHOP. I read up on it from the notes Bernie had given me.

The diagnosis was officially Non-Hodgkin Lymphoma stage four, grade four. I asked if there was a stage five and was told stage five involved a wooden box and a trip in a hearse. Of course, I asked about life expectancy—like everyone does—and was told I might have as little as six months, depending on the response to the chemotherapy. I didn't ask any more, but was determined that six months was nothing more than a guess that didn't apply to me. I would beat it, irrespective of what it took.

I was started on steroids and had to take sixteen of the little red pills every day, which immediately cured the itch on my leg.

The only side effect I experienced with steroids was bloating around my face, which does go away once you stop taking them. Small price to pay and only temporary. However, long term use does have consequences as I explain in the section Roid Rage later.

What Stage? What Grade?

When I was first diagnosed with cancer, I was stage 4, grade 4, aggressive, which meant nothing to me.

After asking and reading up on staging, my stage 4 meant the cancer had spread, as I had it in my spleen, liver, and heart, then with my fourth visit from Non-Hodgkin Lymphoma it progressed into my colon.

High grade would be Grade 4 and meant the cancer spread fast.

If you're wondering exactly what the grades and stages mean, I've explained all the variations below, and although it's interesting to know exactly where you are with your cancer, I wouldn't get too hung up on them.

Stage

The stage explains how large the tumour is and how far it has spread in the body; it ranges from 0-4 and is usually depicted using Roman numerals. (I, II, III, IV) The further the spread, the higher the stage attributed. The usual method determining stage is by the use of scans such as a CT, MRI, or PET scanner.

Stage 0

Abnormal cells have been detected that are not cancerous but could become so in the future. It also confirms the cells have not spread to any other parts of the body. Depending on the location, health, and age of the patient, a watch-and-wait approach may be used, or ideally the entire tumour is surgically removed. This stage can also be referred to as *in-situ*, which means, in place.

Stage I (1)

Sometimes referred to as early-stage cancer, it confirms cancerous cells have been detected, but the cancer is contained and hasn't spread.

Stage II (2)

Larger cancers or tumours that have grown into adjacent tissue are classified as stage 2.

Stage III (3)

If a tumour has spread more deeply into surrounding tissue or advanced into the lymph nodes (but not other organs), it is classified as stage 3.

Stage IV (4)

And this was my stage where the cancer had spread into other organs of the body, which in my case meant, spleen, liver, and heart. It can sometimes be referred to as secondary or metastatic cancer, which means spread to other parts.

This stage is the one most people dread as it's a guaranteed death sentence. Oh, wait, I was stage 4 and over time it also spread into my colon, and I'm still here, so those people saying it means death? Yeah, they wrong.

Grade

The grade attributed to a cancer diagnosis is determined by how the cells and tissue look under a microscope after a biopsy.

Some cells look relatively normal (though still replicating) and are classified as low grade and well differentiated, Low grade cells have a better prognosis and are less aggressive.

Differentiated is one of those words that requires explanation. Developing cells become mature cells with specific functions, and well differentiated cells resemble the normal tissue it originated from, whereas, poorly differentiated or undifferentiated cells grow quicker and spread more, which makes them dangerous.

High grade cells and tissue look abnormal from healthy cells and tend to be more aggressive. They are classified as poorly differentiated or undifferentiated.

Grade 1 means the cells and tissue resemble healthy cells and tissue and are low grade.

Grade 2 is where the cells and tissue are moderately differentiated and somewhat abnormal. Grade two signifies intermediate grade cancer.

Grade 3 cancer cells and tissue look very abnormal as they don't have architectural structure or pattern resembling normal cells or tissue.

Grade 4 cells are the highest grade which grow and spread fast. The cell structure is totally abnormal and aggressive in its spread. I hate to bring it up again, but I was grade 4 and here we are. Bad? Yes. Impossible? Nope.

TNM staging

Depending on the type of cancer you have, the grade and stage method shown above may not be used and instead the TNM (Tumour Node Metastasis) method is used.

The primary tumour is referred to as T.

TX means the primary tumour cannot be measured.

T0 means the primary tumour cannot be found.

T(is) or in situ. The 'is' means in situ (original place). The primary tumour is within the confines of normal glands and cannot metastasise.

T1, T2, T3, and T4 all refer to the size and extent of the primary tumour. The higher the number the larger the tumour or the greater the spread.

The lymph nodes are referred to as N.

NX means the cancer in nearby lymph nodes cannot be measured.

N0 means there is no cancer present in nearby lymph nodes

N1, N2, N3, and N4 all refer to the number of lymph nodes affected and potential spread.

Metastasis (spread of cancer to other parts) is referred to as M.

MX means the metastasis cannot be measured.

M0 means the cancer has not metastasised.

M1 means the cancer has metastasised and spread to other parts of the body.

Friday 3rd May 2002 (Day 1 of treatment)

News came back that my first lymph node biopsy didn't produce a malignant sample and had to be done again, which was a surprise to me, but considering the number of lymph nodes in the human body (500-600), it isn't that unusual.

Now, as I'd already been there, done that and bought the t-shirt, I decided to pay more attention this time and watch while they operated, which turned out to be too much too soon, as it's not recommended if you are scared by the sight of blood as I was. It was a bit freaky second time; watching them lifting parts of you out while you're awake, but other than the blood, it wasn't really a problem.

Once back on the ward I started my first CHOP chemo with Bernie, my chemo nurse.

My CHOP Chemotherapy Regimen consisted of:

C Cyclophosphamide (Cytoxan®)

H Doxorubicin (Adriamycin® or Rubex®)

O Vincristine (Oncovin®)

P Prednisone (Deltasone®)

Plus Rituxan - a monoclonal antibody; just to finish things off nicely.

Not unexpectedly, Dr Kyle was ahead of the curve with the treatment, as Rituimab/Rituxan had only just been made available, and after suggesting it to me, I leapt at it. She already knew my attitude towards cancer, so it didn't come as a surprise I was up for trying anything and everything.

Fact sheets are available for all chemotherapy treatments, and your chemo nurse will usually give you the relevant literature before treatment starts, although asking fellow patients can usually give you a better indication of what to expect and how to deal with it.

If you do take the time to read the list of potential side effects, it will make your head spin as they seem to cover everything and anything. You will be constipated, or have the runs, you'll shrink, or grow taller, you'll lose muscle tone, you'll turn into the Hulk, your hair will fall out, your hair will grow rapidly, etc.

Watching paint dry

Drip, drlp, drip.

Wow, that's a lot of dripping; or is it? There are 360 drips shown above, which equates to one every 10 seconds or to put it another way, one hour of chemotherapy. (yes, some will be quicker and some slower, but taking an average)

Some treatments take six, seven, eight or more hours, so pages and pages and pages of drips.

Now, if you take the time to read each word instead of assuming they're all the same, you'll find one is different, and no, you don't have to check, but imagine if you did, because for some people, that's what they do from the first drip to the last during chemo; and they wonder why it takes so long.

They watch each one fall and have a story as it does. This one will cure me, this one will make me sick, this one will make my hair fall out, this one will kill me, this one…

Divorce yourself from the process and find a distraction such as reading, talking to other patients, meditating, visualising, listening to a podcast or audiobook, watching a webinar or film or program, but don't watch the paint dry.

Yeah, I would have had to check each one as well, so to confirm your genius, it's drip number 299 which has an L instead of an i, DRLP. If you found it, go you, if you didn't, better luck next time, and if you didn't bother looking, you're going to have a much better time with chemo than you imagined.

Saturday 4th May 2002 (Day 2 of treatment)

No problems to report and I was allowed home around five o'clock.

Glad to be getting home, but the nurses had been excellent, and I felt a bit guilty leaving them, although they were probably happy to see the back of me and my balloons.

The do-gooder

Just home and 'The do-gooder' paid me a visit.

Do-gooder - 'a well-meaning but unrealistic or interfering philanthropist or reformer.'

He convinced me the macrobiotic diet was used by a friend of his with great results, so I tried it.

Frankly, if I had to spend the rest of my life eating the seaweed and pulses recommended, I'd rather be dead anyway.

I researched it in the end and found that other than losing weight, it has no effect on cancer, and I didn't need to lose any more weight.

Don't get me wrong, if I were in their shoes, I would probably have ended up doing the same thing, and they've got your best interests at heart, but when they approach you with, "I've got a cure," they should then follow it up with, "I'm the idiot who read on the internet that eating dried dog faeces cures cancer and the government is trying to hide it."

Thank them for trying to help and promise to discuss it with your consultant, then forget it.

If there was a miracle cure out there, don't you think some of the world's richest and most famous people who have died from cancer would have used it? (see 'Celebrities and cancer' later in the book)

The governments of the world would love a quick solution. It would save bazillions.

Unfortunately, it doesn't exist yet, but the minute a break-through is made, everyone will use it.

"You never know how strong you are

until being strong is the only choice you have."

~ Cayla Mills

Complementary Therapy

As the word suggests, this therapy is complementary to conventional medicine and is used to aid recovery and tolerance of the symptoms. It is not used to cure cancer.

It's worth remembering that the belief in something—whether rational or not—can have a placebo effect where the expectation of a successful outcome can be facilitated by the mind.

A practice that might not suit one person, might suit another, depending on beliefs.

As an example, I believe that visualisation helped me immensely on my journey; yet it is considered to have no effect on cancer by most healthcare professionals.

Acupuncture

The use of needles at points on the body to reduce pain or the feeling of sickness.

Based on ancient theories of Chinese medicine, the acupuncturist alters the flow of Qi (energy) along channels called meridians to restore good health by inserting needles through the skin at certain pre-designated points

It is claimed it can stimulate nerves to release endorphins in the spinal cord and brain which in turn relieve pain. Serotonin can also be released by acupuncture which promotes a feeling of wellbeing and is also a pain reliever.

A friend bought me a session with an acupuncturist, and it didn't hurt in any way; unfortunately, it didn't make a difference in any way either. At best, it was relaxing, but if that's all you're after, try meditation.

Aromatherapy

Aromatherapy is the use of fragrant substances, such as essential oils, in the belief that smelling them will positively affect health. Although there is some evidence aromatherapy can improve general well-being, it has also been promoted for its ability to cure cancer. The American Cancer Society states: Scientific evidence does not support claims that aromatherapy is effective in preventing or treating cancer.

Art Therapy

It's a distraction from the everyday cancer presence. The theory is that by being creative through painting, drawing or sculpting, you use parts of your brain not normally in use which can help you deal with your feelings. It's normal to have group discussions or counselling afterwards.

Counselling

By now, you already know I recommend counselling for everyone going through the cancer journey, including the immediate family. Friends and family are great, but speaking to someone who is trained to help can work wonders.

Counselling can help to get your mind around the diagnosis and journey through treatment and help you manage your emotions. It will show different ways to cope with some of the problems that arise during and after the journey.

Can it cure cancer? No. There is no evidence to show it having any effect on cancer, but it can have a huge effect on how you progress through treatment which can have a very positive effect.

Diet and food supplements

In general, cancer experts recommend following a healthy balanced diet. People often ask their doctor about special diets, but there isn't enough clear information to make exact recommendations about what someone with cancer should eat.

Each person's needs are different. A dietitian can give you advice on what to eat and may prescribe supplements if you need them.

Advice from a dietitian can be helpful, as following a healthy diet can help you fight the cancer by providing you with the energy needed. You have to make sure you have enough energy to deal with everything, and in addition, if your taste is affected during chemo, a dietitian can suggest alternative foods that you will get some satisfaction from.

Some alternative medicine practitioners claim diet can cure cancer, but if you think about it rationally, there is no way a change of diet can attack cancer cells. It just isn't going to happen. There is no evidence anywhere to show diet having any effect on cancer cells.

Hypnotherapy

Hypnotherapy can be used in conjunction with visualisation and can help you make positive lifestyle changes and encourage positive emotions.

Massage Therapy

Massage therapy is a structured and therapeutic touch that can help you to relax and relieve tension.

Meditation

Meditation is a method to reflect, and deeply relax and calm the mind, which can reduce fear, pain, depression, and anxiety.

Put simply, it can help you get control of your emotions and understand what you are experiencing and what you may experience in the future.

Sit in a comfy chair or relax on a bed and don't worry about preconceived notions of sitting cross legged (unless that's what you prefer).

At its most basic, all you have to do is concentrate on your breathing. That's it. In, then out, then…

Your mind will wander at the start, but stick with it and time will sort it.

For a total relaxation experience, lie flat (preferably in a dark room), arms relaxed by your side, and just feel the surface below your body.

Concentrate on your head first and feel it touching the surface. Now feel the weight of your head.

Then, move your concentration to your shoulders and do the same thing, feel every area touch the surface and let the weight hold them in position.

Top of your arms next, followed by bottom of arms, then hands, then back, bum, thighs, calves, and finally feet. Let the weight of each area hold them in position and aim to make everything heavier.

Now, as your eyes are closed, you can't see anything; but you can. Look at the insides of your eyelids (yes, I know you can't, but do it anyway). After a minute or so, your eyes will generate black spots, or green, or a kaleidoscope of colours, and all you do is concentrate on what you're seeing.

Once you are totally relaxed, you'll know, then you'll spoil it, then you'll go in again, then you'll spoil it, then you'll…

As with everything, the more you do it, the better you get.

After around ten sessions (which can be as short as say five minutes and as long as you like), you'll be able to achieve total relaxation in minutes after just lying down and taking a couple of deep breaths.

Don't over think it. Just let it happen and smile.

There are MP3 files on my website you can use to start.

Mindfulness Meditation

Mindfulness meditation is slightly different to meditation alone as it focuses your mind on the moment. You become more aware of your breathing, your life and the now.

It can have a calming and relaxing effect that makes you appreciative of life now, irrespective of any other problems.

Music Therapy

Music therapy is the use of easy-to-play instruments (depending on your level of competence) to promote a sense of achievement and wellbeing. It stimulates parts of the brain you may not normally use, which can act as a distraction.

Reflexology

Reflexology is gentle pressure applied to points on the hands or feet in the belief that different areas represent, or are connected to, different parts of the body.

It can aid relaxation and promote a feeling of wellbeing.

Reiki

Reiki is a procedure where a practitioner blows on, or taps, or touches a patient in an attempt to affect the energy in their body.

It can aid relaxation and promote a feeling of wellbeing.

Self-help Groups

Meeting up with a group of people affected by the same or similar cancer and sharing life experiences of before, during and after treatment.

You can read books and talk to doctors and nurses, but the only way to find out how cancer and treatment affects sufferers, is to talk to someone who has made—or is going through—the journey.

The groups are useful as a source of information and sharing as well as encouragement.

Support Groups

Similar to self-help groups with the advantage of having a professional counsellor or other professional in attendance to guide the topic and offer advice, not only on treatment but the psychology as well.

They are frequently organised by hospitals and charities.

Tai Chi and Qi Gong

The use of physical and mental exercise to cultivate the Qi (energy) that flows through the body's energy pathways.

The practice combines gentle, low-impact movement, breathing and meditation techniques.

It can aid relaxation and promote a feeling of wellbeing.

Therapeutic Touch

In therapeutic touch a therapist usually works just above the surface of the body in the belief that healing energy is transferred from the therapist to the patient.

It can aid relaxation and promote a feeling of wellbeing.

Visualisation

For me, visualisation was the use of the mind to target the cancer cells in an attempt to destroy them, but it can be used effectively to help with pain, sickness, headache, pre-planning a procedure, etc.

Used well with an open mind, it is you training your brain to achieve the outcome you want. You have already seen it demonstrated with my endoscopy exam at the start of my journey.

It is useful to promote the feeling you are contributing to your own cure. Studies have shown that an actual effect on the white blood cells can be achieved by this method, but there is no evidence to show it having any effect on cancer cells directly, but other factors make it a worthwhile exercise.

Yoga

Yoga is (usually) gentle physical exercise and stretching, combined with breathing exercises.

It can aid relaxation and promote a feeling of wellbeing.

My Opinion

My opinion on complementary therapy is that as long as you realise it's not a cure, but a distraction designed to make you feel better, where's the harm?

Anything that can take your mind off your cancer or contribute to a better understanding of your circumstances has to be a good thing.

Concentration is a problem

Understandably, we can't really control our thought processes, and as you're probably thinking about the outcome of your treatment and possibly death, your mind is continually working in an attempt to come up with a solution, so concentration isn't something that comes easy during the process.

The way to counter this is with small manageable targets of distraction. Watch television, but only recorded programs you can dip in and out of, so that when you lose concentration, you can switch to something else and return. Same with magazines, books, computer games, or why not try writing; I did, and here we are. Start a novel or short story, and if you become involved, it's surprising just how fast time passes, and you don't even realise.

Set yourself gentle realistic targets, but don't beat yourself up if you don't meet them. Aim for five or ten minutes on a computer game, TV programme, or read ten pages of a magazine or two of a book. Easily manageable goals are the secret. Sitting down with the intention of reading an entire novel that you would have done in the past just isn't realistic, no matter how much you like the author, but two pages or a short chapter?

Keep yourself constantly distracted and give yourself a pat on the back when you beat your target. Don't have a daily target for every hour of the day as you'll be over-optimistic, and you need to allow time for sleep (when the need arises), but instead use hourly targets and modify as necessary as the hours go by. It can be helpful to write activities on little cards that you can shuffle and take them as they come.

Write your progress down and it will give you something to compare the next day and the one after that until everything is back to some sort of normality.

If you ask for sympathy or complain, it's probable the people you talk to aren't undergoing treatment and have no idea what you're going through. "Grab a seat and watch TV," they say, "you've nothing else to do, you lucky thing."

Seriously? If it were only that simple.

When I received my stem-cell transplant, I was locked in a tiny room 24/7 and was going nuts. Sure, I had a TV, but although I tried to watch, my mind quickly lost interest.

During treatment, regular sleep patterns vanish. When you want to sleep, you can't, and when you want to be awake, you need to sleep, and when you are awake, your mind is so mixed up you can't enjoy things you previously enjoyed as you can't concentrate.

It all sounds overwhelming but knowing what to expect and planning how to deal with it can make a huge difference. It's something you can't comprehend until you're out the other side, so make your plans now and don't get caught out.

You need to understand it's the treatment/circumstances, and given time things will improve. It's not you.

Don't stress or allow yourself to get frustrated.

Just accept it and take it one step at a time.

The more potential distractions you have, the quicker time seems to go by, but be sensible, fill your day by all means, but rest when you need it.

Meditation time can help a lot with this, as well as simple breathing exercises where you free your mind to concentrate on nothing but the inhale and exhale and just feel your body working. Visualisation is even better, and both are discussed later in this book.

The secret is little and often and lots of variety.

Try something for as long as you can comfortably stick it, then move on to something else or just rest if that's what you need.

Constipation

Sunday 5th May 2002 (Day 3 of treatment)

I was constipated. Boy was I ever.

Very painfully constipated. Really, really constipated. Awesomely constipated. You get my drift?

I sat on the loo so long straining, my wife thought I had bad sunburn on my face when I eventually came out. I was bright red, and all for nothing.

In fairness, I had been warned it might be a problem and had been given some lactulose home with me, but because of the possibility that diarrhoea might also be a problem, it wasn't suggested I take it beforehand. Wait and see what happens, they said. It'll be a surprise, they said. Some surprise.

My advice is plan for constipation and if it turns out you have the opposite, it isn't going to make much difference, but out of the two—in terms of pain—I'll take diarrhoea every time.

I said at the start of this book there might be some embarrassing episodes, but I'd be honest, irrespective of how bad they might be, so here goes.

The fact is lactulose takes time to work, and constipation is painful, so what to do?

In my frustration, I had a brain wave. At this stage the possibility of using a spoon had crossed my mind, but what I ended up doing was filling a washing up liquid bottle with warm water mixed with olive oil (no, I have no idea where that came from either), squatting in the bath and squirting the liquid where the sun doesn't shine.

What I recommend is you plan for every eventuality based on the information sheets on the drugs and avoid having to do this, but… it did work, and it was bliss.

Every time thereafter, the night before chemo, I always had a large spoonful of lactulose. First thing the next morning, I had another large spoonful, and I also had a breakfast of prunes, lots of them.

Find out if constipation is a possibility for the treatment you are likely to receive. If you ignore it, you will regret it.

Ask your doctor or fellow patients for advice and start your new high-fibre diet, which makes everything move a lot easier.

If you do get caught, as I did, you should immediately call your doctor (don't try to sort it yourself), explain the seriousness of the situation, and ask for immediate advice. If it means a visit to the hospital, then do that.

After I managed to get everything sorted, someone asked me what I thought about constipation. I told them I couldn't give a shit.

Pain rating is 11/10. Everything to worry about. Avoid at all cost.

Another useful tip

This one took time to discover as I'd never used them before, but haemorrhoid suppositories work wonders and probably help to avoid haemorrhoids in the process

I suspect most people won't even know what a suppository is, which is a good thing, but with cancer, things change.

My best description is that it's a little bullet shaped pill, about an inch long, that goes where the sun doesn't shine, and it numbs the pain of haemorrhoids and shrinks them. You can insert one while sitting on the toilet, or kneel on the floor and insert it from the front or back, whichever is easier, but don't take any chances with elaborate positions that require balancing as light-headedness is always a possibility when you're on treatment.

You're probably wondering why I'm talking about haemorrhoids when the subject was constipation, but in this instance it's relevant because the suppository softens the stool and makes it easier to defecate.

Unfortunately, I have to get ever so slightly technical with the technique as just inserting without pushing it through the sphincter means it will pop out immediately, so you have to actually push your finger in a little bit until you feel the suppository pass the sphincter.

Yeah, it's a tad embarrassing to describe, but... the potential for relief from constipation far outweighs my unease.

Hygiene is obviously paramount, and you will need to wash your hands thoroughly afterwards, especially when you find out the suppository cream seems to be waterproof and you need lots of soap to dissolve it, but it's not a problem.

I would advise you to check with your doctor to see if they're okay with it, because there may be complications in your medical history that I don't know about, but for me, my chemo nurse and my consultant both said it was okay and thank goodness they did because it made things so much easier.

Squatting.

No. I'm not talking about taking possession of an empty house.

I'm laying my soul bare here, and even before I begin, I'm embarrassed, but needs must, and if you can benefit from my experience, then it's something that must be included.

As described above, one of the most unpleasant side effects can be extreme constipation which is painful and can cause other problems when you strain too hard, such as literally ripping yourself a new asshole. Sorry, I apologise, and I know this isn't the nicest subject to broach, but, if reading this helps, you'll thank me.

The human body isn't designed to sit on a throne to defecate; it's made to squat. You know, like an animal?

If you haven't heard of this—and let's face it, not many have—Google defines it as: 'Compare sitting on the toilet to a kinked garden hose, it just doesn't work properly. In a squatting posture, the bend straightens out and defecation becomes easier. Assuming the squat position is the natural way to achieve easier and more complete elimination.'

Our ancestors did it, and it's still practised in some countries, but in the 'civilised' world we live in, a toilet is the preferred option; but it makes it a lot easier when you squat.

If you are severely constipated and have been sitting on the toilet most of the day with no results, you'll try anything to relieve the pain, and yes, I ended up trying it, and yes, it works.

It's a complicated and dangerous procedure to try standing on the rim of the toilet and lowering yourself into position, but at the start—when I was still reasonably strong—that's what I did. It also has the added risk of passing out when you're trying to balance and evacuate at the same time, so if fainting is your thing, there is an alternative.

Later on, when the chemo was taking its toll and the energy wasn't there, I used a newspaper in the bath and a load of tissue spread out on top, which works well, but urinate first; and no, I didn't find out the hard way.

It should go without saying that a rigorous clean-up and wash afterwards is necessary.

Plan it out and take your time.

The added benefit is that if you do an ordinary poo, you'll find that sometimes you wipe and wonder why you bothered because there's nothing there. It's a much cleaner process, albeit not in the tray.

An easier way to do it—rather than using the shower or bath—is using a little tray or basin you can buy from any kitchen supply/hardware shop; put folded loo roll tissue on the bottom, do your business and tip everything into the toilet, then wash it with some hot water and it's ready for next time.

Some people are going to say, "I could never do that. That's disgusting."

I would say that what is disgusting is suffering unnecessarily and trying to force yourself because humans do it the wrong way. When you're on chemo, you need to make everything as easy as possible.

Constipation is hard to avoid when you're on chemotherapy, but a change of diet works wonders, and using the lactulose as and when required is recommended. Everyone is different, and your chemo may affect you in other ways, but for me, I always took some lactulose the day before and morning of chemo.

If you can get into the habit of eating prunes for breakfast, they will help free your insides, as well as incorporating roughage into your diet. All supermarkets carry tins of prunes, so just pop the lid and throw 10-12 into a bowl, it's not that bad, honestly.

Ask for and take advice from your doctor or nutritionist.

I'm glad that's out of the way. I can feel my face going red when I'm typing, but not as red as it was when I was straining on the loo.

Haemorrhoids

A royal pain in the ass. (forgive me)

Haemorrhoids (which are also called piles) are swollen veins in the last part of your back passage, the anus. They can be inside the back passage, or more often, they will protrude outside the anus. If they become inflamed or irritated, they can bleed and will usually be uncomfortable, or painful, or extremely painful.

They are mostly caused by straining when you go to the loo or by very loose stools (diarrhoea). Chemotherapy and haemorrhoids go hand in hand, so be prepared to ask the nurses for something to stop the pain the minute they appear, otherwise, they will just get worse.

Particularly when I was receiving my stem cell transplant, I had lots of problems, and it was one of the most common topics talked about by patients on the ward. (fascinating conversational stuff, I'm sure you'll agree)

Some people are initially embarrassed to ask for help when this problem arises, and the only advice I can give is; get over it. The downside is so far down, you will regret your embarrassment. The nurses and doctors have encountered this problem with most chemo patients and won't think twice about it. They may need to look at them, and you will have to lie on your side and pull your knees towards your chin. Yeah, that's what happens, but again, your bum ain't anything special.

Best advice: Watch out for them, expect them, and have the cream and suppositories ready.

Crying like a baby?

Whether it's down to the chemotherapy or an emotional response to the process is something that seems to divide opinion, but for some people, tears can appear without any apparent reason or warning.

I have seen big men crying like babies and, although I don't think I'm in the big man category, I count myself among them as a fellow cry-baby; however, where the word is normally used to describe a whinger, in this context it's related to the physical act of producing tears. Lots of them.

Everything is fine until it isn't. You're all growed up and you don't cry. You haven't since you were at school and then, one day, you find yourself bawling your eyes out. Not a little weep or a stray tear, but enough to fill a swimming pool, and no, you can't control it. You know it's weird, and you know it's not the normal you, and you know you can stop it; except, you can't.

You analyse your current mood and try to determine exactly what's wrong, but can't find out why it's happening.

From wet experience, I've never been able to control it. The good news is that after you finish treatment and come out the other side, it rarely happens, but during treatment, whether it's the chemo or the cancer or the pressures associated with both, or something else, it's just gonna happen. Don't think any less about yourself or see it as any type of failure; just accept it, and if you're reading this and it doesn't happen—lucky you.

But, tears are good. No, seriously. They are nature's way of helping you cope, and when you need a good cry, you should do just that and don't try to stop it.

There are three kinds of tears:

Basal Tears – These keep your cornea lubricated and nourished.

Reflex Tears – When you cut that onion or get something in your eye, reflex tears wash away the irritation.

Psychic Tears – Produced in response to emotional pain, physical pain, stress, etc.

The relevant tears for our purposes are the Psychic Tears, which are related to the area of your brain that deals with your emotions called the limbic system and specifically the hypothalamus, so when the tears start, they also release a natural painkiller called leucine enkephalin, which is the reason people feel better after a good cry.

Of course, it isn't all bad. You'll find yourself crying when your happy, or sad, or when someone's nice to you, or when someone ignores you. For no reason whatsoever you'll cry, but afterwards, when you've changed your shirt and dried yourself off, you will feel a lot better. Then you'll be happy, then you'll cry because you're happy. Yeah, it can be a wet and confusing time.

My opinion is, this phenomenon—in my case—doesn't seem to have been motivated by the emotional response theory as it's still there to some extent (once in a blue moon) well after chemotherapy has finished.

Another little side effect? Maybe not for everyone, but it isn't a bad one.

Expect it and accept it as another side-effect if it does happen, and if it doesn't, it's all good.

Cancer ghosting?

Yeah, it's a funny term; it sounds like cancer is not only in your body but haunting your house as well; it's not that, but it is something that happens frequently, and it's when you have a relationship with someone who you know you can rely on, then you get a cancer diagnosis and they disappear. It's as if you don't exist anymore.

Research conducted by The War on Cancer found that 65% of survivors said they had been ghosted by friends who they thought they could never in a million years have fallen out with or ignored.

The reason is potentially; some people are idiots and think cancer can be transmitted through close contact, or—because you have now decided to be sick—you can't help them anymore, or they're unsure what to say, or your illness has reminded them they're mortal, or... The list goes on and on, but basically, they can't face you. Your BFFL (Best Friends For Life) vanish without a trace.

Some just aren't equipped to provide the emotional support they know you're going to need, so they don't give any at all.

They feel guilty because they're healthy, and you're dying, and even though cancer isn't necessarily a death sentence, in their minds, you've already got one foot in the grave, so it's easier to distance themselves then turn up at the funeral and say great things about you.

The other thing is, you may have thought they were your lifelong, absolute best friend, and you could have been wrong.

Could it be you were just a means to an end? That happened to me. Two of my friends jumped ship when I was first diagnosed. One just vanished and wouldn't take my calls, the other visited me in hospital during my second chemo, and that was the last I saw of him.

The surprising thing is others I knew wouldn't be on my side, rallied around and were exceptionally supportive.

I gotta say, it hurts, especially when you're lying in bed thinking if the shoe were on the other foot; but that's life. Better to find out sooner rather than later.

Years later, the guy who I knew would never let me down apologised when I bumped into him at a chip shop. "I wasn't there when you needed me. I apologise. I just couldn't handle it."

What was the point? It was way too late. I remember I might have suggested he go away. Yeah, I can't remember the exact wording, but the second word was definitely "off."

I invested my emotions in this person, and if they had been where I was, I would have been there for them—100%. Tell me what you need, and I will make it happen.

"*Not getting what you want is sometimes a wonderful stroke of luck.*" ~ Dalai Lama.

I've said it before in this book. Sometimes cancer is what you need. Sometimes cancer is a revelation. Sometimes cancer changes you for the better. And when your friends let you down, it's a harsh wake-up call, but a necessary wake-up call that brings you to the reality of life.

It's better to find out the hard way than not find out at all. That's a strange thing to say, but if they don't have your back when you're ill, they never had it in the first place.

Cut them out of your life like cancer and don't look back.

Granocyte/Neupogen/Neulasta injections

After chemo, I was told to come back the next day to get an injection of a drug designed to make the white blood cells grow again.

Granocyte is used to stimulate the growth of white blood cells after you have received your chemotherapy.

It is injected under the skin, usually around the abdomen, thigh, or upper arm area. Simply pinch some skin and insert the needle at an angle. It's known as a *sub-cut* injection (subcutaneous) as it's injected under the skin and not into a vein. Your doctor or nurse will make sure you are trained in this procedure. (yes, you're going to do it yourself) If you cannot bear to inject yourself, a district nurse or outpatient visit can be arranged for this purpose, but, if you can get your head around it, the injections are easy, and I gave them to myself many times.

The thing about it is, when you inject yourself, it empowers you. You are participating in your own cure. You are actively doing something to beat cancer. You are a superpower.

The training consists of practising on a red rubber ball and simply inserting the needle and injecting the liquid. They suggest you insert the needle in one quick movement, but I found a better way. (Yeah, you knew I would, didn't you?) Being averse to pain, I found that by just pushing the needle against my belly gently and waiting, the skin actually swallowed the needle by itself; no need to pinch the skin and no need to jab it in, which made it a lot easier and meant there was no bruising afterwards. Another tip is to avoid squirting the liquid in quickly, as I found it produced yet more bruising, so instead, I squeezed it in as slowly as I could and stopped occasionally for say ten seconds, then started again. Understandably, the nurses don't have time to wait until your skin decides it will welcome the needle, but when you're at home, you have plenty of time.

If you visit www.cancerology.co/injection you can watch a video where I not only talk you through it, but I inject myself as well just to prove how easy it is.

The one big plus in giving yourself an injection is a) you're one of only a few people who have done it, and b) you're really, really participating in your own cure. The feelgood factor after giving yourself an injection??? It's off the scale.

Like almost all drugs, growth factors may cause side effects. These depend on which growth factor you have and will vary from one person to another.

Later in my treatment, I was changed from Granocyte to Neupogen, and at one stage I also used Neulasta. All these are designed to combat Neutropenia, which is when your blood has lower levels of neutrophils (white blood cells), which increases the susceptibility of infection.

Some people have bone pain: usually a dull ache or discomfort in the bones of the back, pelvis, arms or legs. This is usually mild and goes away when the growth factor injections stop.

Your skin may become red and itchy around the place where the injection is given. This will disappear once the course of injections is over, but the solution is to find a new site each day. Personally, I had no problems with the injection site and it never became red or itchy. I put this entirely down to my more gentle method and could easily inject the same site multiple days, whereas, other patients were constantly showing me their bruises and complaining. (Yes, I did tell them my method and it was confirmed as a good idea the next time we met.)

You may have fever, chills, fluid retention, and breathlessness. Fluid retention may lead to swelling of the ankles or breathlessness, which again, I managed to avoid.

Tell your doctor or nurse if you have any side effects.

Your doctor may prescribe painkillers such as paracetamol or something stronger to help.

My experience was that I used the injection every day until the pain started and then stopped. Maybe I had a high pain threshold or maybe it just took time for the pain to develop, but I did suffer occasionally and had to use the oral morphine, but of course, there was that one occasion where I didn't stop on time and paid the price.

Stick it in my bum

Yeah, I'm betting the headline made you stop and think, didn't it? My first ride in an ambulance was during my CHOP treatment when the bone pain associated with the granocyte injections was unbearable. I had woken up around three in the morning with the pain, and even though my wife brought me oramorph (liquid oral morphine), it wasn't up to the job and an ambulance was called.

When they arrived, I couldn't even get out of bed, and they had to strap me into a chair to get me down the stairs. Once the ambulance started, I discovered that if the driver hit the cat's eyes on the white line, the bumping relieved the pain, so I insisted he drive to the hospital hitting as many potholes and cat's eyes as he could.

The pain was immense, and I've subsequently talked to a lady who had the same experience and even she said it was worse than giving birth, so as guys don't tolerate pain anywhere near as much as girls, you can appreciate the problem.

Once at the hospital, I bypassed casualty altogether—as the risk of infection was too high—and went straight to the cancer ward, which is the normal protocol for all cancer patients.

I was put in a cubicle and told to wait.

By now the pain had me occasionally seeing black with little stars, which is usually associated with passing out, but I couldn't lie on the bed and had begun to stomp my feet as it brought some relief.

A doctor arrived and told me a simple morphine injection in my behind would solve the problem. As he was preparing the syringe, I started shouting for him to stick it in my bum, over and over again. My wife laughed, but unfortunately, I wasn't in the frame of mind to see the humour. Eventually (which was probably less than a minute but felt like days) the morphine was injected and relief arrived.

I was in bed when the curtain was pulled back and the guy in the next bed asked, 'Well, did he stick it in your bum?' The ward that had been quiet on my arrival erupted into laughter, and I confess, even I seen the funny side.

"Not once, not twice, but 17 times I beat cancer.

So fight like you mean it."

~ Lawrence Wray

Should I stop treatment/chemo?

If you're thinking about stopping treatment, it's probably because you're having a rough time afterwards; sickness, mouth ulcers, exhaustion, etc., but this is a question nobody can answer. For sure, I can't answer it, but I suspect if I met you, I'd advise against stopping, but talk to your doctor and take advice from them. Seek a second opinion, but don't let people tell you what they think you want to hear, that is not helpful.

Some people give up because they can't afford the time off work, and that's just stupid. You can't work if you're dead. Wise up.

Some because they have found alternative treatment or believe something else will be better. Be very careful here; you're making a decision when your mind is overloaded and you'll believe anything (because you want to). If you find something wonderful that nobody else knows about, check it. See if I've included it in the alternative treatment section.

I had a friend who had completed four out of six treatments, but it was hard, and she was in hospital more than she was out, so after talking it over with a team of cancer experts—which comprised of her friends and family—it was decided (against medical advice) to stop treatment; after all, she had already finished four of the six so that was probably all that was required.

You might have heard the joke about Paddy Irishman swimming the channel (I'm Irish, so I can tell Irish jokes), and when he was three-quarters of the way across he was exhausted so turned back. Think about it.

Have you ever had a hangover? (If not, skip this paragraph, but if you have, read on.) A hangover where you're on the big white telephone talking to God? Vomiting your guts into the toilet and retching till there's nothing more? Then it comes; "I'm never drinking again." You swear that's it, it's not worth it, then Friday arrives, and your friends invite you over, offer you a drink, and the cycle starts all over, even though you swore you'd never do it again.

The brain is a funny thing; it can control you or you can control it—even though it's the brain doing all the work in the first place—and that's what happens with alcohol, so when you're having a rough time on chemo and swear to stop, it's easier to stop as there is no friend inviting you out for a pleasant time that may or may not end up with a hangover, it's a doctor advising, and a guarantee you're going to feel bad, so the thought of stopping is strong. You might have just started treatment, and everything has come as a shock, but you're stronger than you think. You might be where Paddy Irishman and my friend were and completed more than half the treatment, so grit your teeth and get it over with?

My friend? She stopped treatment, felt better for five months, then when the cancer returned, decided to go back on treatment, but it was too late; the cancer had metastasised, her body was riddled with tumours. She died.

I had begged her not to give up with only two treatments left, but no matter what I said, her husband told her she was suffering too much and he had a good feeling. A good feeling? What the hell does a good feeling have to do with anything? For very obvious reasons, I haven't spoken to the dickhead since, and if he reads this, tough.

I don't have a magic crystal where I can tell you what to do, but there were many times in my journey where my brain said, *give up*, and to be fair I thought about it, for like a millisecond, then said no. The determination came from common sense, and sheer bloody mindedness. Was I scared I might die anyway? Yes, but without treatment I knew I didn't stand a chance with my prognosis as bad as it was.

I have no doubt there are exceptions where somebody has stopped treatment and survived, but I also have no doubt that the number who have stopped and died is way greater.

Cancer is hard. Chemo is hard. Death is harder. Fight like your life depends on it; it does. Once you start, don't stop.

"I have heard there are troubles of more than one kind,
Some come from ahead and some come from behind,
But I've bought a big bat, I'm all ready you see,
Now my troubles are going to have troubles with me!"
~ Dr. Seuss

Sunday 12th May 2002 (Day 12 of treatment)

First sore chemo day. Spent most of the day in bed.

Sick and out of sorts but not sick, if that makes sense.

In other words, having had the expectation of severe vomiting because of the chemo, it didn't materialise.

Nausea and vomiting are caused by the body stimulating the vomiting centre of the brain (honestly, that's what it's called). Vomiting is a protective mechanism designed to eliminate anything that irritates your stomach or small intestine, and signals are sent to the vomiting centre from the relevant organs which makes you vomit in an attempt to expel the offending substance. There is also a part of the brain known as the chemoreceptor trigger zone which detects any problematic substances in the bloodstream and notifies the vomiting centre when anything is detected that is deemed to be potentially harmful.

I asked about this and discovered that if you've abused alcohol (as I had) or drugs (nope), the body builds up a tolerance to toxicity and abuse. When someone has their first bottle of wine and throws up, and then ten years and numerous bottles per night later, three bottles hardly has any effect as their body is used to the toxicity, it's the same with chemo, and when it enters the equation, the body doesn't panic as much as someone who doesn't drink.

It is also usual that guys tolerate the chemo better than the ladies. (Sorry, girls)

Understandably, people don't relish the prospect of constantly being sick, but the first time you vomit as a result of chemo you should think of it like this:

I'm being sick, which means the chemo is having an effect and I'm getting enough.

If it's making me vomit, it means it's working.

You need to turn negative feelings into positive feelings and welcome the fact this is happening, which isn't as hard as it seems. When you vomit try to relax. Yes, I know that sounds silly, but get control of your bodily functions and accept your body is doing its job. Realise your stomach is going to heave and whatever contents your stomach has will exit your throat, so losing some of the tension in your body makes the process easier. Easy is good.

Unfortunately, a side effect of vomiting can be a little accident at the rear end, so a) if it happens, clean up and move on and b) you might consider an incontinence pad. At the end of the day it's not a biggie, but anything you can do to make it easier is good as you don't have the energy to jump in a shower every time it happens.

It's not funny, but cancer is the gift that doesn't stop giving, but… once you're out the other side, you're stronger in every conceivable way in comparison to everyone else.

You don't have to look forward to being sick, but you do need to accept it as a good sign and make it easier on yourself.

If every time you throw up you consider it the worst feeling in the world, then that's what you'll experience and you'll dread it; so please, expect it and welcome it. Turn the negative into a positive and you'll deal with it a lot better.

Wednesday 15th May 2002 (Day 13 of treatment)

It started a couple of days ago when I noticed hairs on my pillow every morning, just a couple at first then progressing to a hairy pillow.

My son started to notice, so being the fun-guy I am, I invited him to pull some out. I thought he would tentatively pull a couple of stray hairs, but no, he grabbed a handful and yanked it out leaving me with a very noticeable bald spot just above my right ear.

It didn't hurt as it was falling out anyway, but it was the first thing my wife noticed on her return from work.

Thursday 16th May 2002

I have big ears that stick out, and ever since I was a child, I insisted my hair cover them, so my hairdresser was very aware just what I wanted every time I went for a cut, but today would turn out to be the last haircut I ever had. Ever.

When I went in, she immediately noticed the bald spot and started laughing, but then I explained the reason for my visit. In fairness, she confessed she had never shaved a head before and had to nip out to purchase a razor.

It didn't take long, and I probably could have pulled it out myself as my eyebrows were also waving goodbye at this stage.

Before we had finished, she had to stop and wipe her tears every couple of minutes.

Emotional stuff, but after she unveiled my new bald-dude look, I went to a shop and bought a bottle of wine and a box of chocolates for her. I suspected I would never need her services again, which turned out to be right.

Hair loss and chemotherapy

Yes… when you get chemotherapy, your hair normally falls out, (not always, but mostly), and some people, when they see the first strands of hair on their pillow think, this is the beginning of the end. They get depressed, they get downhearted, they're going to be bald, they're going to look awful, and people are going to laugh, which of course isn't the case, but it's a general perception and it's understandable.

The thing to remember is that once your hair starts to fall out, it can really only mean one thing, and that is that the chemotherapy is working. It's killing the cells, so your hair falls out, and if it's killing the cells, it's also killing the cancer cells, which is the aim of the game. So, when you see the first clumps of hair on your pillow, you should be thinking, *Damn this stuff's good and it's working.*

Rather than feeling bad about it, pre-accept it's going to happen, and when it does, you should have a smile on your face. You can, of course, throw in a, 'Wow. This means I'm going to be okay,' or something similar, but the fact is the treatment is doing what it's meant to do. So instead of tears, it should be a celebration, and as it's very early on in treatment, you might even have a little bubbly because you'll still have your taste buds at this stage. That's something to look forward to, the loss of taste, which also means that the chemo is working and killing cancer cells, which also means the loss of taste is a good thing too, but a pain at the same time. The next thought in your mind should be that your hair will grow again after treatment has finished, and that's something to smile about. Something to celebrate. So, when you think of it, it's an inconvenience, but really, in the overall scheme of things, it's not a big deal. Not even close.

Guys

My advice—for what it's worth—is wait until it starts to comb out easily or mess up your pillow, and then bite the bullet. Go and have a number one or better yet, just get it shaved. If he/she won't shave you, get plenty of shaving foam, and do it yourself. It's very easy, and no, you shouldn't be able to cut your head with the razor as the skin on your head is much tighter than your chin. When you get used to doing it, it's like combing your head with a razor, if that makes sense.

I've seen a couple of guys who didn't want to say goodbye to their curls, and without exaggeration, there is nothing more noticeable or silly-looking than a guy with tufts of hair randomly sticking out of his head.

Anyway, that's my advice; it's up to you what you do.

Girls

My sympathies are with you.

I know how much it means to you, but it's only short term. It'll grow back again once chemotherapy is finished, with the added bonus you are still alive, so prepare for it from the start and organise a wig if that's what you decide.

Well before you need to have your head shaved, cut a sample so you can match it to a wig if necessary, and if you do go down that route, organise it well in advance of needing it.

You can also wear the wig to the hairdressers and get it cut to your normal style.

Alternatively, just accept it and go bald as many girls do. Personally, I think it looks great and it's also a way of saying, Fuck Cancer. It says you're strong, you're independent, and you're fighting. In some ways, it can make your determination even stronger.

Guys and Girls

Hair loss is not only restricted to the head. Basically, everything from top to toe falls out eventually, and yes, that includes pubic hair, nose hair, eyelashes, eyebrows, leg and body hair. I found out this isn't as bad as it sounds, and if I had the choice, I think it's much more hygienic not to have hair all over your body, but as I say, that's just my opinion.

Nineteen years on and, although I can still grow head hair, I choose to shave my head twice a week.

If you're used to having a full head of hair, you will also notice how warm it kept your head. It's freezing without hair, irrespective of the weather, but eventually, you get used to it. When you're on treatment, you must keep warm, so buy some headwear and make use of it.

And the last thing to prepare for is how white your head is compared to your face if you are even slightly tanned. Not a biggie, but you'll notice it, so if it's going to be a problem, organise some make up to blend in. I really noticed it and felt self-conscious of it, but then I thought, it is what it is, it's cancer, and really, who cares?

Another interesting side effect is you may find your nose runs. When you get out of bed and stand up, some snot may fly out as a result of having no hair to hold everything in. All things considered, it isn't really a problem, but something to be aware of. Make sure you have tissues placed around the house just in case.

Cold Cap

Before treatment starts you may be offered the use of a cold cap, which is basically scalp cooling in an attempt to delay/avoid hair loss on the head.

There are two types of cold cap. One is filled with a cold gel that needs to be changed every thirty-minutes, and one that uses a cooling machine to pump liquid coolant through the cap.

Both types need to be worn before, during and after the chemotherapy is given and your chemo nurse can give you the necessary advice.

On the plus side, a cap may help you either keep your hair for longer or delay hair loss completely, and on the negative side, some people suffer headaches afterwards or symptoms like a brain freeze after drinking a cold drink.

The idea is the cap reduces the blood flow to the hair follicles, which may reduce the amount of chemotherapy they receive.

In fairness, it works with varying degrees from person to person and depends on the type of chemotherapy received.

You will also have to bear in mind there are some chemotherapy drugs that can't be used with a cold cap as it restricts their effectiveness.

Normally you will be given conditioning treatment to put on your hair before using the cap, and it is recommended you comb this through your hair to flatten it before the cap is fitted.

It is also essential to make sure the cap is a snug fit and covers all areas where your hair normally grows. If it's loose on the back of your head, then it loses its effectiveness in that area.

As I haven't worn a cold cap, I can't give you first-hand details, but many women describe the first half-hour of wearing the cap as being the most uncomfortable.

After treatment, it is recommended you do not wash your hair for around forty-eight hours and try to limit washes to two or three times a week using warm rather than hot water.

When drying, simply pat dry rather than rubbing with a towel, and brush very gently using a soft hairbrush or wide-tooth comb.

You stink

One of the minor but unpleasant side effects of chemo is when the drugs are metabolised in the body and eliminated through sweat. Irrespective of how often you wash or how much deodorant you use, your body is continuously producing sweat, which, when modified by the metabolised chemo, can have a disgusting smell.

When chemo suppresses the immune system, the skin's normal response is altered, which means different bacteria that would have previously been routinely destroyed, can now develop.

Washing regularly does help, as well as drinking plenty of water to help flush the chemo. You have a good indicator of how effective drinking water is when your urine is nearly clear. If you notice your urine is dark, it's time to up your fluid intake.

Exercise that produces sweat will also help to reduce the smell as you are expelling a lot more in one go. If you can't exercise, ask your doctor if you could use a sauna or steam bath.

Diet also has a part to play and eating plenty of fresh fruit and vegetables can help as they provide detoxification support for the liver, which is where the metabolism of the drugs initially takes place.

Unfortunately, there is no quick remedy, which means that clothes and bed linen will need to be changed often, but it's a small price to pay, and after chemo, everything will quickly return to normal.

"When someone has cancer, the whole family and everyone who loves them does too." ~ Terri Clark

Sex and cancer

The problem with your sex drive when you're on chemotherapy is; it doesn't exist. (Yes, I will concede that in the mind, sex is still great, but in reality... not so much.)

They say some people can carry on their sex lives when they're having chemotherapy: I personally find that hard to believe because there is no energy. When you think about it, if you're too weak to go for a normal walk, then the physical effort required for good sex means it ain't gonna happen.

Before cancer you may have been a sex god (I was) (*Oh, no you weren't*), but once you have treatment, interest goes and then the ability follows.

The good news is it doesn't last and returns with a vengeance, but for 3-6 months of your life as a grown adult, not wanting sex is going to be a surprise. It's a bit like not wanting to eat for someone who's always had a great appetite and loves food (but chemo will take care of that as well).

For the partner of a cancer patient—especially if they're used to a loving physical relationship—it can be a problem if you take the physical aspect away. It puts a lot of pressure on both parties. One thinks they should perform (but can't), and the other thinks they (the patient) should perform even though they understand that cancer is in the way.

It needs to be discussed, and don't forget there are other ways to satisfy; it doesn't have to be penetrative sex.

Discussing it openly with your partner is a great idea, before, during, and even after treatment, as you are going to be affected and will need time and understanding; and that's a potential problem, because if time and understanding isn't available from your partner, you've hit the rocks as a couple.

It happens to so many cancer patients who were previously in a loving relationship that their partner doesn't have the patience to wait; doesn't have the empathy or the capacity to understand.

As I've said previously, everyone needs to be on the same page, and sex is no different. Of course, for those couples for whom sex isn't a big part of life, it's not so much of a problem.

In addition, you've got to take precautions because if you're on chemo and you're a guy, then there is the potential your semen can have chemotherapy in it. Experts say it's not definite, but it is probable, and in the same way it was thought chemotherapy doesn't cross the brain blood barrier, it clearly does, so you'll need to use a condom.

I would suspect the same is true of females, so if someone is giving oral, chemotherapy might be present.

The major risk is if chemotherapy has affected the sperm and pregnancy occurs as there could be problems, however, the usual problem during and mostly after chemotherapy is sterility.

I am no expert in this as it's not my area of expertise, so as usual I'm going to suggest you ask for help from those who know.

When I was on chemotherapy, sex was great in my mind, but realistically, it didn't happen. I didn't have the energy. But a cuddle was nice if that was available.

"Anyone who has beaten cancer is gifted with a superpower mortals can't understand." ~ Lawrence Wray

The Fabulous Nocebo Effect

I think it's fair to say most people will have heard of the placebo effect, but have you heard of the nocebo effect?

The definitions for the two are:

The Placebo Effect

A medicine or procedure prescribed for the psychological benefit to the patient rather than for any physiological effect. A substance that has no therapeutic effect, used as a control in testing new drugs.

How does this work? You have an illness, and as a result of taking nothing for it, you mysteriously get better?

Weirder still, there have been studies where patients knew from the outset they were taking a placebo and again it worked. Some even asked to be given the pills to use after the trial was over.

If a placebo works, but doesn't do anything, and it works even though you know it doesn't do anything, then why do you need it in the first place?

Nobody can give an accurate reason as it varies from person to person, but the thought is that the expectation of a result motivates your body to provide you with just that outcome.

If you expect something, your body will do everything in its power to make it happen, and it's just my opinion, but throughout my various treatments, I always expected to come out the other side. I always seen myself finishing treatment and being healthy again.

In a controlled test, a group was told to exercise for thirty minutes as hard as they could on static bikes while taking a sip from a cup every five minutes, swilling it around their mouths for ten seconds and spitting it out. The amount of liquid was carefully measured to ensure nothing was swallowed. The test was then repeated two days later, which gave them time to recover. Unbeknown to them, the control groups were split into two, with half getting only water with colouring in it, while the other half were given the same mixture but with added sugar. On the second ride, the cups were switched so everyone had experienced both liquids. The results showed that even though the riders were spitting the liquid out each time, the group with the sugar mix in both tests performed significantly better.

Okay, so not really a placebo test in the truest sense, but the body analysed the liquid in the mouth, deduced that the one with the sugar meant the body would be getting energy from the drink and boosted the performance on the expectation.

Could it then be said that having a positive approach to the outcome from cancer treatment could have similar results? Personally, I think that if you think the cancer is being beaten, then the body will do everything in its power to facilitate your expectations.

This experiment, to me, would seem to indicate the brain has a reserve of power that, for some reason, it only allows you to access at certain times or for certain reasons.

A startling report on homeless people who had died and been autopsied discovered that over eight percent had cancer at some point that had left its mark but subsequently regressed. These included people with lymphoma, prostate cancer, stomach cancer, colon cancer, kidney cancer, and even brain cancer. The deaths were attributed to other causes, but the evidence showed the previous existence of cancer that had never been diagnosed or treated and that had gone away without explanation. The people had survived cancer for years afterwards, and although nobody can explain why, it is assumed that at some stage the brain kicked in and stopped the mutation of cells. I concede the placebo effect isn't strictly in play here, but could it be that the people attributed the discomfort to something less worrying and just carried on, leaving the brain to sort it?

The placebo effect is a strange thing; for example, did you know that if you're in a hospital room with a beautiful view of mountains or a beach, you're more likely to get better quicker, for the simple reason you want to get out there as it looks healthy, and if it looks healthy, it promotes healing so you can enjoy it.

As cancer is known to be caused by irregularities in the DNA, it is thought that once we can perfect DNA restructuring, it will be a major breakthrough in eradicating cancer, and advances in genome research are being made each day that will, hopefully, achieve this goal.

The Nocebo Effect

A detrimental effect on health produced by psychological or psychosomatic factors such as negative expectations of treatment or prognosis.

This is similar to the placebo effect in that your body will try to fulfil your expectations, so when you ask, "how long have I got?" and the doctor gives you a number of months or years, you have to understand it's based on the doctor's experience with previous patients and statistics, none of which apply to your exact cancer as no two cancer diagnosis are the same, and those who have gone before you are not you.

It puts the doctor in a difficult position as they don't know you. They don't know whether you have an attitude to fight, or an attitude of resignation to the assumption of inevitable death. It's not really a fair question to ask, yet we ask nevertheless. You have to realise in most cases, this is the first time the two of you have met, so it's just a guess, nothing more.

For some patients, the nocebo effect can be one of the most dangerous aspects of diagnosis. Even more dangerous than the cancer itself.

Accept the diagnosis and the fact you now have cancer, but do not accept the prognosis that within a certain estimated amount of time you will die.

The problem with the nocebo effect is some patients will write their *Estimated Date Of Demise* (EDOD) into a diary and will actively work towards getting their affairs in order; so much so, that when the date arrives, it turns out to be a self-fulfilling prophecy.

I did the opposite, as although I recorded my Estimated Date of Demise (six so far), I did it to make sure I beat it. It was something to work towards and celebrate.

My most recent estimated date of demise was 7th July 2018 as I was told on 7th July 2017 my bladder cancer had advanced to stage three and I could expect six months to a year. As usual, I ignored it, but if you check my Facebook page, you will see I put a banner up to let everyone know I would be sticking around for a while longer and an Estimated Date of Demise (EDOD) is just a guesstimate.

As with everything in your cancer journey, you should always try to turn potential negatives into positives.

You only have to go back to the start of this book where I told you about my brother getting his diagnosis. He ran up the stairs and had to get a lift down based on how he interpreted what the consultant had said. I made it plain what happened afterwards, and I think this is an accurate illustration of just how powerful the nocebo effect can be, if you allow it.

The Medicine Nocebo

The nocebo effect isn't only about the diagnosis and receiving news; it also relates to the medicine prescribed.

Assuming you read all possible side effects, it can affect how you tolerate the treatment.

If 100 patients receive the same medicine and two of the potential side effects are made up, someone will experience them. Say the two side effects are a feeling of numbness in the left elbow and a tingling in the little toe of the right foot, you can bet that some of the patients will experience one or both of them.

The expectation of a problem with treatment means that something as simple as knocking your left elbow on a door can trigger a long-term effect unrelated to the treatment.

As with receiving an Estimated Date of Demies (EDOD), the body will do all it can to facilitate your expectations, and it can be the same with any prescribed medicine, so read the side effects but don't live with the expectation of problems.

'Give-up-itis' can kill you.

In a study conducted by Dr John Leach, a senior research fellow at the University of Portsmouth, it is the first to describe clinical markers for psychogenic or 'give-up-itis' death.

If you go back in time, people died when someone put a hex on them, or cast a spell, or put a Voodoo curse on them, but we all know that nothing actually happened, it was the expectation of a horrible death that brought about the death, and not magic.

Could it then be possible that a modern day doctor giving an Estimated Date of Demise (EDOD), is similar to someone casting a spell way back when?

People have all sorts of names for Give-up-itis, such as 'Voodoo death', 'psychogenic death', 'psychosomatic death', etc.

Dr Leach said: "Psychogenic death is real. It isn't suicide, it isn't linked to depression, but the act of giving up on life and dying (usually within days) is a very real condition often linked to severe trauma."

A cancer diagnosis with a bad outlook, or even just a diagnosis irrespective of the potential outlook could potentially trigger psychogenic death in some patients, and if not arrested, death usually occurs three weeks after the first stage of withdrawal.

The condition was highlighted in the 1950s by US Army medical officers after soldiers died in the Korean war without any obvious cause. It was given the nickname, *give-up-itis*.

In the case of a prisoner who had served a ten-year prison sentence and was then told his term had been prolonged indefinitely, he died the same day with no visible reason.

There are five stages leading to the psychological decline, and it is thought it stems from a change in a frontal-subcortical circuit that governs how a person maintains goal-directed behaviour.

The condition is reversable if caught early, and something as simple as physical activity or a change in attitude through therapy can trigger the release of dopamine, the feel-good chemical.

The five stages of give-up-itis or psychogenic death are:

1) Social withdrawal—when the patient displays a lack of emotion, indifference, listlessness and becomes self-absorbed.

2) Apathy—which can display when people take no interest in cleanliness or appearance. On awakening, the patient has no interest or energy to prepare for the day ahead.

3) Aboulia—a severe lack of motivation and a dampened emotional response, the inability to make decisions and a lack of initiative. At this stage there is no appetite or desire to drink, and communication skills are non-existent.

4) Psychic akinesia—results in a further drop in motivation. The person is conscious but in a state of profound apathy and unaware of, or insensitive to, even extreme pain, not even flinching if they are hit, and they are often incontinent and continue to lie in their own waste.

5) Psychogenic death—is the final stage of the disintegration of a person. At this stage the patient has completely given up. They may have one last moment of pleasure when they ask for or do something pleasurable as a final reward before death.

From stage four to stage five usually takes three to four days.

So, it would seem conclusive evidence has now proven that participation in your own cure and a positive mental attitude are paramount for anyone facing a life-threatening illness of any type.

The power of the mind over cancer is demonstrated worldwide at least once a week when someone is told they only have a limited amount of time left, but there's a wedding, christening, graduation, or other celebration in their future. Not always, but a lot of times the patient will manage to hold on to attend the function. My question is, if their mind can achieve this short-term goal, why stop there? Why self-limit in the first place?

I wrote this book because people need to be aware that cancer is just a diagnosis and not necessarily a death sentence. But all too often, it is translated into a death sentence in their mind, and once that happens, it becomes a self-fulfilling prophecy. They expect to die, they give up and don't fight, with the result, they die. I have to point out this is based on personal experience with patients on the same journey as me and is not just an opinion. I've seen it happen way too many times.

As I've already said, on six different occasions, I've been given estimated survival times; six months with my first cancer, three months with the second, three months with the third, another three months with the fourth which escalated into three days during the second treatment. On 7th July 2017 I was told six months to a year was the best I could expect, but on the anniversary, I posted on Facebook that again I had beaten it. It's now 2021 and although this is early in the book, it's one of the last things I wrote. I'll be getting more maintenance chemo every three months to hopefully keep my bladder cancer at bay, and if that doesn't work, I might need my bladder, prostate, and ureter removed, and a stoma bag fitted; but if that happens, I'm damned sure it isn't going to kill me either. Ultimately, I never give it a second thought and if I have to face it, then I'll do something about it at that time.

"Cancer is a word, not a sentence." ~ John Diamon

Interviews with the Ologists

I took this one step further by seeking clarification on this nocebo phenomenon from three of my consultants who have treated me on previous occasions. All three were very reluctant to comment, but eventually agreed on the understanding their comments be anonymous.

The first one I asked said she had always found it very difficult when patients ask for an estimated survival time, and she never predicted less than twelve months, even if it was obvious the patient probably wouldn't make it to the one-month mark. The surprise to her was the number of people who probably shouldn't have survived in the short term but did reach the twelve-month mark. Even worse, when this happened, she felt guilty she hadn't given them years to live, but there are no strict guidelines on this advice and it's up to each individual doctor to decide what to say. She said it wasn't an exact science and over the years her method of arriving at an estimated date had changed dramatically from what she had given when she first became a consultant.

The second one said if he thought a patient had only two months to live in his professional opinion, he would always double the time as a matter of routine. Again, he was surprised at the number of patients who made it to or beat the deadline.

The third one said it depended on a lot of things and not just the patient. I asked her to explain, and she told me that from years of experience, the patients who were most successful were the ones who had not only a strong desire to survive, but also a strong support network who were encouraging them. She said when I was her patient, she thought it was a waste of time giving me an estimated date as I wouldn't take any notice anyway. She said she always tries to be as optimistic as possible, but where it was obvious there was no fight left and basically no hope, she tried to be as accurate as possible, which usually proved to be right within five-ten days either way.

The one thing I did learn from all three interviews was just how difficult it was for the doctors, and by that, I don't mean just talking about it. Each death seemed to be a personal failure on their part, and when talking about what I assumed to be recent cases, they all demonstrated regret at the outcome beyond words.

What most patients don't realise is counselling is something doctors use to deal with the death of a patient. It's not just a matter of, "nothing more I could have done," and off for a round of golf. They question if there was anything more they could have done, or done differently, or if there was anything they missed.

All were of the opinion that giving deadlines was a necessary evil as it allowed the patients to plan ahead, but all three expressed surprise at the number of people who did actually die within days of the deadline.

Two said that when they tell someone they have cancer, they can determine—with a fair degree of accuracy—those who are probably going to make it and those who probably won't, based on the response to the diagnosis.

They both had similar views. Those who say, "why me?" or "this isn't fair," are probably the ones who will rely totally on the treatment and won't involve themselves in the process too much; but those who ask, "how are *we* going to beat it?" or "how are *we* going to fix it?" are the ones who will probably make it, as their attitude confirms they're already up for the fight ahead.

"Time goes on. So whatever you're going to do, do it now. Don't wait." ~ Robert De Niro

Can you die of embarrassment?

Technically, no, but on the other hand, yes; well, sort of—let me explain.

My best friend's son was a research chemist at a prestigious American University, and I was always being presented with books his son had written/contributed to, or articles from a newspaper/medical journal. His speciality was cancer research, and he was a genius in his field having invented a modified protein that is still used worldwide.

My friend got a call from his son's wife telling him his son had been admitted to hospital, but not to worry as it wasn't serious. Days passed, and eventually my friend learned the diagnosis was penile cancer. As I had already beaten my first four cancers, he asked for advice. I had no idea, but I knew a lot of people who did, so I asked some questions, and they contacted the hospital in America. The news wasn't good, and I had to tell my friend he should ring the hospital and talk to his son.

The cancer had spread, and the reason was that although he knew something was wrong, he was too embarrassed to go to the doctor due to the location of the problem.

Eventually, I convinced my friend to book a flight and go to America. He arrived three hours before his son died, but at least he did arrive in time to say goodbye.

The fact he was embarrassed and didn't go to the doctor was the reason the cancer was so advanced when they eventually diagnosed it. You can't die of embarrassment, but it can lead to your death.

Embarrassment is something to get used to

I've met patients who were very nervous about having a camera up their back passage, but had it done anyway, and I've also met some who refused. Of course, eventually, it has to be done, but for some people, the dread is too much and they have to be knocked out for it to happen.

When you've got cancer, there are a lot of procedures you're not going to be looking forward to, but they are necessary and unavoidable, so it's better to find a way to accept it's going to happen and live with it. For the doctors carrying out the procedures, they are simply routine, nothing special, nothing unusual. For you, bearing your bum or front bits for inspection/invasion is a major mind melt, so talk to your doctor and express your concerns. You won't be the first patient who has reservations, and you won't be the last. They are there to help and will have a solution or can talk you through everything and set your mind at ease. The secret is to always ask for help.

The way I dealt with it was to think of my mind and body as two separate things. My mind was me; it was my essence that defined who I was, and my body was just a biomechanical device I used to get around. In my mind, my body was nothing more than say a car or van that had broken down. If you can't do this, that's okay. We're all made differently. But if you can, it makes things a whole lot easier.

Sometimes you may be asked if you mind trainee doctors or nurses being present to watch the procedure, and you may be okay with this, or you may not, but ask yourself this question: How are they going to learn if they can't watch real procedures being carried out? Yes. You're a special person and unique in this world, but to someone who is looking at private parts day-in-day-out, you're nothing special and they don't give it a second thought. Once they've recorded their findings, it's as if you had never been there…next patient please.

The journey through cancer and treatment is one of constant mind readjustment. When something is proposed you are worried about, talk it through and think it through. Take your time. You're a lot cleverer than you think.

Spontaneous remission

Sometimes cancer surprises us with an unexpected outcome called spontaneous remission/regression or radical remission/regression.

This phenomenon has been documented for hundreds of years and is now accepted by medical professionals as something that just happens from time to time, with no rational explanation. How or why it happens isn't known, and we have no way to replicate what caused it in the first place.

There are no accurate statistics available as those cured frequently just stop attending their doctor, and those that do continue to attend are put on a wait-and-watch regime, so no clinical papers are published to confirm the outcome.

In the year I was initially diagnosed (2002) the website of the National Institutes of Health confirmed there were at least four articles published on the subject every month by doctors listing cases in all forms of cancer.

In a study on mammography in 2008, it was found that 22% of small tumour breast cancers underwent spontaneous remission.

It is estimated that 1 in every 100,000 people with cancer may experience spontaneous remission, but with the odds so low, is it worth the risk you may be the one?

It's a lottery

You've asked for the statistics for your cancer, and the percentage of survivors is low. What should you do? I'll tell you; you should take the odds given and welcome them with open arms. Even if it's only a .1% chance of survival that still means one person out of every thousand survives. It could be you, but only if you don't give up.

Why wouldn't it be you? If you can give me a reasonable explanation why it shouldn't be you, I'll listen, but as there isn't one, I'm not expecting anyone to contact me.

People do survive cancer. I did. Good people and bad people, tall and short, black, white and all shades in between, male and female, fat and skinny, clever and stupid, etc. There is no determining factor why some people die and some live, unless of course, you give up before the fight has even started.

The phrase 'it could be you' is used in the UK lottery, and every week millions of people enter in the hope of winning. In fact, the chance of winning is officially 1/45,057,474. The odds are massively stacked against you, but they still do it. We'll round it off to a nice even one in forty-five million chance, yet some people lose it when they miss a week as that could be the week they were meant to win; however, when faced with a 15% chance (15 in every 100) of beating a cancer diagnosis, people think it too small and give up.

Does this seem like a rational conclusion?

DEEMS

Before publication of this book, I gave copies to other sufferers with a variety of different cancers and, without exception, they all said it helped them to understand the cancer journey; but what I didn't expect were the requests they meet with me on a regular basis to act as some sort of cancer coach.

One asked me if I would be on their side throughout treatment; but the thing is, I'm on everybody's side, which is yet another reason for the book in the first place. The only person you need on your side (apart from the medical team and family) is you.

Everything you need to know will initially be told to you by the medical experts treating your cancer, and even more information can be obtained from other patients and (dare I say it) from this book.

The fact is **you** will know what **you** need to do, and you don't need anybody to motivate you. The main motivating factor is you already know you need to fight your cancer, and I know that for a fact, otherwise you wouldn't have even made it this far in the book.

You have to participate in your own cure. Help your treatment to work and your body to mend by doing as much as you can to help.

I thought about all the things I had to do during and after treatment and came up with DEEMS.

DEEMS is my thing and it came about as a result of this book, but in reality, it was something I did when I was going through treatment, and yes, you will have to force yourself, but little and often works wonders.

DEEMS is a five-point plan which stands for:

D – Drink plenty of water and keep a note of your intake. During treatment you won't feel like drinking, so take frequent sips and every time the glass is empty, fill it up and start again.

E – Eat frequently. It amazed me how my appetite went completely when I was on chemo as I had always loved food; as my figure confirms. Little and often is the secret. Make small but frequent meals you can either tackle in one go or dip in and out of. Don't worry if it's chocolate/sweets or fruit or steak; as long as you're eating, it's all good. As little as one spoonful at a time will work wonders, as long as you do it regularly. If it gets too much, change the dynamic from eating to simply swallowing. Get the food in your mouth and chew until it's nothing more than liquid, then swallow. Don't call it eating anymore as you already know you don't want to do that.

E – Exercise. You probably won't feel like doing anything, but it's essential you keep mobile and exercise those muscles. I'm not expecting you to run a marathon, but short and (very) frequent walks are good. Aim to do something every hour, even if it's just climbing the stairs or venturing into your garden. When I was at my worst, my goal was simply to keep putting one foot in front of the other; didn't matter how slow, just as long as there was constant (slow) motion.

M - Meditation and especially visualisation (more about visualisation later in the book) is a great way to get your mind around your circumstances and plan for the day ahead. It also helps with the usually inevitable depression or point in the day when something triggers your mood and you feel low.

S – Sleep is essential when you're going through treatment, and you may think it's only something you do at night, but hey, you're special, you're on treatment for cancer, so sleep as and when you feel like it as sometimes you simply won't be able to sleep at night. If somebody comments, do not let them put you off sleeping as required, you're the one that needs it.

It's not just me

The best thing about my idea that 'tomorrow will be better' and 'you have to participate in your own cure', 'DEEMS', etc., is the fact that although it's my story, it's not unique.

I've met many patients resigned to dying, and I've met many determined to fight. I try to convince some there is a fight to be had, but ultimately, if they have no interest, I eventually give up; but when I meet someone willing to take on the fight, the methods they use are—broadly speaking—similar to my own.

Positive attitude, acceptance that bad days happen, forcing yourself to drink, eat, exercise, meditate and sleep, doing everything the doctors advise. We all realise it's not just down to the doctors to cure us; it's our fight as well, and it is that attitude that has meant huge progress for everyone concerned.

And yes, sometimes it doesn't work, but it works 100% better than those who don't try.

It's just a temperature

There are times on the cancer journey when your temperature will spike, and you will realise you need to go back to the hospital, but then your brain will say 'no' because we don't like hospitals. Hospital is not a good place for us to be. We'd rather stay at home and watch Netflix.

Now here's the thing; nobody wants to be in hospital, but if that's where you need to be, it's not negotiable

When you need to go into hospital is not when your brain or feelings decide, it's when your temperature or whatever ails you is important.

I've got a temperature. I'll take it easy. I'll try an ice pack. I'll lie on the couch. I'll drink cold water. I'll...

You have cancer, and you probably have a temperature because you have an infection. Now here's the thing my friend—and I'm not going to beat about the bush with this—infections kill. Wait, that was harsh; let me rephrase that or put it another way in case I wasn't clear—infections kill cancer patients.

If you get an infection and you delay going to hospital, and the infection takes hold, and you end up being hospitalised because you didn't go when you should; there is a strong possibility that because of your weakened immune system and your weakened state, the Grim Reaper could come knocking. Yes, I'm making this sound grim. Please pay attention because it *is* bloody grim. I have known people with cancer who have rang me and said, "I have a temperature; what should I do?"

"Dude, it's a no brainer, get to the hospital right now, do not pass go, do not collect 200, just go."

Then I get a series of excuses why they shouldn't go to hospital.

The bottom line is; there might not be a tomorrow if you don't pull your head out of your ass and go to hospital. It's that serious.

By way of illustration, one of the guys who rang me frequently because he took frequent infections—as I did at one stage and I didn't like going into hospital either—but he kept ringing saying my temperature is 38.2 or 38.5, what should I do? And every time I give him the same advice.

The fourth time he took an infection, he knew better. Then he ended up in intensive care, immediately followed by the morgue. The infection took hold. He didn't go in time. He delayed and excused. He died.

If that doesn't illustrate how serious a temperature is, I don't know what will. As I've said before, it's a very tiny percentage of your life, and nobody's really responsible for the fact that you have cancer. Again, as I've said before, quite crudely and horribly to make a point, suck it up, own it. Get on with it. This is part of the process. Shit happens.

Thankfully, when shit does happen, we have a backup. We have a medical team. We have everything we need. The only thing potentially missing is common sense. So do not delay and hope for the best, or say a prayer, or cool yourself with ice, or take a shower, or whatever. You need antibiotics, you need to get well, you need medical intervention. Go to the hospital. Pack your already prepared case, and go in with the attitude that it's a holiday, and it's going to be really enjoyable because all you've got to do is lie in bed. You'll be waited on hand and foot, they'll put a drip in, which will be really uncomfortable until you remember I've given you distraction techniques and it's a no brainer. There's no hassle, because you are a cancer warrior. You've got the tips and tricks I've given you and I'll keep giving them to you and as long as you use them—guess what—the journey is so much easier.

Before I finish this section I can't stress enough, DO NOT MESS ABOUT WITH AN INCREASED TEMPERATURE. If you need to go to hospital; go to hospital immediately.

Can't eat? Don't eat.

Eating isn't hard, all you have to do is swallow.

When I had my stem-cell transplant, I had no appetite.

I remember calling my wife proud as could be and telling her, "I ate half today."

"Half a meal?" She said.

"Half a digestive biscuit," I replied

Okay, it doesn't sound much, but having been on a liquid diet and drips to keep me strong, it was a milestone, then I discovered that all I had to do was swallow.

I had no appetite, but I realised I had to eat as it was the only way they were going to discharge me, so I started eating. Not for enjoyment as I had done all my life, but with the solitary goal of escape.

It is advised to chew your food at least thirty times before swallowing, but I found myself chewing until everything had turned into a liquid, then all I had to do was swallow. It wasn't food anymore, but a drink. Not the nicest experience, and it felt like an obligation as there was no taste reward, whereas previously I ate to satisfy my taste buds, but as that was no longer an option as I had no taste, it became a chore; but a chore with a goal, and that, I could live with.

So don't think of it as eating, think of it as a nourishment exercise. Eating isn't something you want to do, but nourishing yourself is something your brain can understand. Sometimes, doing something you have no desire to do is simply a matter of reframing. Chew till your jaw hurts, then swallow.

I forced myself to start eating, and before long, the doctors said the drip could be removed.

The lack of taste is a big problem as you experience no satisfaction from the act of eating, but you have to force yourself.

Suck it up and realise it's only temporary, and on the plus side, when your taste returns, the reward is you appreciate your food all the more.

Yes, it's hard, but you realise you're participating in your own cure. You're actively fighting towards success.

Everything in cancer treatment is a fight. It's not easy, but fighting is a reward in itself. It makes you feel better, it helps fight the cancer, it rewards you mentally, and most importantly, physically. The healthier you can make your body (and mind), the healthier it will be.

Give it the fuel it needs to get back to health.

Exercise is essential to recovery

One of the things you aren't going to want to do when you're on treatment is exercise, yet it's an essential part of your fight. The benefits range from fitness, to the effect it has on the mind. The sense of accomplishment is one of the main feel-good factors, and feeling good is a major benefit in dealing with the situation you find yourself in.

Chemotherapy can be a rough ride, but imagine how you'll feel when you do something as simple as taking a walk with the knowledge that *you* are the only person in the world who has just had chemo and is walking down that road or path that day. You're one of a kind. The only one on the planet. Nobody on the face of the earth has your exact diagnosis, and here you are exercising; there is no feeling like it in the world.

Neighbours and friends will see you and comment on your strength and determination, which motivates even further.

Bad days will come, and you might slow down, but always remember that tomorrow will be better. It's as simple as remembering one foot in front of the other is success, you're moving and it doesn't matter how slow or fast, it's all progress.

Walking, or jogging, or running. Whatever exercise you can do will make a huge difference in how you feel about your progress through treatment. You're actively participating in your own cure, and there's no better feeling in the world.

During exercise, endorphins are released in the brain which make you feel better.

It can be something as simple as a walk around the garden or using the upstairs loo instead of the downstairs one. Every time you exercise, you'll feel better, and a pleasant side effect is when you feel hungry as a result, so it helps when you don't feel like eating, and it helps you to sleep, so why wouldn't you do it?

I can remember the first time I left the room after my stem cell transplant; the nurses warned me that I wouldn't be able to walk any distance, but I was determined to at least walk the length of the ward. I managed around eight steps before collapsing backwards into a wheelchair that they knew I would need. Exhausted doesn't describe it, but the next day I didn't need the wheelchair and managed around twenty steps, then forty, then the length of the ward, then a lap of the ward, then two, etc.

Of course, with every milestone the nurses were by my side, but the compliments afterwards were what pushed me to do better the next day, and other patients watched me, then forced themselves to do it as well.

So yes, I've been there. Used to jogging most of my life, then being able to only manage a few feet, but pushing myself and being encouraged made a huge difference in my recovery time.

Set yourself manageable goals and don't beat yourself up if you set yourself unreasonable targets at the start; simply accept that your circumstances have changed, set new realistic targets for the next day and participate in your journey to recovery.

If you ever find yourself in the position where you're completely incapable of exercise, you'll wonder why you wasted the opportunity when you had the chance.

Of course, I have a couple of phrases you can use.

Motion is lotion. - Movement of any kind will improve your fitness, your muscles, your mind.

Movement is improvement. - Exactly the same as above. Everything and anything you can do to keep mobile is gold.

Make sure you say them both before starting any exercise and your brain will do the rest.

Personal Records

It's also worthwhile getting into the habit of keeping personal records, which are not only handy if you need to confirm something with the hospital, but you will see just how well you are doing and, if things get tough, you can refer back to previous days and use them as a guide.

Thermometer

When I was on treatment, I purchased a thermometer you simply insert into your ear, press a button, and you have your temperature. Every morning, afternoon, and night, I recorded my statistics.

The normal range for temperature is around 37°C (98.6°F) but as everyone is different, this may consistently be a shade higher or lower, and can also vary depending on the time of day, age, sex, fluid intake, and the method of measurement. (oral, rectal, ear, forehead, or under arm)

Once a baseline has been established using one method, it is recommended to be consistent.

If your temperature goes above 38°C/100.1°F, you will definitely need to contact your doctor/hospital as it probably indicates you have an infection or fever.

Scales

One of the side effects of cancer is usually weight loss, and although this might be welcome, it's something you need to keep an eye on as too much weight loss isn't good, so morning, afternoon, and evening records are handy to refer to.

Blood Pressure Monitor

120/80 is the goal and it will vary throughout the day, but if it goes up or down substantially, it's something you should seek advice about.

I had an electric monitor that kept a record of previous measurements and indicated if the reading was dangerous. I recently dropped it and needed a new one and found the price has lowered considerably, and the new ones are easier to use and even measure your heart rate.

Oximeter

An oximeter is a little clip-like thing you place over your finger and it tells you what your 'stats' (the proportion of oxygenated haemoglobin in the blood) are. You will probably have had one on your finger in hospital at some stage and I thought it would be good to keep a record along with everything else I checked on a daily basis.

Normal oximeter readings usually range from 95 to 100 percent. Values under 90 percent are considered low and you should tell your consultant if this happens, although, from experience, a couple of deep breaths will get it back up again. (But if that works, you should monitor your breathing and stats at least every fifteen minutes.)

Way back in 2002 when I purchased one, it was a fortune, but now you can pick one up on Amazon or eBay for very little, and it's also worth checking your phone as some of the newer models have an oximeter built in.

Water/Fluid

You may be asked to keep a record of your fluid input and output immediately after chemo, and it is normally recommended you drink at least 2 litres/3.5 pints (UK)/4.22 pints (US) of water every day to help flush out the chemo.

The hospital will usually provide you with a measuring jug and all you have to do is pee in it and record the amount each time.

Some people say you should drink only water and nothing else, but studies have shown that coffee, tea, and any other fluid consumption should also be included.

When you have just had chemo, you may not feel like drinking, but it is essential that you do; so little and often is always my advice. Keep a bottle and glass nearby, take frequent sips and when empty, fill and repeat.

Food

No, I'm not going to suggest you record your output, but it helps to record your input, as it means you can refer back on the days when you don't feel like eating and motivate yourself with the figures.

Sorry to keep repeating myself, but… you have to participate in your own cure. You have to actively get involved. Weigh yourself, take your temperature and blood pressure readings every day and use DEEMS.

The more you do (even if it's just notes), the more power you give yourself, and the more power you get, the better you can cope with the journey.

Taste.

Wow, does your taste change when you're on chemo?

When I was receiving my CHOP chemotherapy, I had a permanent metallic type of taste in my mouth and couldn't taste any of the food I was eating. It is hard to describe it well, but it is a problem if, like me, you like your food. Old favourites, which you know you like, will become unpleasant and very frustrating/impossible to eat.

Again, as if you haven't had enough to contend with, this is where the 'fight' becomes very relevant.

To begin with, you don't have much of an appetite on chemo, and you know the more you eat, the more you have available to throw up, and now, you can't even taste it. What's the point?

The point is that in order for your body to fight the cancer and tolerate the chemo, you have to provide it with energy and there is no alternative other than getting a drip.

You have to force yourself.

I found that burnt steaks or burnt burgers were something that appealed to me, but when I offered them to the wife or kids, they thought I was mad, but I did get some sort of taste from them, which was mildly pleasant.

For drinks, I couldn't beat Bovril. Not something I would normally take, but with a couple of big thick spoonfuls of Bovril in a cup of boiling water, I got my taste fix for the day.

Strong smoked fish was also something I became partial to, but you will have to try different things you wouldn't normally dream of and see if you can come up with something better. I tried everything that was available, but the above is really the sum total of my success.

The spice rack will become your best friend, but be careful. Although you can't taste the spices like you used to and have to use lots, they can easily upset your stomach.

The good news is once chemotherapy finishes, your taste will return, but be warned, it is a slow process, and in my case took a couple of months.

After all my treatment had finished and my taste had returned, I spotted a pot of Bovril in the cupboard and decided to have a cup. I couldn't drink it as it was way too strong and I had to dump it down the sink and start again with a much smaller amount. But on chemo, it was pure gold.

Mouth Sores and Ulcers

Because of the effect chemotherapy has on good cells as well as cancer cells, it is common to develop sores, ulcers or infections in the mouth, throat, or gums, which usually occurs 5-10 days into chemo, and it is for this reason it is recommended to visit your dentist before treatment starts. The hospital will either recommend it or send you to the hospital dentist to have any necessary work carried out.

Mouth washes and creams are available to help if you develop mouth problems, but you should receive a specialised mouth wash when you start chemo to help prevent anything in the first place. Use it frequently, and by that, I mean every time you go into the bathroom and especially if you've just been sick. Again, and yes, I apologise for going on and on, but every small thing necessary is usually something you won't want to do and… Yeah, you already know I'm going to say, this is where the fight attitude is necessary. You won't want to wash your mouth after being sick, but little victories win the battle.

Although it is essential you maintain dental hygiene, you also have to realise that vigorous brushing can also cause problems, so frequent but gentle is the answer, as well as using a mouth wash.

If you do develop problems, they are usually only temporary, and you will be helped with prescribed creams.

Once formed, it is a simple matter of drying the ulcer and applying a smear of the paste onto it using your finger. The paste seems to form a protective cover on the ulcer and is very good.

In fairness, I wasn't bothered too much by sores or ulcers, but the cream definitely helped when they did appear.

If you have a routine dental appointment planned, it is essential you inform the dentist you are undergoing chemotherapy as various problems can arise, and once chemo has started, the risk of infection is too high to carry out dental work.

Use the cream 3-4 times per day if sores or ulcers develop.

Pain rating ½/10 More of an irritation than anything else.

Problems afterwards? None

Teeth.

Unfortunately, chemotherapy can have an adverse effect on teeth and gums.

For me, this meant that due to the high dose chemotherapy, my teeth became loose and—because of the risk of infection getting into the gums—it was decided the offending molars be removed.

Like most people, a visit to the dentist isn't something I look forward to, but on this occasion, the teeth were so loose that after freezing my gums, he simply reached into my mouth with his fingers and pulled them out.

I needed to have my gums stitched, but it wasn't a problem during the removal or even afterwards.

Pain rating 0/10 (you're aware they are doing something in your mouth, but it doesn't hurt)

Problems afterwards? None.

Nails.

Certain chemotherapy drugs, such as doxorubicin, and cyclophosphamide, can make changes to your nails, and they may become darker and develop little ridges. This has happened to me twice during the different regimens and it's not a problem.

The nails will return to normal in a few months, once you have finished your chemo and the ridges grow out.

Chemo-Brain

According to findings published in the Journal of Clinical Oncology, it is known that chemotherapy can impair your memory for at least a few years after treatment, but the study shows this can have an impact for as long as ten years.

The official name for Chemo-brain or Chemo Fog is 'Chemically Induced Cognitive Impairment' (CICI), which is great when you're trying to explain it to someone as they hear the word 'chemically' and immediately jump to the conclusion you're a junkie, but I like watching their reaction, of course, that's assuming I can remember the thing in the first place. Some people replace *chemically* with *chemotherapy* or even *chemotherically*.

Cognitive problems such as trouble with thinking and memory that many cancer patients experience, and a growing number of doctors believe, may be related to chemotherapy.

In a survey of patients who complained of problems, some of the comments were:

"It was like being drunk, without being drunk."

"My brain is different as I now have to use notes for everything, even when I deliver presentations I wrote myself and have presented over and over again. I feel my brain is about ninety percent back, but after eight years, I think this is as good as it will get."

"I walk into a room and have no idea why I'm there or why I went in, then as soon as I'm back, I remember and have to go back again."

"I can have a conversation with someone, and then ten or fifteen minutes later, comfortably have it again, without any recollection of ever having had it before."

From my experience, I can confirm the above are relevant, and by way of illustration, I had my own special moment years ago when I was on a call to my daughter and couldn't remember her name, which would be impossible under normal circumstances. The phrase should have been, "Okay, Danielle, I'll…", but the name wouldn't come, which was shocking and very scary at the time. How could someone forget their own daughter's name? Then the brain provides the answer with a variety of scary possibilities starting with Alzheimer's and ending with Brain Tumour.

I think it is fair to say that Chemo-brain does exist, and is now accepted by the medical profession, but the cause is still in dispute.

Until recently, it had been thought most drugs used in chemotherapy do not cross the blood-brain barrier (a protective membrane that acts as a filter between substances in the circulating blood and the brain) and to an extent, this is mostly true, but although most of the molecules of the substances used in chemo are blocked, some do get through. In fact, many chemotherapy drugs are too big or have chemical properties that prevent them from effectively crossing the blood-brain barrier, and this is one of the reasons why most chemotherapy drugs are ineffective at treating brain cancer.

It is also thought chemo-brain can be caused by the chemotherapy indirectly, as it can cause the body to pump out natural chemicals called cytokines that enter the brain and may cause significant decreases in brain function.

Whatever the cause; in a test of 128 healthy breast cancer and lymphoma survivors, who had survived for an average of ten years after completing their treatment, it was found that patients treated with chemotherapy scored significantly lower on tests than those patients who were treated with only radiation and/or surgery but without chemotherapy.

On some of the cancer forums I'm on, some people have complained that if they had known about chemo-brain before treatment, they would have refused chemotherapy. Seriously? I've had it bad, and I've improved it substantially through understanding and memory exercises. If you get it, you can dramatically improve it, but whining online isn't the answer, however, refusing treatment on the assumption you might suffer something in the future defines stupidity—sure, you won't have chemo-brain, you'll be dead.

It is however widely agreed that the benefits of chemotherapy far outweigh the risks of chemo-brain, since problems appear to be subtle, and can easily be overcome by simply recognising and planning for potential problems.

My advice is to accept it as a temporary problem and don't beat yourself up when it happens. Get into the habit of using the dictation app on your phone or take notes as and when something you have to remember pops into your head; if you don't, the thought may return, but by then it may be too late to make use of it.

When you think of it, I have chemo-brain and wrote this book, and earlier this year (2021) I was on the phone with a company and they needed to run me through a security check to confirm my identity. Name, address, postcode, all okay, but when I was asked the date of birth? "Twenty-fifth of… ahhh… Scorpio... ahhh." The person at the other end of the phone told me to stop winding them up. I went through the months, "Jan, Feb, Mar, Apr, May, June, July Aug, Sept… it's the next one." So only months ago I knew I was a Scorpio, I knew it was the month after September, but no way could I get the word October into my head. The thing was I knew at once what the problem was. I didn't panic, didn't get embarrassed or think I was losing my mind, and I knew the information was there all the time, so it is possible to function irrespective, providing you plan ahead and accept problems might arise but you can deal with them.

Always remember (Yes, we're talking about memory loss and I'm telling you to always remember. Duhhh) it's just a memory problem. It's not like the information has been removed, it's just the method of accessing is problematic at times, but just knowing and accepting that makes it easy to deal with.

There are a number of helpful exercises and videos on the website which will help with the effects of Chemo-brain and also improving your memory.

"Whether you like it or not, you're in the fight for your life."

~ Lawrence Wray

Motivation

One of the big motivating factors for me was when I was given six months to live and my wife pulled out the life insurance policies and said, "World cruise, here I come."

Was she kidding? Yes, I know she was, but…

Anyway, I wouldn't give her the pleasure.

Thursday 23rd May 2002

I received my second CHOP treatment today.

Walking very slowly both going into and out of the clinic due to a combination of not being able to sleep, no appetite, and the lingering effects from CHOP one.

Mind Tricks

Oh, yes. You know it as you look around the waiting room and see all the faces, and you know one of you is going to be next, but which one? Is it going to be you, or the lady sitting opposite, or the old man on your left, or the child sitting beside its weeping mum? Without a shadow of a doubt, it's going to be one of you. Statistics aren't on your side.

People die every day from cancer, and the problem is you don't want it to be you. Anyone but you. Even the kid? Yes. That's the way your mind can work. It's not you as such, it's those deep and dark recesses of your mind where thinking gets done on a subconscious level, where there are no boundaries, and yes, it's hard, but it happens. You'll feel guilty about it, both at the time and afterwards, but sometimes you can't control your thoughts. It's basic human nature. The logic of survival. Why would you feel guilty about it? It's not like you're going to act on the thoughts, or even have any influence as a result. The problem is these thoughts can appear unannounced and uninvited.

Everyone gets them, it's just that everyone keeps quiet about it. It wouldn't be proper to announce to your neighbour that your subconscious has decided it might be a good idea if they pop their clogs next and give you a better chance of survival. After all, you need to be in that elusive tiny percent of people who survive your particular cancer, and the more people who die on your journey, the better your chances.

And, of course, you feel guilty, but you can't say anything because it sounds irrational. It's a thought you wouldn't have if you weren't sick, and it's a thought that if you told it to someone who didn't have cancer, they would think you're some sort of psychopath, but if you do share it with a fellow sufferer, you stand the chance they will have one of two reactions—either, wow, I thought I was the only one, thanks for sharing, or, what kind of a dick are you? Hopefully, they just move away from you and don't call for help or hit you a slap.

The thoughts are there, people, it's just that not everybody a) has them and b) if they do, they won't necessarily want to share due to potential embarrassment.

Losing friends on the journey is gonna happen. It's not okay, but it's okayer than if it was you.

It's a hard thing to get your head around.

Blood Tests ~ What are they all about?

Frequent blood tests are necessary to monitor overall body health and condition of the blood; especially when someone is receiving chemotherapy.

Blood is made up of plasma (fluid) which carries the cells around the body.

Listed here are some of the normal blood tests and their limits, but although you may find them interesting, the only one who knows what the results mean is your consultant, so I wouldn't worry too much about memorising, but they are interesting to compare with when you do get results.

In addition, the ranges shown below do not take into consideration age, sex, or race, and by that I mean a female child's range will differ to a male adult. Someone from Africa will have a slightly different range in some areas to someone from London.

If you want to keep an eye on all your tests, I have a pdf available to print at www.cancerology.co/bloodtests

White Blood Cells

4,000-11,000 is the normal range.

The white cells are made up of two main types called neutrophils and lymphocytes, and their main job is to protect the body against infection.

Red Blood Cells

The normal range for men is 4.7 - 6.1 million cells per microlitre

The normal range for women is 4.2 – 5.4 cells/mcL

Symptoms of anaemia (feeling exhausted due to a lack of red blood cells) start to appear if the count falls below twelve.

Red blood cells carry haemoglobin which gives the blood its red colour.

The cells have an average life of 120 days, during which time they incur substantial damage and are broken down and removed by the spleen.

Haemoglobin Concentration

Haemoglobin is a red protein that transports oxygen in the blood.

Adult male 13.3-16.7

Adult Female 11.8-14.8

Absolute Neutrophil Count

Adult 2500-6500

The risk of infection increases when the neutrophil count falls to around 1,000.

Platelets

Normal range is 200,000-450,000

If the level drops below 20,000, there is a risk of abnormal bleeding.

If the level drops below 10,000, doctors usually recommend transfusions of the platelets to reduce the chances of haemorrhage.

When I had my Stem Cell Transplant, they wouldn't release me until my platelets were over 60,000.

Blood Culture

Microbiologists check the blood for infection, and this is called a blood culture. The blood is given nutrients to encourage the growth of bacteria and if an infection is found, the cultures are treated with different kinds of antibiotics to see which is the most effective before prescribing to the patient.

The blood may also be examined so that certain salts and chemicals in it can be measured, which gives information about kidney and liver function.

This is the test most patients complain about as they want to know the results immediately, but it takes time for the bacteria to grow, then even more time to treat sections of the bacteria with the antibiotics to see what works the best.

Blood samples may also be used to crossmatch in case a transfusion is necessary during treatment.

Blood gases test

This is an unusual one and I've had a couple carried out. The sample isn't taken from a vein, but from an artery in the wrist. Veins tend to be visible and close to the skin, but when it's an artery, mine seemed to be in the middle of my wrist. They do tell you it's going to be painful, but if you relax and accept everything, it's not that bad. Afterwards, I had to hold a little square piece of plastic on the puncture as hard as I could, but that wasn't a problem either.

The test checks the balance of oxygen and carbon dioxide, and also the acid and alkali balance.

Pain rating 2.5-3/10

Accept it's going to be painful, and it's never as bad as you expect.

Specific blood tests for cancers include:

LDH Levels

Lactic Dehydrogenase or LDH is a protein which is a useful tumour marker and can show if the cancer is reducing, spreading or dormant.

This is something your consultant will be aware of and is not normally reported to patients, but knowledge is power and it's worth asking about, although it isn't relevant for every cancer.

PSA

Prostate-specific antigen (PSA) is a marker for prostate cancer and other potential problems such as an enlarged prostate gland.

CA125

CA125 is a protein that can indicate ovarian cancer as well as pelvic inflammatory disease.

BRCA1 and BRCA2 genes

The presence of these genes can indicate the potential for breast and ovarian cancer. The test is an option if your family has a history of certain cancers.

Blood transfusions

Blood transfusions can become a way of life for cancer patients undergoing chemotherapy. The main worry people tend to have is potential for diseases being transferred during transfusion and what the procedure is like.

Unfortunately, nothing in this life ever works 100% all the time, and yes, there has been occasions where blood has been transfused that has been tainted, but in the UK, the Blood Transfusion Service check for hepatitis B, hepatitis C, hepatitis E, human immunodeficiency virus (HIV), syphilis, and for first time donors they also check for the human T-lymphotropic virus before use. If any blood tests positive, it is not used, and the donor is contacted and offered support and advice.

During my time with Non-Hodgkin Lymphoma treatment, I had over twenty transfusions and never had any problems.

Transfusion is a simple procedure where a canula is inserted into the vein to receive the blood, or if you already have a picc or Hickman line attached, that can usually be used. The infusion is a slow process, and for me, the only side effect was a feeling of heat throughout my body during the transfer, but it wasn't uncomfortable or problematic.

"*Don't count the days, make the days count.*" ~ Muhammad Ali

Hospital essentials

Everything you do in life should be with the ultimate aim of reducing stress, and there is no time more important to intentionally reduce stress than when you have cancer.

You're on the journey, treatment has started, and it's probable at some time you will need a trip to the hospital, and the last thing you want to be doing is running around trying to get everything packed while you feel like death warmed up, so pack a case in advance and have it sitting ready. If you're really organised, you can have two cases ready, one for short-stay (overnight) and an additional one for a longer stay. If you go in expecting an overnight and it turns out otherwise, someone can bring your long-stay case when they visit.

In a way, this goes against the theme of this book because I want you to prepare for the best outcome, but I also want you to be realistic, and part of being realistic is being ready for things you don't expect, like an unplanned trip to hospital.

First things first, buy a decent bag or suitcase, one with a lock on it, as even though you (hopefully) know the nurses, somebody else might fancy a look around in it and help themselves to a trinket.

Someone taking a trinket is inconvenient and annoying, but if someone lifts the case itself, it can be a disaster. Most mobile phone companies offer little trackers that can be hidden inside the case and tracked on your phone. They're inexpensive and can be used for loads of other things when not in your case (children/pets/bikes, etc), so it's a good idea to invest in one, just in case. (see what I did there?)

Fellow patients, visitors, someone just walking in and helping themselves, other workers who pop in, etc., are all potential problems waiting to happen; so if you want to keep it, protect it.

The fact you have cancer evokes sympathy in most people, but to others, it means you're just another distracted target. Harsh, but true.

I have a friend who was in hospital for three days and had (yes, had, as in past tense) a beautiful Cartier watch her husband had given her on diagnosis, but, she never wore it through the night and instead took it off before lights-out and placed it on top of her bedside table (not inside a drawer, or under a pillow, or in a shoe, but on top of the table). The second morning, the tooth fairy must have called and lifted it. Who'd a thunk it? Unsurprisingly, the hospital took no responsibility, and again, unsurprisingly, the insurance company laughed at the claim and refused it because no precautions were taken to prevent the theft. So… if you have a Rolex, or Cartier, or other fancy trinket/s; hospital is not the place to show them off.

The contents

This is as comprehensive a list as I can make it, but it's not exhaustive and some things guys/girls aren't going to want and vice versa, so pick what you need and ignore the rest.

It's a long list, so be sensible. There are things you will need, some you might need, and others you'll use occasionally, so plan it out. If you're in a ward with other patients, you're going to have less security, but, on the other hand, you're going to have multiple new friends to keep an eye if you have to nip out. It's a tricky balance as you never know what to expect, so caution is advised.

Let's face it, sometimes shit happens, so if you're rushed into hospital without a chance to grab your stuff, leave a copy of this ticked list on top of the suitcase/bag, and when someone collects it for you, anything not packed will be shown and they can sort it.

You can print this list out with tick boxes at www.cancerology.co/hospitalessentials

Personal details

A sheet of paper with your full name, address, date of birth, hospital number, insurance details (if relevant) and consultant's details printed out so it can be given to the nurses if you're in a bit of a state at having been taken into hospital. Printable pdf at www.cancerology.co/personaldetails

A list of medicines. Yes, even though your hospital should be aware of everything you're prescribed, bring a list anyway, just in case something hasn't been updated. You may think this isn't necessary, but if you have a problem that needs medicine that may interact with another they don't know about, it could save your life. Printable pdf at www.cancerology.co/medicines

A list of any vitamins, supplements, herbal remedies, or anything else you're taking, irrespective of whether you think they're relevant. Again, it could save your life.

Other drugs? Yes, you know what I mean, don't you? If you occasionally indulge in recreational drugs, and irrespective of what they may be: tell the doctor. Let me say that again: tell the doctor.

But… There are no buts, there is either cooperation or potential death as you're trying to hide something. Tell the doctors what they need to know and deal with whatever afterwards, or you could avoid the whatever and the afterwards, if you see what I mean. Choice is yours.

Copies of any relevant notes you have regarding previous days. (You know, the pdfs you downloaded from my site, blood pressure, temperature, weight, input/output, etc.)

There is no such thing as too much information and the clearer the picture for the doctor, the better.

Basic essentials

Pyjamas.

A dressing gown/bathrobe.

Clean underwear.

Slippers.

Thick socks to keep your feet warm, or ones that double as slippers.

Flip-flops for the shower.

Tracksuit.

Loose fitting t-shirts.

Woolly hat/cap if chemo has removed your hair.

Wig, if you usually wear one.

Headscarf/Headscarves.

*An eye mask to help you sleep.

*Earplugs.

*If you use the eye mask and/or earplugs, don't forget you will normally have your temperature/blood pressure taken throughout the night to monitor your progress, so it can be a bit of a shock when someone sticks a thermometer in your ear and you're in the middle of a dream. It might be an idea to ask the nurse to awaken you beforehand. Organise a method like a gentle shake or taking your hand, or if you're like me, you get so used to it you sleep through it.

Must haves

Some cash (just enough for basic needs) and a credit/debit card. You might want to organise a pre-loaded card that someone can top up for you as and when; that way if it goes missing it's only a small amount and you can get another card.
If you're using your main card, write out the contact details for the bank and leave it with a friend/relative you can easily contact as that way you can put a block on it until it is either found or replaced. You can print a pdf for your bank details at www.cancerology.co/bankcard

Phone and charger.
If you forget the charger, it's common now for wards to have spare chargers for patient use, but it's not guaranteed.

Glasses, or contacts and cleaner. If you use separate glasses for reading and long distance, you'll probably only need the reading glasses, but forewarned and all that.

Hearing aid and batteries/charger.

Walking stick.

Headphones/earbuds.
You may want to consider headphones as a hospital preference, as earbuds can irritate, and cushioned headphones also block out any external noise so you can use them turned off.

Spare USB cable. (no idea what for, but if you don't have one, you'll probably need one)

Laptop.

A kindle, e-reader, or tablet.
Sometimes, the air conditioning in a hospital can dry your eyes and make it hard to focus, so being able to increase the text on the device can make a huge difference when you're reading.

Battery hand fan or USB powered mini fan.

Prunes for breakfast.
Yes, I know you're in hospital and they can give you lactulose, but if your body is used to prunes to help with constipation, keep the rhythm.

Hygiene/looks

Toothbrush.
A soft one as chemotherapy can affect the teeth/gums.

Toothpaste.

Mouth wash.

Facewipes.

Facecloth.

Soap/Shower gel.

Electric razor.

Wet razor with spare blades.

Shaving foam.

Shampoo/conditioner. (if you still have hair)

Shower cap.

Hair dye.

Soft Towels.
Most hospitals don't supply towels and if they do, they're like sandpaper.

Hair drier.

Comb/brush. (flexible wide tooth if you're on chemo and still have hair)

Moisturiser.

Deodorant.

Hand sanitiser.

Hand cream.

Lip balm/Chapstick.

Eyedrops. Air conditioning can dry your eyes and chemo can also cause problems.

Soft toilet paper. (Because you can be tender down there and constipation/diarrhoea can be a side-effect of treatment, and let's face it, hospital loo roll isn't going to win any awards for comfort, so treat yourself.)

Moist toilet tissues. (These are also gentle and can make life a lot easier.)

Tampons.

Incontinence pads.

Entertainment

For some, being in hospital for even a day can irritate as the time drags, so some sort of entertainment for a distraction is a good idea.

If you're in for a longer stay (especially something like a Stem-Cell-Transplant) then variety is required as the attention span is severely restricted, so little and often is the answer.

Colouring book/s and pens.

Puzzle books. Sudoku/Wordsearch/dot-to-dot/spot the difference/crosswords, etc
Ideally something you're good at and something you've never tried before or know you're bad at. You can print some sudoku puzzles and crossword puzzles and word search puzzles for free from my website. www.cancerology.co/freepuzzles
If you're already in hospital reading this, ask one of the nurses if somebody in administration can print a couple of pages for you. (Offer to pay, but they probably won't accept unless you start abusing the privilege.)
It's probably better if you put the pdfs on a memory stick clearly marked, but don't forget hospitals can't risk getting hacked, so may refuse to use a memory stick or even accept an email. If they do accept emails, it's usual for delivery to be delayed due to virus checking and other software.

Magazines.

A book of short stories.
Short stories allow you to set a target to finish one a day, and the fact you've completed something is rewarding.

New books.
Yes, more than one is what I recommend. If you have a couple on the go, they engage the mind with different plots and encourage you to find out what happened next. Make sure one is outside your normal genre.

Cancerology. (obviously)

Pens/pencils, and a notebook.
Write a journal, write a diary, write everything that happens to you including your opinion of the doctors, the service, your feelings, moods, hopes, aspirations, dreams, views, etc.
Write the nurses/doctors names and memorise them.
Write what you need to do or change to achieve success and set a plan of action.
Hell, write a book; I started one in 2002 and for a variety of reasons couldn't release it (there was a TV show that came out at the same time that was too similar), but I've rewritten it and it will be released early 2022.

A highlighting pen.

Dictation machine or use the app on your phone to dictate things you need to remember or ideas for a book, etc.

Jigsaw/s
The problem with a jigsaw is it can take up so much room, so if you're in a ward, it's probably not a good idea, but if you're in a room where you can store it until it's complete (and you know you're in for a while), it's a great distraction with a reward at the end.

Knitting, crochet, bobbin lace, etc.
Although it hasn't been a problem when I've been in hospital (as I've watched others knitting in bed), you may need to check with the staff as knitting needles are pointed and therefore potentially dangerous, so might not be allowed.

Treats

Diluting juice for drinking

Some snacks with a strong flavour if you're taste has gone, but not spicy as they could upset your stomach.

Bovril/Marmite, or something similar.

Tinned pineapple.

Crackers.

Nuts.

Popcorn.

Boiled sweets like lemon drops. Something that is going to give you a sensation of taste.

Mints.

Things you can't pack but can use

Audiobooks.

Learn another language or learn to draw, or learn to…
How? YouTube has lots of free courses on anything you can think of, and learning a new skill stimulates different areas of your brain, which, in turn, distracts and stops you constantly thinking about cancer.
Any long-term goal where you see yourself the other side of cancer is motivational.

The MP3s/videos on the Cancerology website.
Breathing exercises, meditations, visualisations, relaxation exercises, memory exercises, etc.

Netflix/AmazonPrime/Disney/Sky access for entertainment.

Personal stuff.

It's also good to have something to look forward to when you come out of hospital, so some personal photographs will remind you why you have to win, but you need to check all this stuff with the hospital and make sure they allow it. Personal pictures that make you smile before you go to sleep and when you wake up; something to motivate the fight, to give you something to fight for, make the smile. Think family, think pets, think friends, think obligations and desires. Not only motivational but just pleasant to have.

Leaving your essentials

From time to time, you will be away from your bed, be it for the bathroom, or a scan, or operation; so if you are in a ward, make friends with a neighbour who can keep an eye on your stuff if you have to leave.

No hospital will take responsibility for your goods; still, you will remember earlier I advised you to make friends with all your nurses, and this is where you can potentially ask one to keep an eye on your goods, or have the curtains drawn around the bed, or maybe keep something valuable in the office until you return from your scan, or operation, or whatever. If you don't make friends with the staff and treat them well… put it another way, if you were a nurse, would you help you?

I can honestly say that every time I had to leave my bed for any length of time (such as an operation), I never left my laptop on the table as the nurses always tucked it away safely for me. Every time.

The most important thing everyone needs to pack

The last thing you need to pack is the most important, irrespective of whether you're going into hospital for an overnight stay or longer, and it's something you're going to have to look for and find and use every minute of every day you're in hospital, and that is your attitude. You need to pack a positive attitude and use it.

Suffice to say, a negative attitude with negative expectations will (more than likely) produce negative results, whereas a positive attitude with positive expectations will (more than likely) produce a better outcome. There is no guarantee a positive attitude will make things perfect, but it does always make them seem better.

"When you come to the end of your rope, tie a knot and hang on."
– Franklin D. Roosevelt

Then I got pneumonia

It's a fact that a lot of people die every year from pneumonia, and pneumonia is one of those things that goes hand in glove with cancer when your immune system is compromised during chemo. It's also one of those words with a silent letter, so you know it's gonna be a sneaky little shit.

I've had pneumonia, not once, but five times, and it's a scary thing because you realise that a) pneumonia kills and b) cancer kills and c) you've got both, so it's like a foregone conclusion; you're definitely gonna die. At least, that's what a lot of people think when they're diagnosed. Of course, you already know my attitude and it was during my first cancer when it struck. I was out walking one night—slow, not a fast walk—when it got increasingly hard to breathe in a short space of time. I couldn't inhale as much air as I wanted to, I couldn't get it all in. My breathing was coming in short laboured rasps. (In fairness, I had been coughing up some gunge over the previous couple of days, and had I bothered to report it and have it analysed, I may have avoided my first pneumonia, so something to watch out for.)

I eventually made it home, but later in bed I really couldn't breathe at all, so we grabbed my pre-packed suitcase, and I was dumped in the car and taken to casualty/ER. We had telephoned during the trip and I was taken straight to a ward and immediately diagnosed with pneumonia. Did I panic? Honestly, no, because a) I was in the right place to have the magic happen, and b) I knew the cancer wouldn't beat me, so I'd be damned if pneumonia would kill me.

I was immediately started on antibiotics and samples were taken to have cultures done. Was it uncomfortable? Yes, mildly, but as I had read everything they had given me regarding potential side effects/problems, I knew what it was and I knew they could treat it.

They got my breathing under control pretty quickly and I was in hospital for only five days, and then I was discharged, and that was my first episode of pneumonia over; all good, back to normal, except it wasn't.

Boy, was I weak? Pneumonia takes it out of you, and I was back to walking like my muscles had gone on holiday and my breathing (although technically normal) wasn't like it had been pre-pneumonia. It took me several months to get back to the stage I had been at before, so keep an eye out and if you start coughing up flem, don't wait, call your chemo nurse. Put a sample into a container and get it analysed as soon as possible.

The second time it visited, I did exactly as I've advised you to do above and when they checked my stats, my oxygen levels were through the floor. Yes, another five days—all expenses paid—at hotel hospital. Throw in a canula, rig up a drip and start with broad spectrum antibiotics until the results of the culture tests come back.

To date, I've had pneumonia a further three times and it's like everything else on the cancer journey; it's like treatment, it's like being sick, it's like the lethargy, it's like... you've done it before, and you can do it again. The problem of course is until you've done it once you don't know what it's like. But I've just told you. And the biggest problem with a diagnosis of pneumonia and especially when you're on cancer is; it's a killer and you've got cancer. Ergo, you're dead. But you've read this, and you know my experience and you know it doesn't have to be like that. I have spoken to a lot of other people who had pneumonia—while on chemotherapy—and you can extrapolate from that, I couldn't have spoken to them had they been dead.

The doctors have your back. Go in with a, 'Here we go again attitude. This is a pain in the ass, but I'll get out the other side and continue the fight.'

The expectation of success is huge. So, as I've said before, don't shake hands with the devil till you meet him. Take every setback—and there will be setbacks—as part of the process.

I have had several exceptionally major things happen, but I'm still here. Don't let perceptions or negative expectations ruin your life; you don't know what's gonna happen till it's happened, and even when it has happened, you don't know how it's gonna turn out.

Live life with positive expectations. Yes, sounds like woo-woo, but it does make a difference.

We need to see you poo

Just another normal day in hospital and as usual and the nurse took my temperature, blood pressure, and stats, then recorded them on my chart; she asked me how I was and then said, "The doctor has said, we need to see you poo."

"Sorry, what?"

"You know? Poo," then she whispered, "excrement."

I said something along the lines of, "Are you right in the head? Not gonna happen." (it's probable there may have been one or two swear words in there)

In fairness, she did look shocked.

Then I said. "They want to watch me having a dump. Are you takin' the piss?" (it's probable there may...)

It was at this stage she laughed, then laughed some more, then shook her head with a grin like a bloody Cheshire cat. "Where did you get that from?"

"You said the doctor needs to see me poo."

The cat reappeared with an even bigger grin. "We need to see your poo, as in what comes out; we don't want to watch you do it, silly."

Did I feel silly? Yes, that would be appropriate. I felt stupid, but then I thought, hang on, why do you want to see my poo in the first place, so I asked.

"We need it for a fecal occult blood test." (Sometimes, you will see it written as faecal instead of fecal, but both mean the same thing: relating to faeces, poo, bum waste, etc.)

"Oh, well, that's okay then," I said, as if I understood.

She then produced a circular(ish) cardboard thing, explained I had to put it under the toilet seat, then go as usual (but don't forget to pee first).

I said, "Wow, sounds romantic. Are you going to buy me dinner beforehand?"

Having spoken to others about this test, the first thing they think of when they hear 'fecal occult blood test' is the word occult. Is the doctor a black magic practitioner? Why the word occult? Well, occult means hidden, and a fecal occult blood test is used to check for blood in the stool sample that the naked eye can't detect.

If blood is detected, you will need a colonoscopy to check if it could be coming from haemorrhoids or a polyp or cancer.

Around 20% of people have polyps in their colon and don't even know it. They are small growths of cells that form on the lining of the colon (large bowel) and are mostly harmless but have the potential to develop into cancer.

This type of test is very effective because polyps or cancers in the colon are often fragile, so passing a stool can damage the blood vessels and cause bleeding; however, as the stool absorbs the blood, it may not be visible to the naked eye.

To test the fecal matter, it is smeared on a test card coated with a guaiac, a plant-based substance that changes colour if there is blood in the stool.

We as humans are a vain bunch who like to be clean and presentable before meeting other people. We wash, clean our teeth, and all manner of other things to conform. We put on perfume or aftershave and deodorant because we like to smell nice, which is pretty much impossible when we're talking about poo, because there is no regime to prepare it for presentation.

It's not going to look nice, and it's definitely not going to smell nice. What seems to be the biggest shock is when you produce the sample, look down at the cardboard and think to yourself, 'you know, I could have done better; that's not the prettiest poo I've ever done'. Yeah, we can be weird like that… or maybe it's just me.

It isn't a competition, and there is no award for best formed or most consistent poo of the day, but I seem to remember producing an excellent specimen I was quite proud of on one occasion.

Then… the embarrassing bit. You have to let the nurse not only take it but see it as well in all its smelly warmishness.

Then it's off to the lab for analysis, but not the whole poo as most people think. What happens is the nurse takes a tiny sample and sends that, then disposes of the cardboard and poo, which begs the question, why take the whole log in the first place?

Because I'm over sixty, I do a home test and post it to be tested. If you need to be tested, they advise you to use cardboard and lift it out and… but all you have to do is slide yourself over on the seat slightly so that your poo hits the porcelain and then reach in with the little spatula provided and you have your sample, then flush.

It's a test that is carried out frequently on cancer patients just to be safe, so expect it and don't be embarrassed; your poo is the same as every other poo the nurse has seen that week.

The Power of You

I'm sorry. I'm not a Christian and I don't believe in God or any all-powerful divine entity. I suppose that doesn't make me a good person in the eyes of some people, and I don't want to offend anyone, (no, really) but here's a thought—I've heard people say, "Don't worry, God will cure you," or "I'll say a prayer and it'll all be ticketyboo." Okay, so I'm ad-libbing here, but if He can cure you, then why did He let you get it in the first place?

It's a win-win situation. If you get cured, it was God's will. If you die, God wanted you home. Really? Ya think?

You have to participate in your own cure.

If you believe in a higher power, go with it, but you have to believe in the power of you. It's what's inside you that can make the difference between a good outcome and a bad one, an easy journey through treatment or a hard one.

Again, I refer back to the placebo effect; if you believe something is going to work for you, then your body will do everything it can to make it happen.

And then I was caught (1st time)

Every time I went for treatment, they did the usual tests: bloods, temperature, stats, blood pressure, but also my height and weight, and as I didn't think my height would ever change, I asked why. The nurse told me the amount of chemotherapy administered was always calculated based on my body mass index. I needed more details (as usual) and was told that the larger my body mass, the more chemo I received. This meant the heavier I was, the more chemo I was given.

That got me thinking.

I've never fished in my life, and I hate the thought of it, but I visited a fishing shop, bought lots of little lead weights and stuffed them into all the pockets of the jacket I normally wore to chemo.

This worked well for two sessions, and I was happy, as in my mind the more chemo I received, the more chance of it eradicating the cancer.

Then the hot weather arrived.

When it came to getting weighed, the nurse noticed my jacket and insisted I take it off as it was so hot. I said I was okay, but she insisted. I removed it and went to hang it over a chair, but she told me to stay on the scales and she would take it for me.

I reluctantly held it out. She took it out of my hand and immediately dropped it on the floor.

Busted.

They weighed it and discovered I had managed to stuff exactly 9lbs (just over half a stone/4.08kg) into it.

I felt like I was back in school again, waiting to be sent to the headmaster's office.

It's not something I recommend as it's dangerous. The chemo is measured for a reason, but me being me…

For some reason, they always checked my pockets after that.

And then I was caught (2nd time)

Tuesday 6th August 2002

You are aware I had a balloon business, but I also had a printing business.

I'm sure you will already know that living in Northern Ireland throughout the troubles (bombings, kneecappings, protection rackets, etc) meant that at some point nearly everyone came into contact with undesirables, and I was no exception, so in the interests of full disclosure, here goes.

I was approached by some unsavoury people who enquired if I would like to start printing money for them. Initially, I refused, but after some threats were made, I complied.

Don't get me wrong, I didn't want to do it, and I could use the excuse cancer had muddled my thought process, but I started printing for them on a small scale.

It turned out I had a talent for it, and we rapidly moved from small scale to large scale, but in my mind, all I was doing was printing little pieces of coloured paper, and what they did with them was their business. I never used them myself as I was too scared of getting caught, and I felt guilty about it, but excuses aside, I knew it was wrong.

The Police too agreed it was wrong and, at around ten o'clock in the morning, they paid me a visit.

After they discovered over £300,000 in fake notes, they invited me to take a trip in their nice car with blue lights and fancy horns.

I was arrested and hit the national newspapers, TV, and radio.

Okay, I was a naughty boy, but due to the intimidation and cancer, I was let off with a suspended sentence and told not to do it again; but it wasn't all bad as the raid had also confiscated over £17,000 in real money and, at the sentencing, the judge decided to pass it on to a youth club. At this stage, I was in the dock thanking my lucky stars and should have kept quiet as that was what was expected, but a youth club? I said, "Excuse me," to the judge and my solicitor gave me a stern look, but me being me, again, I couldn't keep quiet. The judge asked me if there was something I wanted to say, so I told him that as I was suffering from cancer, I thought the money should go to a more worthwhile cause, like a cancer charity. Thankfully, he agreed.

Needless to say, the pressure on the family/marriage increased and I was unsure if I could face going for my final chemotherapy, but then I received a call from one of the nurses asking if I was okay. I explained my reservations and was told I was being silly and to complete the course, after all, it wasn't like I had hurt anyone.

On reflection, and indirectly, I did hurt people. People who were passed the money for goods and services and were left out of pocket, so hopefully, this book may go some way to repaying my debt to society in some small way.

It's funny now looking back, and especially when the subject of a criminal record comes up and I say, "I have one," and they jokingly ask, "How long did you get? They never quite expect to hear twenty-four years, then they ask, "What did you do?" Again, they never quite expect to hear, "I was a printer." Nobody ever considers a printer could break the law, after all they're only putting ink on paper. Yeah, it's a funny one now, but not at the time.

Still, as Interpol said they were the best counterfeit notes they had ever seen, it's a bit like a recommendation. Does that allow me to say, I'm the only printer in Ireland recommend by Interpol? I'll take it anyway.

It would be fair to say I go to extremes and being arrested for being the biggest counterfeiter of Euros in the world is rather extreme. Still, by way of illustration, it works, because for others, it can be something as simple as having your shopping drop out the bottom of the bag, an accident, or having your car repossessed, or mortgage arrears, blown fuse, or…

All sorts of things can and will happen on the journey through cancer that can trip you up, and all of them are unexpected, and because you're under so much pressure, small problems are perceived as huge.

It would be stupid to say you have to be prepared for the unexpected, so I'll just say, yeah, be prepared for the unexpected.

There is no other way of saying it; it's a stupid phrase; a better way of saying it might be when the unexpected happens—and it has a tendency to do just that—don't overreact; realise what it is and find a path through it.

There are many things in life that a knee jerk reaction will make worse, so a deep breath and count to ten, or one hundred, or one thousand; whatever it takes to realise that looking back a week or month from now will leave you wondering what all the fuss was about.

The first thing to ask is, what is this trying to teach me? Is it as bad as I think?

Sometimes the lessons are worth the lesson, if that makes sense.

Be prepared. That's all I'm saying.

Wednesday 10th August 2002

Due to the pressure on my family from my printing adventure, we decided a holiday was in order for my wife and kids, so off they went to Disneyland Paris for a well-deserved break.

Left home-alone, I thought: Well, at least it can't get any worse. Oh, you shouldn't ever think that.

"You don't see faith healers working in hospitals in the same way that you don't see psychics winning the lottery every week." ~ Ricky Gervais

Palmistry, clairvoyants, fortune tellers, astrology, etc.

Okay, maybe this section will dent my credibility somewhat, but I had visited palm readers and clairvoyants over the years, and to some degree I believed in them, or hoped they were right; but none of them ever mentioned cancer or a period of illness in my projected future, so naturally when it arrived uninvited, my faith in them was somewhat dented.

Anyway, one night just before I was diagnosed, I was out walking with the kids and noticed a red coat lying on the road tight to the pavement. We went over to investigate, and found it wasn't a coat at all, but a little white dog covered in blood and scrapes. He must have been run over by a car. Couldn't just leave him there like that, could we? So, we bundled him up and it was off to the vet.

The next day the vet reported the dog had looked much worse than he actually was, but was obviously abandoned as he had had to cut the collar off him because it was so tight and was choking him. He also asked us to come and collect him.

Now, my son, Jordan, had asthma and was allergic to animal hair as it brought on a fit of coughing and usually a visit to the hospital followed, so a dog was out of the question, but the vet said that unless we collected him, he would have to dispose of him.

We collected him.

He was brought back on the understanding he would be an *outside* dog and wouldn't be allowed in the house at any time, but you know kids, and of course, he was allowed in.

I was diagnosed with cancer a couple of days later and admitted to hospital for tests and chemo, during which time the dog went missing.

I had got it into my head that as long as I had 'Rascal'—which is what the kids named him—I would be all right, as I could take him for walks as the books recommended, and he would keep me fit and help cure me, but where was he?

I went into hospital for a couple of days, but when I came out, he was still lost. Then I got a phone call. Rascal was found and was only a couple of hundred yards up the road at a neighbour's house.

We immediately went and got him from a Mrs Kitson, who, as I said, only lived up the road. We started talking and, without any warning, she was telling me things about myself and my cancer; but without any input from me.

I stopped her: not because I didn't like it, but because I wanted her to slow down and tell it to me in a way I could absorb and remember.

It turned out she was a clairvoyant, and if not for Rascal (my cancer exercise partner), I would never have met her.

We hit it off, so I arranged an appointment where I could relax and record what she said.

She told me lots, and so far, everything (good and bad) has come true. She offers you the choice of hearing only good things or hearing everything; I choose to hear everything, and she didn't charge me anything in case you're wondering.

She also gave me a good luck charm: a blood charm she called it, and of course lymphoma is a blood disorder, which begs the question, how did she know I had a blood disorder? I had only just found out and none of the neighbours knew. Anyway, for the first time ever I wore a necklace, and on it hung one of the ugliest little dudes ever seen, but I wouldn't let anyone take it away from me, it brought me luck and I felt invincible when I wore it. The nurses teased me about it, but I wouldn't take it off.

My consultant at the hospital had hoped the cancer would be cleared up with the first CHOP regimen, but Angela (Mrs Kitson) had told me it would come back repeatedly and I wouldn't be cured for years, but she also said it would never kill me. After hearing this, I had no worries. I took everything as it came, safe in the knowledge that eventually I would be better, and guess what? It worked. (well, until bladder cancer visited me, but so far 2021 has shown no recurrence)

I remember Dr Kyle (my consultant) telling me the cancer had returned for a second visit, and I told her I already knew that was on the cards as I had been told in advance. A (very) short argument ensued as to why I was consulting with another doctor, but once I explained, we had a laugh (or to put it another way, she thought I was nuts).

The funny thing is, I was also told about my dad's death, and that three gentlemen from the government would be paying me a visit about something serious, but not to worry, as everything would work out okay. If you read the section, 'And then I was caught (2nd time)', you'll understand, as there were two detectives and a UK counterfeiting expert involved.

Later in this book I debunk alternative therapies, and it would be fair to say that someone offering to foretell the future should be included in this category, and I agree, but I can't get my head around how accurate she was. For some reason, she seemed to be the exception to the rule.

Fortune telling and associated practices are said to have originated when P T Barnum (the famous circus owner) compiled a list of things to say to people when reading their palm, or crystal gazing, or whatever method of reading was used. The list was used to great effect when a class of students were interviewed by a fortune teller and asked their date of birth from which he could predict their future. After a time, he returned to the class and called out the names for each of the students to collect a personalised written reading about their future. Once everyone had read the predictions, they were asked to complete a questionnaire about the accuracy of their reading. The figure came back at a very positive 97% accuracy. At this point the students were invited to swap their *personalised readings* with another classmate, which was when everyone discovered that with the exception of their name at the top of the page, all the readings were identical.

The list included:

You have a great need for other people to like and admire you.

Disciplined and self-controlled outside, you tend to be worrisome and insecure inside.

At times you have serious doubts as to whether you have made the right decision or done the right thing.

There are times when you just want to be left alone to contemplate life, and you're a serious thinker.

You prefer a certain amount of change and variety and become dissatisfied when hemmed in by restrictions and limitations.

You don't think of yourself as a lucky person, but you know you are.

You have a tendency to be very critical of yourself.

You pride yourself as an independent thinker and do not accept others' statements without proof.

You have found it unwise to be too frank in revealing yourself to others.

You know what your lucky numbers are, so you should write them down and use only them to do the lottery.

At times you are extroverted, sociable, affable, while at other times you are wary, introverted and reserved.

You have a great deal of unused capacity which you have not turned to your advantage.

Why do you hold yourself back? You know what you should be doing, but you seem to be reluctant.

While you have some personality weaknesses, you are generally able to compensate for them.

Some of your aspirations tend to be unrealistic.

Security is one of your major goals in life.

The problem with my reading was it was so precise, and as none of the phrases above were used, I can't explain it.

If you regularly read your horoscope in the paper, stop and read each prediction slowly and you will find they are not as accurate as they seem and are relevant to anyone reading, irrespective of their star sign.

All of the above Barnum phrases are relevant to everyone, and even if they don't fit exactly at the time, your mind will interpret a meaning for you, as you want to believe you haven't been duped.

My advice is you make your own mind up and proceed with caution. I suppose best advice would be that if you have a reading done, look out for the standard phrases used in the list above, and if they're used, you'll know it's nothing more than a rehearsed scam, and if you are constantly being asked to confirm questions, walk away.

When I had my experience, I couldn't get a word in until she was finished.

"*When you've beat cancer once, there is nothing you can't do, and that includes kicking cancer's ass again.*" ~ Lawrence Wray

No instruction manual

I don't really need to tell you this because you know it instinctively, but a reminder never hurts.

Two identical people going through the same procedure on the same day can have two different experiences. One will say it was easy, while the other will say it was the hardest thing they ever had to do. The question is, why?

The answer is programming, or attitude, or expectation; call it what you will.

Your brain believes what you tell it; that's part of visualisation and pre-programming yourself for a procedure like I did with the endoscopy test (and at that stage, I didn't even have a name for it).

I'll say it again; the brain believes what you tell it, so if you tell it that the procedure will be the worst thing in the world, your brain has an expectation that it will be, so it facilitates your expectation. Tell it that everything will be ticketyboo, and... yeah, you already know the answer.

Some people might say, I'm not built like that, I've got total control over my brain. Well, let me tell you, you're the only person on the planet who does.

The human brain is a three-pound muscle (actually, it's an organ, but think of what it can do and you'll probably agree that muscle is a better term), which is potentially the most powerful computer in the universe, but definitely in our world, and it comes without an instruction manual.

When you think about it, the human race is self-limiting; you have a child who learns to crawl, walk, and talk in one or two or maybe even three languages, all before school starts. It learns to control its bodily functions, can play games on tablets and phones, and the intelligence level is sky-high.

People who have suffered an injury and had to learn how to walk/balance again can tell you just how complicated the process is, yet kids do it naturally. Then we send this little bundle of brains to school to be taught, and the teacher says, “Do you think you could colour in the nice picture without going over the lines?”

The kid’s brain is probably thinking, be serious. I can walk. I can talk. I can play a video game better than you, and you’re asking if I can colour between the lines?

We don’t challenge the human brain. We lower expectations after spectacular brain growth. We don’t understand how powerful it is and how we can program it, which brings us back to, I’m not built like that, or my brain doesn’t work like that; but it does.

Ever watched a sad movie and cried? A horror movie and jumped? You’re crying or jumping at light on a screen that isn’t real, but... once you’re immersed in the film, your brain believes what you tell it (what it sees in this case). It’s that simple, and it happens to everyone.

If you pre-programme your brain for a good outcome, it will try to fulfil your expectations; if you programme for a bad outcome, it will try to fulfil your expectations.

If you remember when I suggested to myself the doctor would say I was the best patient he ever had; you may have thought I was laying it on a bit thick, but it’s what I thought, and more importantly, it’s what my brain expected, so the procedure couldn’t have been easier.

I have spoken to loads of other people who have had the same procedure and would never want to go through it again or would like to be asleep for it because it was the worst thing in the world.

Your subconscious does not know the difference between reality and imagination.

If you pre-programme your brain before any procedure, or something you're not looking forward to, and prepare for a pleasant experience, it makes things a lot easier, and it's a simple formula; for example, if you have a week to prepare for the experience, then two or three minutes a day of seeing a good outcome in your mind will build a positive expectation. Then, two days before, spend seven to ten minutes preparing, and on the day itself, spend as much time as you can reinforcing, and guess what, easiest thing in the world. Trust yourself. Trust your brain; it has your back.

People don't think they're as smart as they actually are; they self-limit, they self-restrict.

Use what you have between your ears and let it work for you. It will do what needs to be done, if you let it.

The ultimate cancer mindfuck

Yeah, it's a great title for this section, but you might want to read this and then give it to your carer; because that's really who it's aimed at, although you need to be aware as well.

Dear, Carer, it's that day you say it, or at least think it. *He/she (the sufferer) would be better off dead.*

This is an example of how far a diagnosis or cancer experience can push someone. I call it the ultimate cancer mindfuck, and that's not an exaggeration.

It doesn't matter the relationship: spouse, brother, sister, parent, or child; someone is having the worst time of their life and the outlook is bleak. Someone you care about is suffering and the end is definitely in sight, then the phrase pops into your head, *they would be better off dead*? Which is immediately followed by guilt.

The first big problem is that unless you have psychopathic tendencies, the thought of killing another human being or even wishing them dead would be abhorrent to you, and you know that in your wildest dreams you would never consider it. Yet, boom, the thought has appeared. Your brain has come up with a solution to both their problem, and your problem. Their problem is they are suffering and going to die anyway, and your problem is it's breaking your heart watching them suffer. Your brain has solved the problem, albeit in a rather harsh way, but for all the right reasons. It's not done because the insurance money is gonna be great; it's not that. You might joke about it, I did, but it's not that, it's something deeper, and ultimately it comes from love, which is strange because it conflicts with itself.

How can you love someone and wish for their death?

As the sufferer, you can understand this by flipping it 180 degrees. You're healthy as can be, and your carer is dying from cancer; what would you do?

I'll tell you: it's unanswerable. You're not where they are, and you can't condition your mind to think like they are currently thinking. You don't have their perspective. You haven't lived through their timeline.

But, even worse. Irrespective of the carer's best wishes, the sufferer survives.

How can this be worse?

Well, it's not; it's a good thing, but not so much for the carer. Although they have the successful outcome they initially wished/prayed for, they now feel guilty because their brain provided the logical solution where you would be better off dead. And there you have it; The ultimate cancer mindfuck.

Sometimes—in their mind—they have already buried you and started a new life without you, and everything is planned out to the last detail, but then you survive (you annoying shit) and deprive them of the idyllic future they had designed for themselves based on your demise. The realisation life might be better without you and the guilt at that thought can really mess with their head.

Then come the mind questions. I wanted him/her dead, and if I had got my wish, they wouldn't be alive now. I'm a bad person. Am I a psychopath? I'm twisted. How could I have thought such a thing?

They second guess themselves and don't realise they were right all along. Their thinking wasn't flawed; it's just that sometimes, things happen nobody expects.

It's the stuff that ruins not only relationships, but minds, and it's nobody's fault. But because of the magnitude of the potential solution—death—it becomes the defining thought; the biggest mistake (that didn't even happen in the first place and was never a mistake to begin with).

It can cut them to shreds for being a good person.

The word mindfuck is horrible, but it's not horrible enough for someone caught in this situation.

Cancer kills, cancer restricts, cancer is hard, but the little shit has more tricks up its sleeve than any magician. It seems to take pleasure where it can get it, and that means collateral damage is not only acceptable, but a requirement.

If it can't kill, it can screw with everybody's mind. Nightmares, sure, throw a tick on the blackboard. Marriage break-up, another tick. Suicide, another tick. It is relentless if you don't understand it; if you let it win.

Pay attention to this section. It's only 794 words, but read it again and let others read it. It might just be the most important advice in this book. It could save your relationship; it could save a life, it could save someone's sanity.

Ultimately, the cancer mindfuck is nothing more than perception.

There is no big revelation, but… there is; and if you understand it, you reduce its power.

Cancer screws with everyone. The person with cancer, and everyone they know.

Yeah, I did it

Thursday 15th August 2002 Last day of treatment.

Finished. That's it, my whole CHOP treatment is finished. I had six in total and throughout the whole treatment, I waited to vomit as predicted, but it never happened. I had felt bad and took a couple of infections, but no big deal, and on the day, everyone wanted to know about the fake money and it wasn't a problem; in fact, they treated me like I was some kind of celebrity.

Friday, 16th August 2002

The wife and kids were coming back from holiday the next day, so I decided to make sure everything was tidy.

In the afternoon, my dad rang to say he was sick, so I drove to his house and found he was worse than just sick and had to call an ambulance.

He was admitted to hospital with suspected renal failure.

What a month August was turning out to be.

Saturday 17th August 2002

Around nine o'clock on the Friday night, the hospital called to tell me my dad had deteriorated and could I come at once.

When I arrived, he was unconscious, and I sat with him and talked, holding his hand. At around one o'clock in the morning his breathing started to labour, and the nurses explained there was nothing more to be done.

At one thirty-two, he died.

When I returned home, I knew I should get some rest, but understandably, it was elusive. I went for a walk and around four hours later, while doing yet another lap of the neighbourhood, my wife and kids arrived to find me slowly walking down the road.

Again, after having a relaxing holiday, they returned to more pressure.

Annus horribilis

In a speech to the Guildhall on 24th November 1992 to mark the 49th anniversary of her assession to the throne, Queen Elizabeth II famously said:

"1992 is not a year on which I shall look back with undiluted pleasure. In the words of one of my more sympathetic correspondents, it has turned out to be an annus horribilis."

Annus horribilis is a Latin phrase that translates into 'horrible year', and I think 2002 was my version.

In May 2002, I was diagnosed with Non-Hodgkin Lymphoma and given six months to live, then in August I was arrested, and then my dad died. I guess, looking back, it was also the month the rot started in my marriage. Not only did my dad die, my marriage did as well, I just didn't realise it at the time.

But even with all that going on, I kept pushing myself to work through a total of seventeen cancers so far, and I'm still here.

...and, of course, 2002 wasn't finished with me just yet. November would turn out to be another kick in the ribs.

Keep Up To Date

As with a lot of factual books, things change over time; new procedures and therapies become available and the never ending list of new wonder drugs on the internet keeps expanding, so with that in mind, I will be constantly updating the book and bringing out revised versions, but in between editions—and only for those of you who have purchased this book—I will be adding additional updates on my website until I have enough to bring out another edition.

The reason for this is simply to be fair to my readers who bought the book in the first place. I don't think it's right for someone to purchase a book and then find out that it has been updated and the author expects you to purchase the new edition.

I have also uploaded videos, MP3 recordings you can download and keep on your phone or computer, as well as sample PDF Input/Output charts, Memory Exercises, Daily Obs Charts, and others you can simply open and print.

All you have to do is register on my website to gain access at. www.cancerology.co/free-stuff-for-my-friends

No, I didn't forget to put a full stop at the end as this is the exact address you will have to type into your browser, and as the page is only available to people who purchased Cancerology, you won't find it on google.

Once you're on it, it will tell you everything you need to know to get access.

"Cancer may have started the fight, but it has stepped into the wrong ring." ~ Lawrence Wray

Hello, hello, I'm back again. Did ya miss me?

Wednesday 20th November 2002

Is it back again? Yeah, must be my magnetic personality.

Thirteen weeks and six days from my last treatment, I was diagnosed with my second visit from Non-Hodgkin Lymphoma.

I had my last CHOP treatment on Thursday, 15th August 2002, and although I had no official confirmation I was in remission, things had been going well, and we had no reason to assume otherwise.

After some weeks, my back started to itch and turned into a rash which spread to the front of my body, and again I visited my doctor, who prescribed hydrocortisone cream to clear it up.

My Haematologist, Dr Kyle, had already organised a PET scan to check the cancer was indeed under control, but when I attended the hospital, they were reluctant to do it as it shows up blood in the body, and as I had a rash, the readings might conflict, but I convinced them and they did it and advised me to see my doctor that afternoon as the rash was bad and needed to be sorted immediately.

I made an appointment with my doctor on my return and was prescribed a cream for Scabies, which is a skin infestation caused by small parasites called itch mites, which burrow extensively through the superficial layers of the skin and irritate it with their waste products. Such mites are usually transmitted by close body contact with another person; hence, Scabies is most common where crowding and unsanitary conditions prevail. It is important to treat all affected family members at the same time, or re-infection is likely.

Not a nice thing to have, and it doesn't sound very hygienic; however, of course, I didn't have it. I had cancer.

I waited the next couple of days to see if things would clear up, but they didn't.

At this point, I'm going to remind you again to seek a second opinion if you're not totally satisfied with the diagnosis, and also point out that having already been through treatment, I should have gone straight to my consultant at the chemo centre to have it checked, rather than at a local surgery. Learn from my mistakes.

I had started to suffer mild sweats and tiredness again, so the thought had crossed my mind that the cancer was back. I made an appointment to see my Haematologist.

No surprise then when she told me she had the results and the cancer was back for round two; however, a big surprise lay in store as I had—in my naivety—assumed I would be put back on the CHOP programme and things would be just like before. Not so. The survival figures were reduced substantially for relapsed Non-Hodgkin Lymphoma, and I was told my chances of survival were now down in the 10-15% range.

Bad news, but what were the options? There weren't any; I would take the percentage.

The plan was to hit the cancer with CHOP again for two treatments and then move onto a new regimen called ESHAP.

I searched for the statistics relating to my Non-Hodgkin Lymphoma and discovered that for my stage, the survival rate was estimated at 15% at best and I can remember telling my wife the good news. She smiled and tried to encourage me, but her face told me she thought I'd probably be in the 85% who didn't make it, but in my mind, 15% was wonderful odds.

I'm a glass-half-full kind of guy and it's always served me well.

PET Scan

PET stands for Positron Emission Tomography, which is different from other scans as it relies on a radiotracer that is injected about an hour before the scan. This type of scan produces excellent 3D results for analysis.

Once injected with the radiotracer, you must relax and keep as still as possible to allow the tracer to circulate throughout your body as movement can affect the distribution. Once I received my injection, they pulled the curtains of the cubicle and turned out the lights. I did what I was told and went to my *happy place*.

It's not as hard as you think to keep still, and the more you do it, the easier it gets. If you think you're going to have problems, they can give you medication to help relax you, but it means you won't be able to drive afterwards.

Due to the tracer, it can not only indicate tumours, but also determine the exact size and show if the cancer has spread to other parts of the body, including lymph nodes and blood.

Pain rating is only ½/10. (simply as a result of the radioactive injection) Nothing to worry about.

Problems afterwards? None really, except if you are going to be visiting an airport within days of your scan, you might trigger the radiation monitors, so if an airport is on the agenda, make sure to bring your appointment letter with you to confirm you have just had a scan. On the plus side, you can tell all your friends you're radioactive.

The Outgoing Guy.

Now, although most of you don't know me personally, I can assure you that I am a very outgoing type of guy, and most things will never get me down. The last cancer most certainly didn't as I was sure I would beat it.

I was driving home from the hospital after the news and thinking about what was happening, when I suddenly found myself crying uncontrollably and had to pull my car off the road onto the grass verge. I had conjured up a picture in my mind—from where I know not—of my daughter (only twelve) walking down the aisle with her husband-to-be, and me nowhere in sight (presumably dead).

This was not like me, but it did get the better of me and I had to telephone my wife. She got out of work immediately, and we met up, and I cried some more.

This depression (for want of a better word) lasted roughly 1-2 days, after which I got my head around the whole thing and started feeling normal again, determined to beat the cancer by whatever means necessary.

Death Thoughts

Do I think about death? That's a question I get asked frequently and the answer is, "Yes. All the time."

Every night I go to bed, I wonder if I'll wake up in the morning, and every morning I open my eyes and say, "Yes, as expected." Cancer changes your thought process. You've gambled, and even though you've beat it, you are very aware it could pay another visit with more determination next time. As a result of cancer your chance of heart attack, stroke, etc., are increased, but you ignore them. The hardest battle has already been fought and won.

Heart attack? Shucks, no. Not gonna happen. I didn't fight this hard to collapse and die. Find someone else.

One of my favourite phrases is: I didn't come this far, just to come this far. Think about it. Make it your phrase as well.

I have no doubt at some stage I will die (no really), but it will be when I'm ready and not before. I've so much I still want to do, and I'll be damned if I'll go without a fight. It's what has kept me alive so far.

"*You have to believe tomorrow will be better, until one night you're in bed thinking, 'Today really was better. You know what? Tomorrow will be better'.*" ~ Lawrence Wray

Tomorrow will be better.

I don't know where that statement came from initially, but I've been using it since my first cancer. Being realistic, tomorrow might not be better, especially if you're just at the start of chemo, but there will be a tomorrow where it does start to improve.

If you expect a bad tomorrow where you'll be sick or weak, then you'll be sicker or weaker than you would have been had you not expected it.

If you expect a good tomorrow where – although you might not be 100% – your health won't be as bad as previous times, then it won't be.

You condition yourself.

If you expect to win the game, you have to see yourself winning.

It's your mind, and only you can control your thoughts and expectations.

Now, at this point, you might be thinking—This guy goes through all this and he never has a bad day?

You'd be wrong.

I've had plenty of them, but the 'good' tomorrow always arrives.

Bottom line? If you think you're gonna die or things are going to be bad, you're probably right.

Set yourself up for success

Before you go to sleep at night, make a point of programming your mind for a good day tomorrow. Yeah, sounds like woo-woo, but… if your last thought is, 'today was horrible, I don't want to repeat that again,' your brain will assume tomorrow will be the same. You'll wake up in a state of dread, and that feeling will stay with you throughout the day, and everything and anything done to you will be a thousand times worse, simply because you expect it will be.

Before you go to sleep, think of the positives. A nurse or doctor you have confidence in, how well you gave blood, how well you're coping compared to someone else, how tomorrow will be better, etc., again… your brain (It's way more powerful than anybody gives it credit for.) will make an assumption about how tomorrow will be, and as you're inputting good thoughts, it will make a point of looking for things to celebrate tomorrow. Life gets easier if you assume it gets easier, and, unfortunately, the reverse is also true.

The Christian Visitor

When you're suffering an infection during chemo, you can't be in the general ward for fear of germs from other patients, so you get your own room. TV, bathroom, shower, etc., all included at no extra cost, but it means that other than nurses and doctors calling in from time to time, you don't get to have a conversation with anyone. It was usual to read at least one or two books each day, so on the bright-side, I did educate myself a bit.

One evening, a lady I didn't think I even knew, came to visit. She sat down beside me and asked me how I was and how treatment was going. We talked for a couple of minutes before she realised she was in the wrong room. I must point out she was elderly, but at the same time, she seemed to have all her wits about her; it was just a simple mistake.

I suppose even though it had been a mistake, she felt obliged to enquire about my health and didn't just rush off to the correct room, so we talked for another ten minutes. For me, it was welcome company, but as she was leaving, she asked me if I would mind if she lit a candle for me and said a little prayer.

I said anything would be appreciated, thanked her and off she went. When she was gone, I thought about it and decided it was the nicest thing anyone had ever done for me. Something as simple as lighting a candle for a complete stranger and wishing them well, brightened my day no end.

I'm not a Christian, and after having spent months in hospital thinking about death and what comes next, I never arrived at any conclusion about the hereafter and I'm still none the wiser, yet her comments meant so much.

I would say that if I had to define a Christian, she would be my example.

Twenty Three

Cancer. Will it kill you, or will you kill yourself?

The Bad News

There is no magic potion. No magic wand. The fight with cancer is yours alone.

I've watched twenty-three people die from cancer since my initial diagnosis, which makes me ask: Why did they die and I'm still here? People who had a less severe cancer than me, people who were younger, older, fitter? I think this book might have been the reason I was spared. Is that a fact? No, it's a supposition and a nice thing to believe. But I believe there must be some reason.

The one thing you can take away today is you're reading a book written by a guy who is sixty-one years old, who got his first cancer when he was forty-one and was determined that irrespective of what they threw at him he would come out the other side. He had a positive mental attitude and was sure he would beat it.

The next line out of your mouth should be, "If he can do it, then I can too."

I counted all the people I have met on my journey who have died since I was first diagnosed in 2002. Hopefully, I haven't missed anyone, but at the time of writing, it was twenty-three. I wrote down all their names, types of cancer, treatment, and both how they died and their attitude towards their fight. Four of them really stood out.

One of them was a guy I talked to nearly every day as he owned a fish and chip shop adjacent to my shop, and I was a frequent visitor at lunchtime. He was a chef and had leaned on a hotplate until his hand was fried and didn't feel a thing. At the hospital, they discovered the cancer and admitted him, but he was only kept for less than a week before being transferred to a hospice. He had an advanced brain tumour and didn't have a choice in the outcome. Unfortunately, it was discovered too late and there was nothing that could be done.

Another one fought like a warrior, but just wasn't strong enough. He was my best friend and was seventy-two at the time. He was a moderate drinker and had been a serious smoker in his youth when it wasn't considered to be a harmful pastime, but when he discovered the dangers associated with smoking, he gave up immediately. He went 'cold-turkey' and said it nearly drove him crazy due to the hairs in his airway growing back after they had been burned away by the constant inhalation. We trained both mentally and physically before the operation and he went in with a 'Let's beat this,' attitude. He got through the operation and was doing well, and then an infection set in. I visited him on what was to be his last day and he was in good spirits, but I had just left the hospital when I received the phone call that confirmed he'd had a stroke and had passed away. It was unfair, but that's life.

A heart attack took the third one after diagnosis but before treatment had begun, and although she was ready to take on the fight against the cancer and had a positive attitude, there was a history of heart disease in her family and it just happened.

Pneumonia took the fourth one after only the second chemo session. She was eighty-one years old and was very frail to begin with as she had a lifelong problem with asthma, but chemo didn't slow her down in any way. When she lost her hair, a bright purple wig let people know something was wrong. She always looked forward to 'meeting her new friends' at the hospital and had even taught one of the nurses how to knit. A combination of ill health, cancer, and living in an old house that didn't have central heating or even double glazing didn't help, but she was determined to live her life, her way. I think if we could have convinced her to move to a home, the result might have been different, but at her age, she was set in her ways.

If I hadn't been so involved with cancer myself, the total would only have been four people I knew, but going through treatment means you can't help but connect with other sufferers.

Two who shouldn't have died.

In 2004 I had a stem cell transplant. Four of us went in at the same time—only two came out.

Due to the seriousness of the procedure, we were each given our own room that had positive air pressure to avoid the possibility of airborne germs. Visitors had to wash before coming in and put on gowns, masks, and gloves.

Prior to the start of treatment, we were allowed to visit each other and compare war wounds. I met a guy who we'll call John, and he was convinced he wouldn't make it. I was stage 4, high risk, aggressive Non-Hodgkin Lymphoma and had already been through it twice with different chemo regimens. He was stage two, low risk and it was his first time. I told him that out of the four of us, I was statistically the least likely to make it, but I was damned sure I would. He remained negative, and no matter how hard I tried to convince him otherwise, he was convinced he wouldn't make it.

After a couple of days, treatment started and we weren't allowed out of our rooms. On day seven, I asked one of the nurses about him, and although she gave a standardish answer of, "Sorry, I can't discuss other patients," the look on her face told me. When the next nurse came in, I said, "Sorry to hear about, John," and he replied, "Yes, he just seemed to give up."

My opinion—which I offer with no medical training or experience—is the cancer didn't kill him; he killed himself. He expected it. It became a self-fulfilling prophecy.

Another patient who we'll call Jane wasn't as negative, but was nowhere near as positive as I was, and she died within three weeks. Again, it was her first cancer and a lower stage than mine.

You have to participate in your own cure.

You can't just lie there and expect the doctors to do everything.

And the big one: if you expect a bad outcome, that's probably what you'll get.

The other seventeen?

Without exception, I have found all of them had an attitude where they expected to die or didn't want to fight.

Different cancers were involved. Some bad, some not so bad, some easy, but all came with a perceived death sentence that was only realised because of their belief.

And yes, I agree, I could be wrong, but when I made the list I allowed for severity of diagnosis, spread of cancer, stage, and especially attitude, and I'm convinced that in the majority of cases there is no room for doubt.

Please don't think it's easy to write this about deceased friends; it's not, but I honestly believe they simply gave up as soon as they received the diagnosis, and if you're reading this and it's making you think, then it's worthwhile.

This is the main reason this book is so very important to me. Seventeen people dying might well have been reduced substantially if only they had adopted a fight attitude. If only they had participated in their own cures, things might have been better.

Tough Love

This book is your wake-up call.

Yes, I know it's human nature to sympathise with someone who has cancer, but that's not what this book is about, and if you've got cancer, then it's reality you need.

Cancer is the ultimate wake-up call. It makes you focus on your life. It messes with your thought process. It transforms you from a rational person to a mind-mess, and while it's understandable, it isn't helpful.

A cancer diagnosis is unfair

Of course, it's unfair. If it were like say a driving test, you would be prepared. You would have had numerous driving lessons and studied the highway code and sat mock exams. When you went for your test and they asked you to identify a sign, you would know it because you previously studied all the road signs. You would have already driven in a car park and on the road, reversed, used the gears, brakes, etc. But, with cancer, it's like a grotesque clown jumping out of a box and shouting, "Surprise". It scares the hell out of you.

Most people are diagnosed with cancer and it comes as a shock. They're not prepared for what comes next, and that's when the mind goes into overdrive. You can't sleep because your mind won't rest, and thoughts of imminent death are foremost; then, your mind starts to explore whether or not it has any experience and, unsurprisingly, it does. A friend, or relative, or character on a TV show has had cancer and died, which means you're going to die too, irrespective of what your consultant has told you.

That's where this book comes into its own. It's a handbook on how to deal with cancer, the treatment, the side-effects, and the mental stress and strain not only on the sufferer but the family as well, and it's told in a frank and realistic way by someone who has first-hand experience of what it's like, not just once, but multiple times.

Tea and sympathy is lovely and—at times—necessary, but you've just been signed up for the fight for *your* life.

At the minute, the best thing we have to fight cancer is surgical removal of the tumour/s, drugs that will make you sick and radiotherapy that will burn, but they are all tolerable, so if you're going to beat cancer, this is your best option. And, yes, it's only my opinion, but it's based on personal experience that has worked for me.

I don't want or need to be your friend, but if we met face to face and you weren't fighting, I'd like to be the one to give you a good shake, and that's what this book is trying to do.

It's a disgrace that people just give up whenever there is still a chance at life, and I've proved that over and over again.

The Good News

At age twenty-three, one of my friends was diagnosed with Non-Hodgkin Lymphoma. It was discovered when it was well advanced, and he received the same news I had been given; six-months to live. We went to lunch and talked for over three hours, and once he knew I had been in the same position, he decided to stop worrying and fight. We discussed what he could expect, diet, exercise, chemo, attitude, and through the treatment he was constantly asking for advice.

Afterwards, he said if he hadn't known someone who had been in the same position and survived, he would have given up long ago, but he figured if I had survived, then he could too. Thankfully, he only had one visit and has been in remission for the last six years.

Even More Good News.

Another friend's husband was diagnosed with colon cancer and had decided to let nature take its course. Cancer ran in his family and everyone in his circle not only agreed with him, but encouraged him to plan his funeral and get things in order. (What a bunch of dickheads.)

His wife called at my house and simply broke down as her family and friends were all convinced there was nothing that could be done to change his mind. I didn't know the guy but paid him a call the next day. We immediately fell out and he asked me to leave.

I have no idea what changed his mind, but that same night, he too called at my house. From reading this book you already know I speak my mind, so another conversation started, only this time, he decided that if I had beaten it with a much worse diagnosis than him, then he would fight. He signed up for the operation and chemo and I went with him to his sessions. Depression hit him hard, but we talked it through, got him help, and he stuck with his treatment. His final scan was clear. Three years on, he's now counselling other sufferers through a charity.

I suspect some might object to my comment about dickheads, but think about it. In all probability, if he had stuck with the negative expectations and planned his funeral, he would probably be dead; and that's not my opinion as I let him read this section before publication and he insisted I keep it.

Yes, even more.

I was introduced to a guy who had been diagnosed with throat cancer and decided it wasn't worth fighting as they were going to cut out his tongue and half his mouth. He had lived a sorry life, smoked like the proverbial train, been in and out of prison, drank all day every day, and had frequently used hard drugs. He had been unemployed for years and just spent his life in a local bar from it opened until it closed.

The question was, is this a life worth saving? Did I want to get involved? Did I have the right to even consider these things?

I had been asked to help, so I gave it a go.

After several hours spent shouting, screaming, threatening, and crying, he eventually agreed that as I had been through it (twelve times, at that stage), he would give it a go.

Yes, he lost most of his mouth, but they reconstructed it and he looked okay. Yes, he hated the treatment. Yes, he's still alive and has found God, given up drinking, smoking and drugs and now has a job as a cleaner.

There have been others, but the biggest motivating factor to fight cancer is to talk to someone who has survived. Invariably, you will find they're just ordinary people that don't have any superpowers, but you will find they all had a positive attitude towards the outcome. The one common thread is each one will freely give advice and be on your side.

Once you're in the cancer club, it seems to be an unwritten rule you help others, it's just something that comes with the diagnosis and it's a responsibility you can't shirk.

Going through treatment, it is unusual if one of your fellow sufferers doesn't die, and the first death is always the worst, but sometimes, it can also be the best. I apologise in advance to anyone reading this who has just lost a loved one, but when you're the patient and another patient dies from the same disease, it makes you realise just how bad cancer can be, and might just change your mind-set from that of a cancer sufferer to a cancer fighter. It can be the wake-up call that flicks the switch that turns your flight-or-fight mechanism to the fight mode and keeps it there. Their death can—in a way—be your salvation.

Yes, I know this sounds very harsh, but cancer is a very harsh disease. It doesn't take prisoners; it takes lives, and it ruins families.

Without looking too hard, you're going to meet someone when you're getting treatment that has had it before and beaten it. Talk to them. Listen to what they have to say. Take their advice.

Think about the next time you don't have the energy to get out of bed. Are you going to force yourself or let the cancer win? Get up. Make the effort. Sit in a chair. The first time someone tells you they admire your attitude you'll move up a gear. You'll want to hear it over and over, and you will. All you have to do is participate in your own cure.

During the final edit of this book I received a call to let me know one of my friends had been diagnosed with colon cancer. It's the gift that doesn't stop giving.

"*Attitude is a little thing that makes a big difference.*" ~ Winston Churchill

A Positive Approach

I've mentioned the idea that a positive attitude can help in the journey through treatment before, but I'm not suggesting it can have any effect on the cancer cells and cause them to stop growing or die, no, what I mean is the attitude towards treatment and the eventual outcome can motivate you to participate in your own cure by making sure everything the doctors tell you to do is carried out, and by doing that you can affect how your body deals with treatment, and in many cases this can have a dramatic effect on your immune system, which is one of the main weapons to eradicate cancer cells.

I think my experience with the endoscopy test illustrates just how powerful the mind can be, but most people will have heard about someone with a terminal illness who has hung on until a baby is born or someone has promised to visit turns up.

People can hang on for weddings, then once they're over, they die. Some make it, some don't, but it's sometimes possible to delay the inevitable with will power.

I used to be in the wedding business and by now you know I say what I think and don't regulate my views, so I totally disagree with this practice, but it illustrates just how important and determined the mind can be.

With regards to any special event, but especially a wedding; should it be postponed?

Okay, the wedding goes ahead, and everything works out well, except that before, during or immediately afterwards, the cancer wins.

All the wedding anniversaries for evermore will be tainted with the memory of the death.

Can the honeymoon still go ahead?

Will the couple feel guilty/responsible?

Be pragmatic, whether you're planning the wedding or the one with the cancer.

I remember a wedding where the father of the bride gave his speech, sat down and died. Another where the father of the groom was wheeled into the reception, had the meal and died during the couple's first dance.

Think about it.

The easiest option is to postpone the wedding. Harsh, but realistic.

Happy New Year

Thursday 2nd January 2003

First day in hospital to start my ESHAP treatment, and it turns out I'm also the first patient to receive the treatment in Antrim hospital. Special or what?

Today was an easy day.

I arrived at the clinic at 9.30am for my appointment and had my usual blood tests; unfortunately, my veins were playing up, and the nurse had trouble finding a good one. My consultant became aware of this and advised I get a PICC line (Peripherally Inserted Central Catheter) installed in my right arm as my veins were not in an ideal condition, and it would make it easier to get further treatment through the line.

I had to get an extra blood sample taken for a kidney function test before the PICC line could be fitted, and once the results came back, I was told everything was okay and they could fit it.

The problem with chemotherapy given through a cannula, is the vein can become inflamed (phlebitis), which is painful. Another problem is the veins become hard to find and tend to move about, making it harder to insert the cannula.

Over time and with repeated chemo sessions, the chances of developing problems increase due to the length of time the cannula is in place, the type of drugs being given, and the size and location of the cannula.

Some chemo patients also develop hard veins or chemo veins, which means the vein can become hardened and in extreme cases, can make it hard to straighten your arm, which is when a PICC line becomes invaluable. Once treatment has finished, the veins do return to normal, but it can take time.

The solution is to insert a permanent line that will distribute the chemo throughout the body more efficiently.

When I went to have my PICC line inserted, the nurse put cream on my inner arm where the elbow bends: it's the same cream sometimes referred to as 'Magic Cream' by kids and parents. This cream has two functions: to help the nurses locate the veins by making them stand out from your arm, and to freeze the area necessary to insert the line. It is applied to your arm and left there for thirty-minutes to allow it to work.

I then lay on a bed and stretched out my arm to have it cleaned, ready for the line.

A trolley was wheeled in which had everything on it, and of course, being the inquisitive type, I reached over to touch the line and the nurses nearly had a fit. They are meticulous when it comes to sterilised equipment, and everything prepared for the procedure would have had to be replaced if I had contaminated it. The advice is—ask, but don't touch.

The time taken to insert the line was about twenty-minutes and I can honestly say I was aware they were doing something to my arm, but it didn't hurt, and I felt absolutely nothing inside where the line was going.

After it was installed, I had to have a chest x-ray to confirm accurate placement as apparently it can be too long or short, or even (rarely) go in the wrong direction. Mine was perfect.

The only other thing necessary is a tiny butterfly type attachment which is stitched in place to ensure the line cannot be pulled out accidentally.

At this stage in my life, I had never had a stitch in my skin, and without exaggeration, I was petrified at the thought of it, but after talking to the doctor, and seeing just how big a fuss I was making about something so small, I took her word it would not hurt. I was pleasantly surprised, and embarrassed to have been so scared.

I was given an instruction sheet and advised to apply heat using a hot-water bottle wrapped in a towel to the upper arm for twenty minutes, four times each day to avoid phlebitis. I found it a brilliant way to relax, and I listened to a CD for 20-30mins while it was on my arm. The only problem is it can be so relaxing, I sometimes fell asleep, and woke up with a cold hot-water-bottle. It is recommended this routine is followed for the first seven days.

Throughout the day, eating and everything else was completely normal.

I would suggest the only thing you need initially watch out for is the line snagging on your clothes when you are dressing or undressing, and even though the site will be covered with a waterproof plaster, you should take care when washing/drying the area.

The PICC line must be kept dry at all times, so consult with your doctor or nurse about your hygiene.

PICC Line - Peripherally Inserted Central Catheter

The procedure involves inserting a thin line into the vein of your arm, which runs up your arm, around your shoulder, and down to just above your heart.

Just above the heart??? Panic? Okay, so here's the thing; the PICC line is extremely similar to a cannula, with the only real difference being the length, so if you've had a cannula fitted, a PICC line just goes further and the distance required is calculated, so it's not like it's going to go through any valves in your heart.

This means any chemo or other medication you will be receiving can be easily administered through the line, and you will not need any further injections or cannula inserted. Don't get too excited though, as blood samples are still taken in the usual way.

The line can be left in place for up to twelve months.

Pain rating 0/10 (you're aware they are doing something to your arm, but it doesn't hurt)

Problems afterwards? None.

After treatment had finished, they removed the line and I asked if I could have it. (yeah, I'm funny like that) Fully stretched out, my PICC line was just over 26 inches and I still have it.

I have a video showing a Picc line and explaining it further at www.cancerology.co/piccline

News just in. Sex and masturbation is good for you.

No, it's not fake news.

Research from Harvard University confirms masturbation can significantly reduce the risk of men developing prostate cancer.

The research (which involved 31,925 men over an eighteen-year period 1992-2010) concluded that those who ejaculate only four-to-seven times a month are at greater risk than those who achieve orgasm twenty-one or more times a month. (5+ times per week)

Ejaculation, whether through sex or masturbation, is protective as it rids the gland of cancer-causing substances and may help to ease prostate inflammation.

In 1992, the study assessed men aged 20-29 and 40-49 and asked them to complete a monthly ejaculation questionnaire. Of the 31,925 participants, 3,839 developed prostate cancer.

The findings, which were published in the European Urology Journal, concluded that the men who reported a higher frequency of ejaculation were less likely to be diagnosed with prostate cancer.

Then, I woke up dead

Yes, this did happen; well, sort of. (I wasn't really dead) At this stage you're probably thinking I've lost the plot, but I haven't—honestly.

You go to bed, have a good night's sleep, waken up and sit on the edge of the bed, but something's not right. You're there, but you're not there. I remember the first time it happened, and even though I was able to sit up, I felt nothing, and everything looked hazy and foggy, and although I could focus, everything was surrounded by white air. I remember the thought hitting me, 'Shit, I'm dead.' What other explanation could there be?

I knew I had muscle control, but I couldn't feel the bed beneath my bum or the carpet beneath my feet. I reached down and felt my legs, but neither my hands or legs acknowledged the touch. I was numb from top to toe.

I said out loud, "Okay, what happens next? Where is my welcoming committee?" I looked around expecting to see those who had preceded me, but nothing. Then regret hit me with, I wish I had, and again I spoke aloud, "My book, I haven't finished my book." Yeah, that was what was foremost in my mind. Strange me. I suspect most people experiencing this will have the 'I wish I had' thought, and nothing focuses the mind like the realisation you've left everything too late.

Then I slowly began to feel the carpet beneath my feet, and when I touched my legs both they and my hands sent the normal signals to my brain, then the fog lifted.

Scary stuff, but it's explainable. It's called sleep paralysis.

It can happen just after falling asleep, or, as with me, when you wake up. Sometimes visual, auditory, and sensory hallucinations can appear as well as a feeling of pressure on the chest, which immediately leads you to think, heart attack.

When we are sleeping, the body is in a relaxed state and the muscles do not normally move, which prevents injury due to acting out dreams, but on awakening with a disruption or fragmentation of the REM (Rapid Eye Movement) sleep cycle, which is the deep state of sleep, this relaxed state is still present, even though you are technically awake. With sleep paralysis, the transition from REM sleep is out of sync with the brain, with the result that full consciousness is there, but the body remains in the paralysed sleep state associated with REM, so even though (on this occasion) I had muscle control to sit up, there was no sensation of weight or touch.

The phenomenon is more likely when a person is under stress, such as just having received a cancer diagnosis.

Sleep paralysis isn't a common side effect of a cancer diagnosis, but I bring it up as knowledge is power, and if it happens and you immediately recognise it and don't panic, you'll thank me.

It has happened a couple of times since, once to a lesser extent, and one where I couldn't even sit up, but knowing what is happening means you can take whatever time necessary for things to right themselves (which they will), without the associated thoughts that you've died.

If you experience sleep paralysis, recognise it for what it is and don't panic.

Roid Rage, Prednisone (Steroids), Mood Swings and Temper Tantrums

In a lot of cancer protocols, prednisone is prescribed as it's effective in autoimmune diseases such as lymphoma.

Prednisone is a type of medicine known as a synthetic glucocorticoid and is a corticosteroid, which shouldn't be confused with the anabolic steroids that bodybuilders use, or more correctly, abuse.

Your consultant will advise when you should take your steroids in conjunction with your other medication, but morning seems to be the recommended time as it reduces the potential for sleep problems.

Used to treat a variety of diseases, the dosage for cancer patients is far above that for most other treatments, which means the potential for side effects is greater, and as it's being taken when the body is weak, it's even more of a problem.

As with all medicine, you should tell your doctor if you experience any symptoms such as a fever, chills, sore throat, ear or sinus pain, a cough, pain passing urine, mouth sores, confusion, excessive thirst, breathlessness, changes in eyesight, black poo, dark vomit, or excessive pain with headaches.

Some of these you will experience anyway, but if they are worse than normal, it's time to seek advice.

Side effects can include:

Insomnia, which means it's harder to sleep when you want. My experience on chemo was exhaustion most of the time, so when I couldn't sleep, I simply did something else until sleep arrived (which usually wasn't long).

Hair growth. This sounds like a good thing when you're on chemo, and especially if you've lost your hair, but it has no effect on chemo patients. Sorry.

Facial swelling or mooning is when your face swells up to resemble a full moon. I had this, and it's hard to explain to everyone how you've lost weight everywhere else and your face contradicts it, but it's not sore and will disappear when you stop taking the steroids. It's not something that happens straight away but develops slowly over time. It's not painful. You just look a bit weird.

Increased appetite. Unfortunately, this doesn't seem to happen so much when you're on chemo and you still have to force yourself to eat.

Night sweats can appear, but if they've already been a symptom of your cancer, they're nowhere near as bad. I didn't experience them when I was on steroids, although other patients mentioned the problem as they thought it was a bad sign.

Acne can appear, but it's not a huge problem.

Headaches are listed but I never experienced them.

Weight gain is also a potential side effect, but if you're on chemo, it generally doesn't happen.

Muscle weakness can slow you down if you allow it, but it's one of those side effects that only win if you let it. You have to force yourself to exercise in some way.

Fluid retention. Your feet and ankles can swell up. I did experience this side effect slightly in my ankles, but it wasn't a problem and cleared up quickly.

Mood swings can and do appear and they can be major. Although mentioned in the warning sheets, there isn't enough detail to prepare yourself for when they appear.

From the list above there was no side effect that gave me any real problems, with the exception of mood swings.

It's usual when visiting your doctor to be stoic, and when asked if you have had any problems with the treatment the answer is usually toned down, but the biggest problem with mood swings is you don't even realise you have a problem. Friends and family will not only notice, but suffer the consequences, and although this can be excused as a side effect of having cancer, it's actually down to the steroids. The problem is you have a free pass, and they don't call you out on it when it happens, so it escalates.

When you don't get a strong enough reaction to a question or comment, sarcasm progresses to cutting remarks designed to hurt: after all, you're the sick one, so why shouldn't everyone have a dose of unhappiness?

I had been on antidepressants earlier in my life due to business stress, so I suppose I was the ideal candidate to suffer mood swings provided by prednisone, and that could excuse it in some people's minds, but it shouldn't be excused.

When you're in the middle of a battle with cancer, your mind is affected, irrespective of the prognosis. Your mind is muddled, prone to negative thoughts, and yes, mood swings; then throw in a drug that exacerbates the problem and it's a recipe for disaster.

Learn from my mistakes. Be aware mood swings are a potential problem, a big problem… a really big problem, and if they appear, own them.

From a family's point of view, this sudden change in demeanour can be tolerated, up to a point; but it can be one of those problems that can break a marriage, or relationship, or friendship, simply through ignorance of the problem.

For me, I think my marriage started to collapse as a result of both mood swings and external pressures. Anyone who knows me will tell you I can be sarcastic, but not in a hurtful way, but, looking back, the biggest arguments I had with my family were when I was on steroids.

Silly little things annoyed me that would have previously gone unnoticed, but when I mentioned them and received no consideration of the magnitude of the problem that didn't even exist, I frequently lost my temper.

I misunderstood their confusion as not taking me seriously, but, of course, there was nothing to take serious in the first place.

It got to the stage where I dealt with it by going into a huff and not speaking, but if I didn't get to that stage, all hell broke loose. Shouting, screaming, breaking things, punching walls, being an asshole, etc.

Violence has never been a part of my life and I'm not prone to physical outbursts. Before cancer, the last fight I was ever in was in the school playground as a kid, but there was one occasion. I wrote the event in my diary. Two big words in capital letters. YOU BASTARD.

This is one of the worst sections I have to write as it will always be a painful memory, and one that could have been avoided if I'd known about the potential, but as I've already said, as the writer, I have an obligation to tell you what you might expect and suggest ways to deal with it or avoid it altogether.

I did have bouts of anger during treatment which were unrelated to the diagnosis, and yes, I broke things, and at one stage my daughter was making a lot of noise and after repeatedly telling her to keep it down, I lost it. As parents, we didn't hit the kids, but I rose from my chair, walked over and thumped her on the arm; only once, but once is one time too many. Her eyes filled with tears and she simply said, "Thanks, Dad."

I think she was shocked more than anything else, and there was no bruise the next day, but below the two words I wrote: I hit my girl. I made her cry. I still have the diary and I still regret it. It's an experience I don't recommend, so pay attention.

Yes, I regretted it immediately and tried my hardest to make up for what I did, and she reassured and said it didn't matter, but it did. It mattered to me. Irrespective of forgiveness and understanding, you'll never forgive yourself if you do something as stupid as I did, or worse. It happened before I even knew it happened, but I still think that given information, I might have removed myself from the situation rather than letting it get out of hand.

I have laid myself bare, and you can judge me how you please. I'm not proud of what I did, and I hope you know that. I'm not happy with it, and if I was you, I would think I was a shit, but it was the only time I ever raised my hand to my daughter.

Had I been given a book that explained the potential for roid rage, then not only would I have been wary of situations that could trigger my temper, but I would have explained everything I'd learnt to my family as well, so they could have calmed the situation in the first place; but nobody tells you.

It's not the doctor's fault as they rely on warnings from the manufacturers, and they don't have the time to explain all the potential side effects that by definition, may or may not happen, and nobody can predict the effect it can have from patient to patient.

Now, cancer doesn't much care who it tries to kill, so it follows that the mild-mannered village vicar might be affected much less than someone who has an aggressive demeanour anyway. Where I lost my temper and struck my daughter once, someone who is aggressive by nature would probably take it a lot further. So, although I'm harping on about being warned and telling the family about its potential, it is something that could save everyone a hell of a lot of trouble.

For anyone previously diagnosed with depression or any other psychiatric disorder, they should be working with a psychologist while on the drug, but regardless of previous mental history, it should be explained to both the patient and carer how mood and temperament can change.

Prednisone can exhibit as euphoria, anxiety, anger, and depression, and the feelings can bounce back and forward in succession without reason.

I reached out to others on treatment while researching this book and asked for comments:

"One minute I was normal and happy, then as if a switch had flicked, I became so sad I wept."

"I hate the steroids; I've been on them with my treatment and it's the worst part of chemo for me."

"My husband is on them and it isn't him anymore. He's so moody, says nasty things and thinks I'm attacking him. At one stage our son had to take him outside to calm down and afterwards neither of us even knew what the argument had been about."

"Steroids are the worst!"

"My husband says it's okay one minute, then he simply walks into a darkness where he can't even stand himself."

I asked for comments, and I received floods of them. It's a problem.

Over caution is advised and silly little arguments can't be tolerated as they get out of control and cause bad feelings, resentment, and hurt for everyone concerned. The phrase, 'you have to be cruel to be kind' is relevant. It's much better to walk away and diffuse the situation.

Logic dictates that you can't hold someone responsible for their behaviour if it was a side effect, but human nature doesn't work like that. Some can forgive, but some can't, and while understanding in advance can help minimise, even then it can be a step too far that ends a previously strong relationship.

Not everyone will experience problems and hopefully you don't; but learn from my mistakes. Rage and temper problems can ruin your life, so it's worth preparing just in case. 'I beat cancer but lost my family', isn't something you ever want to say.

When one person has cancer, the whole family has it as well.

There is nothing worse than surviving cancer and then having to attend the funeral of your relationship.

One of the most important things to remember when someone in the family has cancer is that everybody needs to be on the same page, which probably doesn't mean what you think it means.

For most people—and especially the person with cancer—it means the family must rally around the patient and understand that they are the most important person in the family circle and that anything they need, want, or desire must be provided before anyone else is considered. Because, after all, they're the one with cancer.

This is a recipe for disaster.

When I say everybody on the same page, I mean everyone—including the cancer patient—has to be on the same page as the rest of the family.

The family suffers as well.

The mental pressures and stress and worry relating to the potential outcome is the most extreme pressure most people will ever experience, then throw in financial pressures, and cancer can easily rip a family apart.

Nobody tells you these things, and it's impossible to plan for because—especially when you're the patient—it's understandable that you don't have the capacity to think outside your own problems.

For the family, it's understandable that they don't want to worry the patient, so they can't even talk about it.

I've been there, and I have made the mistakes. They are costly mistakes.

The fact is; the cancer patient can and will take everything into consideration if it's explained clearly and rationally. Empathy isn't a one-way street.

I knew I did it, but I didn't know I did it

As a result of writing this book, I now have a greater understanding of what I went through (and what I put my family through), but I was oblivious for years and didn't know what I had done. But that's not entirely true, for the simple reason, I always kept a diary, and during the writing of Cancerology I referred back to them and discovered that at least every week while I was on treatment I had an argument with my wife, or family, or friend, or neighbour, or someone else. The entries were all similar: I had a fight last night, or I had an argument last night, or I fell out with the wife last night, or I went to bed last night and nobody spoke. On a couple of occasions, I put in what the fight was about, and frequently very minor things had happened that normally wouldn't have annoyed me, but for some reason I kicked off.

The answer to this problem is to be aware it can happen, and that means knowing about it before the fight/argument takes place, and I know I've said it before, but it's worth stressing that the whole family should be made aware of the potential problem and not just the patient. It's not going too far to say that when a cancer patient kicks off, he or she isn't really aware of what is actually happening.

The easiest way to diffuse the situation is to have something in place that everybody understands, so that when a safe word is used (Red Curtain or Black Cloud or Uncomfortable or whatever) or other mechanism deployed (Time out signal, hand over eyes, hands over ears, etc.), both parties realise it's time to take a step back, to stand down and breathe. It's something that needs to be agreed on in advance, and something so strong it can't be ignored, irrespective of the temperament. Promises have to be made that can't be broken. Once triggered, both parties are on time out with the cancer patient being left alone to sort it out themselves, and although it sounds harsh—the poor cancer patient left alone with a muddled mind—I wish I had known about this technique. Given a couple of minutes of thinking about what triggered the safe word or signal can prevent a world of hurt.

It could be something as simple as producing Cancerology and saying read the relevant section, and at that stage remove yourself from the equation; go for a walk, change rooms, go into the garden until everything gets back to normal. Don't get me wrong, this isn't easy to do, but an understanding by all parties that the problem exists in the first place should make it easier to deal with.

It's possible that if I had bothered to read my diary at the time and when I was calm, I might have noticed a pattern and asked for help, but I didn't. Yeah, bloody hindsight is great.

Irrespective of demeanour or potential for problems with attitude, a lot of cancer patients start keeping a diary, some for the first time ever; but it's a good idea for a number of reasons, the main one being you can look back and notice patterns of behaviour, and if you do need to seek help you have a written account of the problems encountered. It's also good to write about when you had a good day, and again, so you can refer back to it and know the good days do exist.

The secret is not just keeping the diary so that years later you can reflect; no, the secret is you review the previous day the next day, the previous week, the previous month; see what you wrote in the cold light of day and modify accordingly or seek help.

Record keeping is only worthwhile if you learn from your mistakes. Write everything down, what happened, your feelings, your interpretation of what others felt… everything, then study and learn. Don't be afraid to share and ask for help understanding.

Being open and willing to learn is a power. Being open and willing to modify your behaviour might save relationships.

I don't think I need tell you, but I messed up big time and ruined lifelong friendships through ignorance, so learn from my mistakes; you don't want to look back and realise you could have easily avoided the problems if only…

Suicide. It's a funny story, well, sort of, but not really

For some extremely strange reason, I have no entry in my diary about one of the most serious events during treatment.

Thankfully, I do have records from my doctor which show that only eight days after the episode with my daughter, I tried to commit suicide and was admitted to hospital. It's referenced with the description: [X] (I've no idea what the 'x' means) Deliberate drug overdose/other poisoning. Opiod – impulsive. Oramorph and Diclofenac. I remember taking the oramorph (oral morphine) and nothing else.

So, a suicide attempt and only once; but let's face it, if you do it right, once is enough, but I didn't (do it right, that is).

I have no memory of why it happened; probably as a result of yet another argument, but I do remember opening the cupboard where the morphine was stored and drinking the remainder of one bottle, then opening a new one and drinking that as well, then I got in the car (and yes, I've often wondered if this was the equivalent of being under the influence, but as it happened immediately, I'm not sure it would qualify, still, you have to wonder) and I drove to a cul-de-sac less than half a mile away, parked, and waited for the inevitable.

I remember being frustrated as I couldn't get a song on the radio that I wanted to die to, but I've no idea what that song might have been, I just remember being annoyed.

Time passed and nothing happened. I didn't feel weird, I kept looking at the time which was going extra slow. I walked around the car a couple of times then ventured further, but when I came back the clock hadn't moved.

Exactly half an hour later, which felt like a day, I was sitting behind the wheel wondering why nothing was happening. I remember feeling weird and deciding that as I hadn't died yet and it didn't now seem likely, I should return home, but… I did realise I shouldn't drive.

Having left the house in a hurry, I hadn't brought a phone, and although I wasn't far from home, I didn't feel like walking, so I looked around, picked a house, and knocked on the door.

The guy looked at me and I burst into tears, then explained I had tried to commit suicide by overdosing as I had cancer, and my wife hated me, and my daughter hated me, and my dog hated me, and my flowers hadn't bloomed, and I had forgot my phone, and I needed to call my wife to tell her I had failed to kill myself and could she come and pick me up.

He let me use the phone, then just as he started to offer some words of wisdom, his wife appeared.

Now, me being in an emotional state and stoned out of my head, I noticed she was pregnant, then I started crying again, then I apologised profusely for bringing trouble to his door and especially as his wife was so heavily pregnant.

"What?" he said.

I pointed to his wife.

He shook his head. "She's not pregnant."

I said, "Oh. Oh, shit. Sorry."

I made a quick exit just as my wife and kids pulled up.

I was taken to hospital, given the once over, admitted overnight and told to bugger off home the next day and not be so silly again.

I have to confess that at the time I again gave no consideration to what I had put my wife and kids through, and it was years later when it came up in conversation I discovered I was seen taking the oramorph, so they knew my intentions when I drove away. I can't tell you how everyone felt on that night when they were driving around looking for me knowing time was ticking, but I think you can imagine that for yourself.

Suicide is selfish, but when you are that low, you don't consider anything.

I can't imagine what it must be like to have a patient you've done everything in your power to keep alive, and then find out they've tried to kill themselves.

But, as with all things in life, it's not that simple.

When I returned for more chemo, I mentioned it and asked if they knew about it. Unsurprisingly, the answer was yes, it was in my notes.

I confess to being embarrassed and we discussed it. One of the phrases used was, "You're not the first and you won't be the last."

It was explained that depression and medication can have all sorts of side-effects, which we have already discussed, but again, which patient is covering up, which patient is struggling, which patient is just about to…? The fact is the only one who can help you, is you.

If you have thoughts about ending your life, don't be a dick, don't bottle it up, don't think you're stronger than everyone else and do not think you're not worth it. Get help, which is easier said than done because when you're thinking about it, you're also thinking nobody can help, but give yourself a break.

Had I been successful, you wouldn't be reading this. I wouldn't have opened a business and employed people. I wouldn't have convinced others to have chemo, and they would probably be dead. There are loads of things I would never have done that I got to do.

"*Suicide is a permanent solution to a temporary problem.*"

People who survived a suicide attempt were interviewed weeks later and most were confused as to how the problem that prompted the attempt even motivated them to consider suicide in the first place.

Now that you know about the potential for suicide, make a promise with yourself that you're special and you have a problem that can be sorted. Give yourself a chance.

If you do have suicidal thoughts, GET HELP. Like… now. Not tomorrow, not the next day, not when you return to hospital, NOW. This second.

Pick up your phone and talk. This is not something you can sort by visiting a website. Call one of the numbers below and tell them how you feel and give them your medical details, then… listen. Just listen. That's all I ask.

UK 116 123

Ireland 116 123 or 1800 247 247

USA 1-800-273-8255

Canada 1.833.456.4566

New Zealand 0508 828 865

Australia 13 11 14

I've listed numbers for (mostly) English speaking countries as it's what this book is written in and where I'm assuming it will be sold, but every country in the world has help available.

If you're somewhere and don't have the number, call the emergency services.

…and if you've done something stupid (like I did), call an ambulance right away. You'll worry about the consequences, and you'll worry about how people will react, but if you're dead, it won't matter, and ultimately, it won't be the problem you assume it will be. Give yourself a break. Take the fucking help.

I have a saying. I didn't come this far, to just come this far.

Adopt it, use it. Don't let me down.

Shingles

Wednesday 24th December 2003

T'was the night before Christmas... and I had shingles.

Without any exaggeration, they are painful.

I had chest pains for a couple of days to start with, then on Sunday morning, at around 4:00am, the pain was unbearable, and of course I immediately thought I was having a heart attack.

The symptoms I had were like someone holding you in a very tight bear hug; one where you couldn't breathe in.

I got up, and at around 6:00am I went to Antrim casualty to get checked. At this stage, I had no visible marks on my body; no itch or anything.

I was diagnosed with muscle spasms, and after extensive investigation which included x-rays and ECG tests, they gave me painkillers and tablets to stop the spasms, and off I went.

On Monday, the pain got worse and small marks started to appear; so late in the afternoon, I decided to pay a visit to Fern House (Chemo Clinic), at Antrim Hospital, with the hope of seeing my consultant, unannounced. I had been warned about the possibility of Shingles by the nurses at Belfast City Hospital after the Stem Cell Transplant. Non-Hodgkin sufferers are very susceptible to Shingles.

Yes… it was shingles. They had developed even more overnight, and I could hardly walk with the chest and back pain.

I was prescribed antibiotics and painkillers, and after being on the medication for two days, I wrote in my diary: Two days of pills and painkillers and I am in a lot less pain; the tablets are working.

After two weeks, the rash had virtually disappeared, although it was still itchy in one area, but the pain had totally vanished.

If shingles is a possibility for your type of cancer or treatment, keep an eye out and if you suspect that it might be starting on you; see your consultant immediately.

Shingles

People on chemotherapy have a 40% increased risk of developing shingles.

Shingles are caused by a viral infection and usually appears on the left-hand side or right-hand side of your torso. It presents as a painful rash of tiny blisters and bubbles.

It's caused by the virus varicella-zoster virus, which is the same virus responsible for chickenpox. If you've suffered chickenpox as a child, the virus lies inactive in nerve tissue near your spinal cord, and years later the virus may reactivate as shingles.

Pain is the first symptom of shingles. It can be very severe or mild with a tingling sensation that feels weird, but you know it will get worse, and this is the time to call your consultant. Not your doctor, either your consultant or your chemo nurse.

The rash can develop quickly and is a delightful collection of little blisters that itch like hell, and when you scratch, they bleed, and you can't lie on your side because of the pain. It's not nice. The good news is that although it is painful, you can get painkillers and depending on your chemo regime, you probably will have oramorph at home, but you still need to get checked.

Shingles are contagious, so if you know anyone suffering, stay away, which also means if you have them, you're contagious as well and can easily pass them on.

If you have a blood cancer such as Hodgkin lymphoma or non-Hodgkin or leukaemia, you have an increased risk of developing shingles.

Best advice I can give is if you feel any unusual pain in your torso, and even if it's not bad, don't wait and see; get it looked at immediately.

Pain rating is 8/10.

Problems afterwards? None.

Make friends with your podiatrist/chiropodist

Podiatrist ~ A person who treats the feet and their ailments.

Which name, you may ask, well, the funny thing is the names are interchangeable, and there's no difference as both describe a foot doctor.

In the UK and Ireland, we use chiropodist, while internationally, it's podiatrist.

They treat infections, bunions, ingrown toenails, heel pain, sports injuries, and any other foot problem.

Not long before this book was published, I went to see a podiatrist because I had an ingrowing toenail that was causing me hassle, and by that, I mean I had tried to cut it and made it worse, so it punctured the nail bed and infection set in.

Within a couple of days, the toe had swollen to twice its normal size, was bright red and painful to touch. I assumed my immune system (the one battered by chemo) would kick in and everything would be okay; after all, it was just a nail, but all through the night my leg was in agony. The following morning, I had black marks going up my leg, so I called the doctor and he said to come straight away. It turned out to be blood poisoning.

I was prescribed a course of antibiotics and given antibiotic cream.

Within a couple of days it got back to normal and I went to see my podiatrist, who told me cancer patients nails change after chemotherapy, and one of the problems is they curl in at the edges, which gives you an ingrown toenail.

So it's worthwhile making friends with your podiatrist and occasionally getting checked just to make sure everything is okay. You can develop little ridges on the nails, which are not the same as the ones you develop on your fingernails during chemo but are long term side effects. They're not painful, and you can only really see them if you're told about them beforehand, but they are different.

Pay attention to your nails, and if you notice curling of the nail on the bed, get it checked, as the infection I had could have developed into something serious if not treated.

The good news is that if your nails do start to curl, they are straightforward to fix. No injections required. You just sit in the chair and the podiatrist trims them back into shape.

"*Just because your pain is understandable, doesn't mean your behaviour is acceptable.*" ~ Dr Steve Maraboli

Gaslighting

If things get really out of control, something strange can happen, and it's called gaslighting, and while I agree the term isn't strictly appropriate in the circumstances, it takes the carer to the same destination.

It is defined as; 'the manipulation of another by psychological means into doubting their sanity.'

Personally, I disagree with the idea of the goal of making someone doubt their sanity in these circumstances, as the ultimate goal from the perpetrator's point of view is to hurt and punish the carer for the fact they don't have cancer and lead a normal life. Life is unfair, and the only ones available to take it out on are often those closest. We always hurt the ones we love.

Male, female, young, old; it doesn't matter, and the worst thing is you may not even be aware you're doing it.

You keep pushing the boundaries with statements like, 'you would be better off without me,' or 'it would be better for you if I were dead,' in an effort to completely control the carer, make them feel guilty, punish them for being healthy. Slight hints at first, but the more tolerance, the more you push, until finally, you can't think of a way to go any further. The ultimate destination is arrived at when suicide threats/attempts appear in the equation.

I remember once when my wife arrived home from work, I was sitting on the couch with a bowl of pills. Looking back, I was a complete asshole, but… at the time, it made some sort of convoluted sense. Did I have any intention of swallowing any of the pills? Well, from what I can remember and from my diary, I'd had a shit day, that wasn't really a shit day, just another day doing nothing, so, somehow, in my fucked up mind, I decided to wait until she came home and start swallowing them as fast as I could. Now, looking back at it from 2021, I have to ask why? Why wait, Lawrence? Where's the benefit waiting until your wife came home? Did you really intend to swallow the pills, or were you just doing it to torture? I suspect I could excuse it as a cry for help, or blame it on steroids, or… Ultimately, I have no excuse and I don't really know why I thought it was a good idea. I don't think I intended to swallow anything, and when she lifted the bowl, I didn't try to stop her. I didn't feel anger, or relief: I just sat there, numb. Yeah, it sounds weird, but yet again, consider how my wife felt. I didn't, because I had cancer and she didn't? Because I had cancer and the world sucked? Because… Honestly, I've no idea, but if she had had cancer and I came home to find her sitting with a bowl of pills, I would wonder if she loved me; which I've only just realised writing this years later.

The problem is that when going through cancer, you have so many thoughts that objective self-analysis isn't possible, and even if you do realise you're pushing your carer away, you're too embarrassed to ask for help from a doctor or other professional, as you know—without researching or asking—that every other cancer patient is doing the same thing; they must be, you can't be the only one, can you? The patient is too wrapped up in matters of day-to-day survival to consider the consequences of their comments, and as it's generally only when the control escalates that it becomes a problem, it's a lot harder—if not impossible—to sort out.

If you haven't heard the term or even considered this behaviour a possibility, please don't think you're immune.

It's doubtful if I would have been in a frame of mind to listen to advice when my worst episodes occurred, but I do know that given the information before things got out of hand would have made me stop and think. Knowledge is power, and knowing about a potential problem before it occurs can allow you to watch out for the signs and reign yourself back before saying anything that starts you on the road to trying to control your carer.

Over time, the patient's thought process bends as they go to higher levels in an attempt to achieve their goal, and the problem is the goal also moves every time it looks like it may be achieved. The fact is there is seldom a specific goal to accomplish in the first place. It's an idea in the mind of the patient that even they don't understand.

Patients, who have never lied before, start to tell blatant lies, and even though both parties know it's a lie, it's used to set up a precedent where nothing they say can be trusted. It's a method of keeping someone unsteady and confused. They will say things they later deny, which also makes the target question their reality, and even though they know what really happened, doubt sets in which is accompanied by frustration, anger, and general upset at why they find themselves being treated this way when their sole target is to simply help the patient.

Over time, as the limits are tested and boundaries moved, it becomes tiring. It starts to wear the recipient down, which can ultimately change the dynamic between patient and carer so much that the carer ends up needing professional help to explain what they are experiencing.

Every now and then, and without any notice or expectation, the patient will say something positive to the carer, but the sole aim is to confuse. They praise you, you drop your guard, and the next comment has even more negative impact when they revert, as they've previously praised. All this sounds very premeditated, but from my experience, it's just done on the spot, no planning to praise or pre-planned comment to follow with any expected outcome, and that's where it's so hard to follow professional opinion on gaslighting as they argue a plan has been in place all along, but no, it's just something that starts and escalates and gets out of control. It becomes the norm, and to a degree is accepted by both parties; until it isn't.

Carers need to be aware that occasional treatment can influence a patient's mind, and a temporary change in attitude can appear immediately afterwards, which can be excused, but, if allowed to get out of control, it moves from a temporary state to the norm, which is when it becomes necessary to get help.

The biggest problem is that (mostly) the behaviour is a slow process that increases over time without the knowledge of the perpetrator, but the results can be disastrous.

People in the ugly category aren't in the ideal position as the long-term outlook is the possibility of eventual death, but it's better than being in the bad category; however, because it's a rest-of-life state, the chances of gaslighting over time can build.

It's only normal that at times circumstances overwhelm and the 'why me' question appears, but you need to realise it's not your fault and, more importantly, it's not the fault of any other person.

If you reflect on something you shouldn't have said, you should make a point of apologising as soon as possible, and work out a way to deal with future potential problems. A solution might be something as simple as a code word where the carer uses it and you both stop talking for a minute and think things through, and if silence isn't possible, the carer should remove themselves from the situation until things have calmed down.

When someone refuses to talk to you, it's generally acknowledged something has been said that has gone beyond what is acceptable, and given time to reflect and thinking about how it was received will guide you to avoid repetition and escalation.

It's also worth remembering that not everyone will have problems with a chronic diagnosis. For most people, the fact they keep surviving motivates them on towards better things, with no issues.

If cancer becomes a way of life, you have to accept it for what it is and get on with it. Make realistic plans that won't cause problems if you are sick and don't just look at everything from your point of view without considering what others are having to sacrifice to help you on your journey.

It's the drugs

While we all accept our bodies renew themselves every seven to ten years, we don't seem to accept that our personality and intelligence is also changing, renewing, and improving.

90% of the atoms in the body are replaced yearly, yet the perception is the brain occasionally works well and never improves, which isn't the case.

Every morning you wake up is a new you, depending on the experiences of the previous day.

In the example above, where I went completely off the rails, this can happen to anyone on chemo when pressures and medication screw with our reality and expectations, our hopes and dreams…and especially our perceptions.

Before diagnosis I was a different person. During treatment I was a different person. After treatment I'm a different person. Everything changes, depending on circumstances.

Mild Mildred can quickly turn into Mad Mildred if something triggers it, and although Mild Mildred is still inside, Mad Mildred has taken control to prove just how messed up your thinking process is. So in a way, it's probably a bit like possession.

The person you were before a cancer diagnosis doesn't exist anymore (temporarily), and the person in the middle of treatment doesn't exist after treatment has finished and the drugs are out of the system.

In everyday life, people fluctuate between mind states. The shy kid at school who is now a politician, actor, musician, etc. An introvert who is now an extrovert. A negative person can change into a positive person. We all change naturally throughout life, but a cancer diagnosis isn't natural. An Estimated Date of Demise isn't natural. Chemotherapy isn't natural. Having your hair fall out isn't natural.

When something like cancer hits and throws a lifetime of experiences at you in one week, the brain scrambles to catch up. It's no wonder people go off the rails.

If someone had told me I'd try to commit suicide by overdosing on morphine, I'd have told them they were nuts; same with a bowl of pills. Just not possible before cancer, but…

And this is where Cancerology comes into a league of its own, because although doctors and pharmaceutical companies will give you leaflets and explain a potential side effect, nobody will tell you about the potential for this sort of nonsense because it's not caused by a single drug.

Most drug regimens are usually made up of 3+ drugs (RCHOP is 5), so it's a mixture of all the side effects combined, plus the mental pressure as a result of the diagnosis, and the treatment, and the potential for a bad outcome, and financial pressure, and family pressure, and... You and your entire family are living in a pressure cooker.

Let's say you're on five drugs.

Drug 1 will make your face turn red.

Drug 2 will make your face turn blue.

Drug 3 will make your face turn yellow.

Drug 4 will make your face develop vertical stripes.

Drug 5 will make your face develop horizontal stripes.

Take one, and you know what to expect, but put them together and what have you got? It ain't bibbidi-bobbidi-boo. It's completely unknown as each person will react differently.

For example, what happens to a person on two drugs: one with constipation as a side effect and the other with diarrhoea?

Is one more likely than the other? The answer is, we don't know.

The surprising thing is, if the person only reads one leaflet, the chances are very high that they will experience that side effect, because it's what they expect.

But if the person reads both leaflets and assumes one will cancel out the other, then, to a degree, that's what will probably happen.

Most doctors are unaware of the extremes because most people never own up when something happens. I have spoken to other cancer patients, and the most frequent response I received was, "I thought it was just me."

'Jekyll and Hyde' was another frequent description.

Can you imagine a warning leaflet saying, 'As a result of being on this regimen, you may turn into a complete fucking headcase?' Who's gonna want that?

But the thing is, if you know the potential is there, you can—to a certain extent—take back some control if the occasion arises.

But even better, if the carer/family is on the same page, they can watch out for anything untoward, and then you guys talk it through (or they call for help). Either way, as long as it's being dealt with before it gets out of hand, it's a win.

Imagine a guy waking up with somebody at the bottom of his bed who says, "Today, you're going to be exceptionally sick, your hair's gonna fall out, you're going to be tired and lethargic and mixed up, and at nine o'clock tonight you're going to die.

I think we can all relate to the thought process of the person hearing that news, but it's the same news a cancer patient receives at the start of treatment. Different timeline, but basically, the same.

The guy in the bed, you can forgive because you know that if it were you, you'd go a bit nuts. But... it is you and every other cancer patient.

Everyone I talked to who had experienced extreme behaviour said they did things they didn't even think they would be capable of; they woke up the next day wondering what the hell happened.

The big surprise came when I said to one of them, "What did the doctor say when you told him?"

She said, "Oh God, no, I didn't tell the doctor."

I said, "Don't you think you should?"

And then it hit me: I didn't tell my doctor.

"Hey, Doc, you're never gonna believe what happened yesterday. I was sitting on a couch with a bowl of pills ready to commit suicide and I wanted my wife to watch me eat them."

I didn't tell that.

That would be embarrassing.

I think it's fair to say at some stage, everyone screws up, and that also applies to family members and the carer.

I wrote this and thought, *honestly, do I really want people reading this when I wouldn't even tell my doctor*, but I decided there wasn't a choice. So irrespective of how embarrassing it is to admit, it's essential I do tell you, so you can avoid it.

In the same way the body renews itself, my mind, understanding, demeanour, outlook, etc., have all changed for the better, but it's a process that takes time.

And then, one day, it's all over.

No. Duhhh. Not like that. I'm talking about the treatment.

The journey was long and hard but now you're out the other side and life is tickety-boo; except it's not.

After months of everyone coming to see you and doing things for you, it gradually stops, and all of a sudden, it's as if you're not special anymore.

When this happens (and it will), be thankful. Let everyone get on with their lives.

Survivor's Guilt

Through my cancer journey I have met other sufferers who have been worse than me and survived, I've also met numerous others who had a much better prognosis and they died. Why?

You may have occasionally thought, 'why me?', when you were given the diagnosis, and now, in a different context, it's being asked again.

After you've finished chemo and been given the all-clear, you have time to worry about other things, and considering you've spent months worrying about yourself, you need something to occupy your mind, so you start wondering about your success.

'Why did I survive?'

Unfortunately, I can't answer this with any startlingly illuminating statement, except to say that some things are just meant to be. But you also know you met it head on and fought, so is it really a surprise?

Hopefully, this book has strengthened your fight attitude; so, if you expect the best, are determined, and you do everything in your power to work towards the best outcome, you have nothing to be guilty about.

But… Yeah, it’s still going to be there to some degree, so you end up with some guilt and all this experience fighting cancer. Now, could it be that the way to lessen your guilt would be to help others? Just a thought, but you already know just how motivating it can be when you meet other survivors.

On my journey through treatment, I met a schoolteacher who had just met the man of her dreams and had plans for the rest of her life, but she died. I also met a guy who had been involved with the paramilitaries in Northern Ireland and had been what people would consider a horrible man, yet he survived.

There is no good reason why. It just is.

But it’s all good afterwards, right?

I know loads of people who have been through cancer, come out the other side, and they give a little cheer, “Yee-ha, I’m cured.”

Then the phone rings: “Is that you Lawrence? I’m depressed. I don’t know what’s wrong with me. I mean, I should be on top of the world because...”

It’s the expectation that once treatment finishes and you get the all clear, the world suddenly turns tickety-boo on the very day you get the news. No more hospital, no more injections, no more chemo, no more sickness, no more tiredness, no more clouds in the sky; it’s back to better-than-normal. Yeehaa.

Well... unfortunately, life isn’t like that after treatment, much as we’d like it to be, because, although you beat cancer and expect to feel on top of the world, your body is still paying the price and will continue to do so for quite a while.

When the expectation is unrealistic and you can’t achieve it, you get depressed because you feel you’re not good enough.

The secret to coming out the other side of cancer is to take it easy. I have a friend who was fat but lost it all when he started jogging, then he took cancer, but thanks to the determination that helped him lose all the weight, he beat the cancer and life returned to normal; only it didn’t.

He called and we met, and the conversation went something like this.

Him: "I met an old friend when I was jogging and I couldn't keep up. He called me an old man and told me to push myself."

Me: "And you were pushing yourself?"

Him: "Yeah, I was trying as hard as I could."

Me: "So he made you feel bad?"

Him: "Yeah, really bad. I can't seem to get it back."

Me: "Well, we discussed this. It's going to take time to get your fitness back, but it will come back if you persevere. The next time you're out and meet your friend, stop, have a chat and in the conversation say you're stronger than you hope they'll ever need to be. Word it like that and make sure to include the word hope. Make them ask why."

He looked at me confused.

Me: "Ask him if he's had stage three cancer and had a bit of his lung removed. I'm assuming he probably doesn't know you've had cancer?"

Him: "No."

Me: "Don't you think his attitude would be different if he did?"

Him: "Well, yeah, but I don't want to use it as an excuse."

Me: "Then you say; meet me here in a year when you've had part of your lung removed and had chemo and your hair fall out and you've had depression and no energy and had all the hassle that goes with cancer and you're putting your life back together and see if you can beat me then, because others with the same disease as me didn't even make it through to the race."

Him: "Really?"

Me: "Or... you could just forgive your body, forgive him, mention cancer in passing and move on?"

Him: "So, I just take it easy?"

Me: "In every realistic way. Keep pushing and it'll happen, but in its own time. If you think about it, you're the only person on the planet jogging that trail after having had part of your lung chopped off. How special are you?"

His face lit up in a smile.

I didn't tell him to realise what he'd been through, I told him to tell his friend what he'd been through and in doing so it made him realise the extent of his experience. We tend to take cancer one day at a time during treatment, which is what I recommend, but that means that once it's all over we don't realise just how hard it has really been. It's like, yesterday was okay, so everything that went before is forgotten. It's a good thing in some ways as it's a coping mechanism, and in some ways not so much.

You're not going to magically transform into superman/woman after treatment, but in reality, that's what you are, only you can't see it yet. You're in a league way above mere mortals who live day-to-day without problems, and once you accept that, you are gifted your superpower.

"*When they said, chemo will be hard. I said, Good, bring it on.*"
~ Lawrence Wray

Cancer number 3

Cancer was becoming a habit of mine as it returned for the third time.

My consultant suggested a stem cell transplant, which was described as bringing out the big guns, and if this doesn't fix it, nothing will.

Yipee. Why didn't we do this at the start?

It's very similar to every other type of chemotherapy I'd experienced prior, except that this one would be the highest dose it was possible (theoretically) to survive, which meant I had to stay in hospital for an extended stay in a little room with positive air pressure.

The air is filtered and pumped in under pressure so that if anybody opens the door, airborne germs can't get in as the air already inside rushes out to be replaced by more filtered air.

Before they were allowed in, visitors had to wash their hands and put on a mask, apron, and gloves.

Stem cell treatment is boring. Other than the routine check-ups, you're on your own.

The actual process is not that much different to any other type of chemo. They pump it in, then wait, and if you don't die, they infuse you with your stem cells, then it's a waiting game.

My transplant was an autologous stem cell transplant, which means it was my own stem cells instead of ones from a donor. The big advantage of using your own cells is there is no chance of rejection. (graft vs host disease, where the body rejects the transplant)

A transplant from a donor is called an allogeneic stem cell transplant, which risks the body rejecting the new cells.

Once the new cells have been transplanted, it's just a matter of waiting until they repopulate the body before they can release you.

It's been described as similar to rebooting a computer. They switch you off and completely kill your immune system, then bring you back to life again, and that's why it's high risk.

As I've said in another part of this book, four of us went in; only two survived. It is a tough regime.

But the two who died were convinced before they started, it wasn't something they expected to finish.

The biggest problem I had was a lack of concentration; it would drive you up the walls—if you had the power to climb the damn things.

It's boring.

However, unlike the two previous treatments, I was eventually sick. Big healthy gut-wrenching heaves that tore at my insides.

After going through CHOP and never being sick, and going through ESHAP and never being sick, stem cell kicked my ass.

But the first time it happened, my first thought was, great, something is finally working.

I didn't complain about it. I welcomed it

My biggest problem was infections in my Hickman line. Once I got one cured, I got another. I never had an infection with my PICC line, but with my Hickman line, ooh yeah, it went all out to be a nuisance.

All told. I was in a couple of days short of three months.

It did take a long time.

Stem cell transplant has a very high success rate, but unfortunately, I wasn't included in that statistic, and my cancer returned for a fourth visit.

Would I recommend a transplant? Absolutely. Yes.

Pain rating: I'm going to go with 0/10

Frustration rating: Has to be 11/10 Avoid.

Femoral Line

Nearer the time of the Stem Cell Transplant—and providing you are eligible for an autologous transplant (cells or tissue obtained from the same individual), you will need to have your stem cells harvested and frozen for use later. This is done by inserting a femoral line/catheter into your groin area.

It's nothing to worry about and the procedure is painless.

A femoral line needs to be in place prior to your stem cell collection in order to ensure sufficient blood flow to carry out the procedure.

A femoral catheter has two tubes leading into one, placed into your femoral vein, which is located in your groin.

The procedure usually takes around twenty minutes and should not be painful as the area is well frozen with a local anaesthetic. Complications are rare, but as with any surgical procedure, a certain element of risk is involved, which will be discussed with your doctor/nurse prior to the procedure.

Once in place, the catheter will be well secured with a waterproof dressing. It will remain in place until your stem cell collections are completed. (usually 2-3 days)

As you will be going home each day with the femoral catheter in place, it is important that you:

Keep the area dry - No baths or showers while the catheter is in place.

No strenuous exercise.

Avoid periods of prolonged standing.

Driving is not advisable while the catheter is in place, although I did it without any problem, but the risk is the line can come out due to excessive leg movement.

In the unlikely event of the catheter falling out whilst you are at home, it is important you are aware of the necessary first aid measures that should be taken.

Press firmly on the area of the bleeding.

Lie down and maintain pressure until the bleeding stops and for a further ten minutes.

Remain lying down for a further hour.

Contact the hospital for further advice.

If your femoral line falls out and you are unable to stop the bleeding by pressing firmly, you will need to call an ambulance rather than trying to contact the hospital.

To extract the stem cells, you will be connected to a cell separator machine, which is basically a pump that filters the stem cells out of your blood and stores them in a plastic bag for freezing.

When the stem cell collections are completed (which took three sessions for me), the nurse will remove the femoral catheter and a pressure dressing will be applied to the site. You will be required to remain lying for one hour after the catheter is removed. The dressing can be removed the following day.

All in all, it's a painless procedure, except of course for the initial jab to freeze the area, but having gone through all the chemo, we won't worry about that, will we?

Pain rating is 0/10.

Problems afterwards? None

Hickman Line

A Hickman Line is similar to a PICC line, but it's more direct and has greater capacity. I had mine fitted before starting my Stem Cell Transplant.

The procedure starts in the morning with a lot of x-rays of the neck before anything happens, and once a vein has been confirmed as suitable, the line can be fitted.

At approximately 2.00pm I was given antibiotics before going to get the line fitted. I was wheeled into an operating theatre and transferred from my bed to a table, X-rayed for the final time, then the area was anesthetised, and they made their incisions and inserted the wire (which precedes the line). Everything was going okay until they started pushing and shoving in order to get the line in. I am assured this is quite normal, but the procedure can be harder to complete if you have muscles around the area. I didn't think I had any muscles left, but I must have had as the process became very uncomfortable. Not excessively painful, apart from the odd nip, but uncomfortable sums it up adequately.

My head was covered with green paper, which was made into a sort of tent that was open behind my head and the radiologist was having a chat with me. After a couple of grimaces, she asked me if I wanted further sedation. I indicated it would be most welcome, and unfortunately, that's all I remember. I woke up around 5.00pm with a headache, and a slight pain in my neck. The nurses got me headache tablets and said the pain would reduce before the end of the night.

I felt a lot better quickly and at around 8.00pm everything was back to normal.

The line was in continual use and was not a problem, except for the odd infection.

The two lumens (two input lines with connectors), hang outside the upper chest wall and are used to connect to the saline and chemotherapy drip bags. You have to be careful not to pull or wet the line, but other than that, there's nothing to watch out for.

Pain rating is 2ish/10.

Problems afterwards? For me, I had frequent infections, but they were manageable.

Taking the line out again can either be a very straightforward or quite difficult process, and I know what you're thinking, but for once, I had the latter. I sailed through everything else, and right at the end, this final process turned out tricky.

The usual and expected method is simply to apply a gentle pulling pressure and out it comes, but mine took a lot of pulling, which ended up with a small incision being made to finally release it.

The area was completely frozen anyway, so I didn't feel anything, it just took a lot longer than expected. I received four stitches in the incision, and that was that.

Pain rating is 0/10.

Problems afterwards? None

Sleeping tablets

It was during my stem cell transplant I was first given sleeping tablets. I had had sleepless nights previously on the other two treatments, but it was simply a matter of waiting or doing something else until sleep arrived, but stem cell transplant is different; I couldn't sleep at all. I could close my eyes, but only minutes later, I was awake, and it was frustrating, or to put it another way, it was driving me up the walls.

One of the nurses suggested a sleeping tablet, and although reluctant to try anything I may become addicted to, I gave in. I asked how long it would take to work. She said, "Give it 20-30 minutes max, and you'll be out for at least eight hours."

Sounds good. Give me one. Four hours later, I was tossing and turning, expecting sleep that never arrived. Instead, I stayed awake all night with a sleeping tablet in me. It didn't affect me. Was it the chemotherapy? Was it me? For whatever reason, it didn't work. But of course, later on that day when people came to visit, I was nodding off in the middle of conversations. The minute they left, I woke up again; the minute another visitor arrived, I fell asleep. It could have been they were boring me to sleep, but no, I think it was down to the sleeping tablets.

That night we tried again with yet another sleeping tablet; definitely 30 minutes this time, a guaranteed eight hours solid. No problem.

It was a repeat of the previous day. It didn't work.

Third day, I refused. I couldn't go through that again.

That night I didn't have much success with sleep either, but what changed was that I didn't have the same problem during the day. When people visited, I could stay awake, but I did have a snooze when they left. That night, as expected, no sleep, because I think in my mind I expected it, so I thought to myself, if you can't sleep, you can dream, and although you can't dream while you're awake, you can meditate. I went to my happy place as if I was in a scanner, and I found that if you really get into it, it turns into a dream; yes, as in sleeping.

I had already arranged with the nurses to check and see if I was asleep when they did their rounds. The following night when the nurse came back on duty, I asked her, and she said from three o'clock, you were in the land of nod, and that was the last time I ever took a sleeping tablet.

Again, it's one of those things in cancer. You can take control, rather than the expectation of not being able to fall asleep based on one night's bad experience. It's back to the tomorrow will be better idea.

I'm not going to say I never had another night where I couldn't sleep, but I always managed to fall asleep after going skiing, or scuba diving, or water skiing, or climbing up the Cave Hill with somebody interesting (Rocky or Jack Reacher or Hannibal Lecter).

I always wind up with a friend I've never met, and we always talk about something interesting; sometimes they were asking me about treatment, sometimes I was asking them about their films or gigs or whatever, depending on who they were, but eventually, I always fell asleep.

Just because you're stoic, doesn't mean you're strong

Stoic - a person who can endure pain or hardship without showing their feelings or complaining.

During all my treatment this word sums me up nicely. I was polite, never complained, and when asked if I was all right, I always confirmed I was, and this even went on during stem-cell transplant when the expectation was my demise by virtually all the doctors as a) I was on my third diagnosis b) I was very weak and c) the cancer was advanced. On top of this, John (not his real name and who I told you about earlier in twenty three) had died exactly seven days into treatment, so realistically, what chance did I have? But this thought only appeared now and again, and when it did, I told it firmly to please go, or more precisely I told it to fuck right off. But, sneaky little turd that it was, it kept niggling.

I'm sure you've seen medical dramas on TV where a doctor will say, "Keep the patient on 45 minute obs (observations) and let me know if there's any change." Well, all patients on stem-cell transplant are checked like clockwork (literally), so I expected my visit. The nurse checked my temperature, blood pressure, pulse, stats, etc., and made the relevant notes on the clipboard at the bottom of the bed. Of course, they aren't as clinical as that and always have a chat to see how you feel, how you're coping, how… We chatted for 5-10 minutes and she left, which was when the damned thought appeared again.

Dude, what chance do you have? I mean really? This is cancer number three and you're weak and you're old and you're ugly and...

I burst into tears, which is what you tend to do anyway when you're on chemo and feeling sorry for yourself, and, by the way, there's nothing wrong with the occasional doubt or need to console yourself. It's all good.

Anyway, I'm sitting on the edge of the bed bawling like a baby when the door opens, and the nurse returns and says, "Did I leave my pen here?"

Now, call me jaded, or call the nurse clever, or suspicious, or say it was just one of those things, but whatever, I was caught. Yeah, this seems to be a theme for me.

When the tears are flowing it's hard to talk, and the more you try, the more determined the tears are to stop you.

She sat beside me, threw her arm over my shoulder and held me tight. (That's what nurses do. They shine)

When I could eventually talk, I said *it* just hit me and had been niggling me every now and again, but not to worry.

But she did, and she called another nurse to finish her round and sat with me explaining how it would have been unusual if I hadn't cried.

I asked if she came back to catch me out and received a shrug and a smile.

We talked for a good half-hour and I realised that although crying is healthy, being stoic all the time and bottling everything up is neither expected nor healthy.

I never thought I knew better than the doctors, but I did hide stuff occasionally and tell the odd fib, but knowledge is power and with experience I can confirm that if I had to do it again—and with hindsight—I would have been a lot more open about how I felt and what was happening to me.

When I did get help and knew I wasn't the only one, it was a weight off my shoulders, and although the thought did return (frequently), it never affected me as much as previously.

Counselling - A waste of time?

All the way through CHOPS and ESHAP, I didn't need counselling, so why should stem cell transplant be any different? I had already extensively read books on lymphoma and studied all the web sites, so what could a counsellor tell me that I didn't already know?

The answer is lots.

During the stem cell transplant, I lost all interest in my computer, TV, newspapers, even reading books. I couldn't concentrate and seemed to get my time in by snoozing, or more often just looking at the wall. Now, after a while, looking at the wall is going to drive you nuts, especially when you're in a small room on your own, and that's what happened to me.

My wife suggested I talk to a counsellor and I said I would give anything a go, so we asked the nurses to arrange it and waited to see what happened.

The Ulster Cancer Foundation had a counsellor who worked full time from the hospital, and she came to visit me. Her name was Ruth Potts, and we just sat and talked; but she took in everything I said, analysed it, and found little problems I didn't even know I had. She started explaining what I was feeling and why, and suggested ways I could improve my lot without having to do too much. We had a couple of sessions, and each time I felt much better after talking to her, and after taking her advice things became a lot easier. There was nothing I couldn't talk to her about, it was fantastic.

You're probably wondering just what she said that made such a big difference. The fact is, she said so much, and took time to explain what my mind was interpreting and how that influenced my mood, etc. (Everyone is different, but this book touches on all the things we discussed, so all you have to do is look out for the problems I have highlighted, and if they appear, recognise them for what they are and read the relevant section again, and maybe even get someone else to read it as well, so everyone is on the same page.) At times I suspect she had to repeat things to me over and over, but she took her time and accepted my condition, and all that helped immensely, but the biggest thing was something as simple as explaining how my attention span was considerably reduced, and how trying to read as much as I used to simply wasn't possible, which frustrated and tormented; instead she recommended taking little bites at watching TV for a target of say five minutes instead of an entire program, then five more reading, five more at a crossword, then back to the TV. Constant small distractions that I could give attention to for a short time without getting frustrated. There were times when I would have gladly jumped out the window to end the mental torment, but this very simple method made a huge difference, and that's what counselling does—it doesn't have to be a huge revelation that startles, it can be something very minor that sorts a major problem.

That's the funny thing with cancer; it's a major problem, and treatment comes with its own set of problems that always present as major because of your mindset and lack of experience, which is where I was. Although there can be problems that require medical/specialist intervention; a lot of the time it's minor problems that appear as major, so try to stand back and rationalise before jumping to conclusions or making decisions.

For what it's worth, my suggestion is make friends with your counsellor right at the start of any cancer treatment and talk things through. It was the best thing I ever did. It's something I should have done from the very first treatment, but nobody told me. It's why I'm here and it's why she's so important.

I'm sure there are others, but the two names I've seen most often in Northern Ireland are the Ulster Cancer Foundation (now Cancer Focus NI), and the Macmillan Cancer Nurses. Worldwide there are other charities that provide counselling for a range of cancers, and also those that provide for specific cancers. The American Cancer Society in America, and The Canadian Cancer Society in Canada are two I've heard great things about in the various forums, but all you have to do is ask your cancer nurse for recommendations.

My friend, Ruth, is the reason you're reading this, and unfortunately, she died of cancer shortly after we met. For years I had done balloons for the Ulster Cancer Foundation, and I met her every year at the Pink Ribbon events they organised, and then one year she simply wasn't there. I turned up as usual and when I was told, I cried. Her cancer had spread and took her. Without her input, I suspect I would have died as well. Something as stupid as simply talking to someone can have such an impact, yet we resist it. It's a sign of weakness.

Listening is a sign of intelligence.

Using available resources is intelligent.

You fool yourself with phrases such as:

It's a failure to ask for help.

I'm strong, I don't need it.

I'm being silly for no reason, I'll sort it.

There are loads more, but the fact is this is the hardest thing you'll ever encounter. I made all the excuses because I knew better and I was strong; I was an idiot.

My advice is good, but the advice you'll receive from people who are involved in your everyday care is way greater; listen to them. Take advice from other sufferers. Take advice from your carers, nurse, and doctors. Take advantage of their positivity and experience. Take advantage of your own positivity. Take advantage of my positivity. Move it forward in your own mind.

Just a little wind

What is that smell?

Cancer being the fun guy it is, likes to play silly games, and one of the games—or should I say tricks—was when I had my stem cell transplant and was at my weakest as I'd just had the high dose chemotherapy to kill everything, basically unplug me and turn me back on again like a computer reboot. I felt bloated, but I knew that as I had been to the loo a couple of times already, I was empty, there was nothing that I could, you know, produce. There was no accident waiting to happen as it was just air, so I thought, *okay, there's nobody here. I'm in a positive pressure room so immediately all the smell will leave. I can't go wrong. Hey, I'm in a win-win situation.*

So, I let out a fart. It was a big fart, and as expected, there was no poo. But water? Liquid? Poowater? Yes, copious amounts of liquid came out. And it came out so quick and so forcefully—I mean, I was able to stop once I realised, but by that stage it was already way too late.

I had been lying on my side and thankfully had my pyjamas on, otherwise I suspect the wall would have been redecorated.

I'm lying on the bed with a dirty nappy, except I wasn't wearing a nappy, no, that was the job of the sheet.

At age 44, what do you do? And the worst part of it, of course, isn't the fact you've done it. The worst part is, you've got to own up to it. Excuse me, sir. I think I've shit myself.

I managed to get out of bed and avoid dripping on the floor by using the sheet, then slowly clean myself in the little ensuite. Then I had the unenviable task of contacting a member of the hospital staff to say, "Hey, guys, you never believe what I just did."

I waited, and I waited, and I waited some more until a nurse came and I said can you give me five minutes, and then another nurse came, and I asked for another five minutes, then eventually a male nurse came. Yes, people, I'm that age where I preferred to have a male nurse see my attempt at a Rorschach picture in shitwater on my bed. (Rorshach pictures are those inkblots you're supposed to make sense of.) A female nurse wasn't something I could have handled at that stage. The word embarrassed doesn't start to describe the feeling you have when at that age, you have messed the bed. I knew my face went red, because I thought I was going to pass out with the heat.

He quickly had it sorted and assured me that virtually all the patients at some time or another had the same experience and the same embarrassment as me, and it was nothing to be embarrassed about.

I already considered my body to be nothing more than a biomechanical device to be inhabited and knew it can occasionally let you down, but wow, this was a big one.

Sometimes we can't control what the body does. For example, when you're on a night out and you've drank too much alcohol and you throw up, you can't control it, you can't stop and say to your body, "look, hang on, this is rather inconvenient, can we do this later?"

When you're on chemo and your body is weak, it's a recipe for disaster, and at times you have no control over what happens.

Unfortunately, analysing this situation, I did of course have the option to get up with a belt and braces approach, go to the loo, sit down and fart there, and I bet you any money had I done that, all that would have happened was a fart, because that's Murphy's Law, isn't it, or Sod's Law, or Cole's Law? Whatever. The one time you take a gamble it bites you in the ass. This whole section seems to have been about my ass, but there you go.

So, it's a very strong possibility that at some stage—whether you're at home or in hospital—you will have an accident. If it's in the hospital, they have plastic sheets below the bed sheets, so it doesn't matter too much, but be prepared in case it does happen. You can buy plastic under sheets very cheap from Amazon or Ebay and put one under your bedsheet, and if the worst comes to the worst and it happens, for example, in the middle of the night, it's an easy clean. Take the sheet off, give the plastic sheet a wipe with a moist tissue and dump the sheet or wash it next day. It's not the most pleasant thing to do, but compared to having to replace a complete mattress, it's a lifesaver.

I know it's not a nice thing to either think about or discuss, but it can happen so easily. I hope it doesn't happen to you, but if it does, you're not the first. Yes, it's a first for you, but give yourself a break, your insides aren't normal, your body isn't normal, hell, even your brain is messed up, so be aware of the possibility and if it happens, shrug and sort it, and if anyone says anything, don't take any shit. (sorry, couldn't help myself)

Did I get caught out again? No, but… I did use the loo, just in case, and several times when I was sure I was wasting my time, it turned out I wasn't and had I gambled, I would have lost.

Friday 9th July 2004

I had another PET scan, just to make sure everything was okay, it was just a routine check-up after the stem cell transplant and I felt fit and well, so no worries. (or so I thought)

Monday 26th July 2004

I telephoned Fern House to see if they had the results of my PET scan.

I spoke to Dr Kyle's secretary and she told me Dr Kyle wanted to see me. Sounded worrying. Why not just give me the results over the phone—unless they were bad results?

Thursday 29th July 2004

I had my bloods checked and went in to see Dr Kyle. She had the results of the PET scan, which showed it was back again. She explained no more treatment could be offered with the goal of beating it as there was nothing they hadn't already tried, so I was now on the palliative care track with them just trying to make me comfortable for as long as I had. Wow. Just when you thought it was safe…

"At any given moment, you have the power to say: This is not how the story is going to end."
– Christine Mason Miller

Palliative care is the end

Palliative care is defined as: care for the terminally ill and their families, especially that provided by an organised health service. The word palliative is defined as: (of a medicine or medical care) relieving pain without dealing with the cause of the condition.

The problem is that palliative care doesn't necessarily mean imminent death, although that is the generally accepted meaning, and in my case that was exactly what it did mean.

The thing with being told you're being put on palliative care is that it's much worse than being given an Estimated Date of Demise (EDOD), because it formalises things. It means the doctors are going to try and make you as comfortable as they can until you pop your clogs. Die, in other words. So, is it actually worse? Because you know you are definitely going to die anyway, it's just the matter of when. But with palliative care, the assumption is you are going to die sooner rather than later, and you're probably never going to leave the hospital, and that doesn't have to be the case.

SPOILER ALERT: I'm not dead.

Feeling annoyed more than depressed, and definitely not ready to accept the time scale—which was maximum three months with a good wind—Dr Kyle did offer me a glimmer of hope when she said, "Strange things can happen, and you're the type of person they would happen to." (Damn right. Nail on head. Couldn't have said it better myself.)

I took the news and went home, but I rang her for another appointment as I needed to know more about my treatment options, history of others in the same position, etc. She agreed to see me within the hour, so off I went, all my questions written out. (you will remember early on I recommended bring a friend or a dictation machine)

Very negative vibes from her, (I suppose she didn't want to get my hopes up, as she knew from experience I would latch on to anything positive and treat it as a foregone conclusion), but she had already consulted with other haematologists and decided to start IVE treatment, followed with Rituximab. I scurried off home to do my internet research on IVE.

Hard to believe after everything; and considering my bloods are normal, and I feel good, dare I say, I look good and I'm definitely not at death's door. Bummer. What can you do? I know, I'll organise a holiday.

Thursday 5th August 2004

This was the day I threw caution to the wind and went on my final holiday—ever. One week in Spain. When I arrived, I knew I'd done the right thing as the heat enveloped me and seemed to immediately start healing me. I brought lots of self-help and meditation books with me and practised my visualisation, which I had started getting into in a big way.

Visualisation

Right from day one of diagnosis when I had the endoscopy test when I used visualisation for the first time, I knew this thing I had (I didn't know there was an official name for it), changed my life, so I started to investigate the phenomenon of visualisation on the internet and from the various councillors, and then I discovered PacMan.

In the 1980s, kids with stomach cancer had been involved in a trial where half of them were told to visualise PacMan inside their stomach, running around and eating all the cancer cells. They did this for fifteen minutes every morning, afternoon, and before bed. The results showed the children who visualised had a much easier time when going through treatment.

Clinical tests have been carried out with patient's bloods being analysed after visualisation, and a measurable increase in white blood cells detected, and other tests have been done while patients are being scanned, which again showed positive results.

With practice, visualisation can help patients deal with fear of medical procedures, nausea, pain, stress, anxiety, and depression. It improves the ability to cope, improves confidence, hopefulness, motivation, and quality of life.

The fact is you feel you're contributing to your cure, as changes in immune activity on the cellular level have confirmed.

Doctors say visualisation can't cure cancer, and that attitude—irrespective of how positive—has no effect on the cancer cells, and while I agree with both these opinions, the practice does make you feel a lot better. Patients who participated in trials produced significant differences in their white blood cells compared to patients who didn't visualise, so it does have a measurable effect on the body, and considering injections are used to boost the white blood cells after chemotherapy, visualisation can work in conjunction to achieve even better results.

There is a power in words by using them to take control of attitude and feelings. Remember when you were a kid and a teacher/parent/friend said you weren't trying, or you were lazy, or even better, stupid. Remember the feeling that evoked? That feeling of dread in your stomach. That's the power of words translated into feelings. Still not sure? Remember when someone embarrassed you and for some reason your face heated up and went red. Words have a huge effect on how we feel physically, and if your face heats up, that's blood, you know, the stuff with all the good cells pumping around your body, so why wouldn't words/images have an effect at a cellular level?

Visualisation is the use of words and your imagination to create the perfect outcome in your mind.

There is no downside to using visualisation as it can't do you any harm, and at the very least it will make you feel better.

We can do a test now if you have the time. This is best done if you prepare yourself by relaxing on a chair, closing your eyes, and getting a friend to read the next part to you slowly or getting the recording from my web site http://www.cancerology.co/lemon although you can do it yourself if you concentrate on the content, rather than the words.

The Lemon Imagery

Imagine a plain white plate with a large lemon sitting on it.

A bright vibrant yellow lemon on a blindingly white plate.

There are beads of water on the lemon as it has just been brought out of a fridge.

It's so ripe you can actually smell the lemon fragrance.

You reach out and touch it.

It's cold, and wet, and the skin has little bumps.

You stroke some of the water off it, still feeling how cold it is and the little bumps on the skin.

To the right of the plate there is a sharp knife with a wooden handle.

You pick up the knife and hold the lemon with your other hand, ready to cut it down the middle.

When the blade touches the lemon, it slices through the skin easily and a huge squirt of lemon juice escapes into the air.

The smell is an aromatic bitter lemon smell that fills the air.

As the blade reaches the bottom, the plate is filled with juice and the smell is wonderful and fresh.

You take one half of the lemon and cut it again into a quarter and then cut again, more juice squirts into the air.

By this stage your hands are covered in juice.

Now, put the knife down and lift the juiciest piece up to your nose.

Take a deep breath through your nose.

As you inhale, you can smell the sharp fresh citrus scent filling your nostrils.

It's the most intense lemon aroma you've ever encountered.

Now touch the lemon to your lips, all the while noticing the sensations of cold, wet, and a bitter expectation on your lips.

Open your mouth and put the juicy lemon flesh between your teeth.

Now bite hard on the lemon.

If it has worked (and it usually does), you should have screwed up your face before you reached the bite, and if it hasn't, then maybe visualisation isn't going to work for you.

For most people, the act of biting the imaginary lemon stimulates salivatory glands and makes the mouth water, usually accompanied by a shiver.

If you did have an experience similar to biting a real lemon, then you have the mind-set to use visualisation to its full potential.

There are a multitude of various methods to try, and it's a matter of trial and error until you find one you're comfortable with, or do what I do and make your own, after all, you know your mind better than anybody.

Depending on just how freaky your imagination is (and the freakier the better) you can see your body lying on a slab with a coloured light sweeping over your limbs. It's green over the parts you know to be normal, but changes to a wonderful and powerful gold colour when it passes over the part of your body where the cancer is and starts killing the rogue cells. (pick your own relevant colours) As it passes the cancer area, you feel an intense heat. It's extremely violent in the most pleasant way. It's on your side. It's killing the cancer cells and making you well again; in fact, better than well. Repaired better than new, better than you've ever been.

Yes, I know some of you will think this is woo-woo, but what's the harm in giving it a go?

As it worked for me, nobody will convince me visualisation can't play a massive part in the journey through treatment and beyond, and you should at least give it a go.

I have recorded some MP3s with relaxation/visualisation techniques which you can get from my website for free if you register. You can download them to your phone or computer, plug in a set of headphones, lie back and relax as you listen. Use them with my best wishes and as I add more, I'll send you the links.

More details are shown at the back of this book, but in addition to the MP3s, there are also printable PDF files for fluid input/output, pill charts, daily stats charts, etc.

Now for the weird one. This one is mine. Don't ask where it came from because I don't know.

Have you seen the film 'The Terminator'?

In the film, the baddie has the ability to regenerate or modify his body using liquid metal.

If you've ever watched the film, they use this shiny liquid metal a lot. It's called The Mimetic Polyalloy, also known as the polymimetic alloy, which is a type of liquid metal compound applied to advanced Terminator series. (and no, it doesn't exist in real life)

I took it as mine and visualised it encasing my spleen, liver, colon, and heart (where the tumours were), and when it was silver, it stopped the cancer spreading, which was my default setting 24/7, but when I used it in my visualisation, I powered it up so it pulsated bright red as it was killing the cancer cells and their blood was flying everywhere. Occasionally there was a 'splat' on the inside as a tumour exploded.

Although this was all in my mind, I felt great afterwards. I accepted the diagnosis, just not the prognosis I was at the end. I exercised, ate, relaxed, took my meds, and everything else the doctors recommended, but visualisation gave me an intense feeling I was actively participating in my own cure and could expect a great outcome.

Eventually, I dictated it onto a cassette recorder (remember those?) and just sat/lay down and listened to it, over and over.

I tried various methods and this one was when I was on palliative care and wasn't expected to live, so use it, don't use it, it's up to you, but for me, I believe it was what made the difference between living and dying.

Wednesday 25th August 2004

This was the first day of my IVE palliative care regimen.

Veins, where have they gone? Bernie, my chemo nurse had a terrible time locating any veins that could be used for my new chemo regimen. I held my arms under warm water, then hot water, we rubbed them, we tightened the band, and then eventually she found one on the back of my right arm, and after successfully getting a cannula in, the vein collapsed. Time to tear the hair out? Shucks, I don't have any.

After more hunting around for an accommodating vein on my left arm, we found one and it worked perfectly. I was started on my old favourite, Rituximab, after a saline flush and a couple of preparation drugs; however, all was not well, and after about ten minutes I started to get stomach cramp. I hadn't eaten breakfast and thought that was the problem, but it got worse, then my throat started to close, and my nose blocked up; all this within minutes of the initial stomach cramp. I sat up abruptly and the nurse next to me asked if I was okay, so I explained my problems, and she called the sister who checked my charts and discovered that although I had had Rituximab before, I had always been given a hydrocortisone and piriton infusion in preparation, and this time I hadn't.

They pulled screens around me and the thought, 'The Final Curtain', did cross my mind, but I didn't panic as I knew they would be able to sort it. All I needed was a hydrocortisone bolus (a large dose of a substance given by injection for the purpose of rapidly achieving the needed therapeutic concentration in the bloodstream) to relieve my symptoms: just a simple injection into the line and about ten minutes later, everything was back to normal. As a result, they decided to slow down the IV, which meant they couldn't give me the first chemo drug as there was no time, and as it's a three-day regimen in succession, they couldn't start tomorrow (Thursday) as that would mean a break of two days, and as Monday is a bank holiday… you see where I'm going here.

It's worth remembering that in all professions, mistakes do happen, and although this was an uncomfortable one, it wasn't intentional. Once everything was back to normal the sister did come to apologise, but by this time I had already sorted everything in my mind, and although appreciated, it wasn't necessary. Just another blip on my journey.

Chemo veins

After receiving intravenous chemotherapy, your veins will probably start to give problems, the biggest one being they are hard to find, which means sometimes you will go through multiple attempts to get one suitable.

Depending on your nurse or doctor they may recommend using hot water running over the area, or a hot towel, or various other things, and you'll find each has their own method that works for them.

For me, putting on a blood pressure cuff never let me down, but… it's not standard hospital procedure in a lot of hospitals, so you might have to convince the nurse to try it, but usually, it's at the discretion of a senior doctor or consultant.

A light slap can make the veins easier to find in some cases, but ask for advice first as it depends on the area. This one is a problem because medical staff were previously allowed to do it until some idiot screamed abuse and the practice was abandoned due to potential litigation, but if they allow you to do it to yourself and have a witness absolving them, it can work very well.

Isn't it a disgrace that someone doing their best for you is vulnerable to an accusation of abuse by simply helping?

Blood samples taken from the back of the hand worked very well for me, but it's a painful area for most people, but not when you use distraction techniques, and one jab as opposed to three or four attempts is way better.

Best advice is to accept it's going to happen and talk to your nurse about what has worked previously, or what they recommend.

Three days

It was a Wednesday afternoon and my wife had just arrived. As usual, I was lying on top of the bed, eyes closed, practising my visualisation. I heard her say hello to the nurses, then the door opened; but as I was in the middle of blasting my cancer with my mind, I didn't intend to open my eyes until I had finished; then I heard my consultant asking her for a quick word.

The gist of it was that the cancer had advanced into my colon, but even better, my organs were shutting down (which I thought was probably a bad sign), and I would have to be put on dialysis immediately.

My wife asked what all this meant and was told that if I didn't start dialysis, I wouldn't see the weekend, and considering the cancer was now in my colon, things were dire, and she better prepare for the worst.

Suddenly, my eyes opened, and I sat up; turned out I wasn't as interested in my visualisation as I was in the conversation. The look on their faces confirmed their assumption I had been in the land of nod.

I said, "So I'll be dead by Saturday?"

"Well..." I then got a lengthy explanation about dialysis, and cancer, and colon, blah, blah, blah, but things weren't looking good.

"What's the point?" I said, "If I'm going to be dead before Saturday and this is Wednesday, what's the point?"

After everything I had been through, I couldn't accept that this was it. The end. I got angry, I swore (a lot), then ended it with, "I'm not going on fucking dialysis and I'll bet you a pound to a penny, I'll be here on Saturday."

The consultant left and I had a very difficult conversation with my wife.

Now, I had just got bad news, but imagine having to go home to your kids after your husband has been given three days to live.

What do you say when they ask, "How's Daddy?"

And if you say, "Well, at the minute, he isn't good."

"He's not going to die, is he, Mommy? You promised Daddy would be okay."

How does anyone deal with that?

Where is the pressure relief valve?

And yes, it's understandable that the patient—me, in this instance—is going through mental turmoil, but of course, me being me, I'm saying, screw this and singing Gloria Gaynor's I will survive over and over, convinced there's no way this is the end for me.

But for the family—of which there is absolutely no thought being given—they are literally in a hell on earth.

When you look at it through a wide lens, it's no different from any other day because we're all under threat of death at any time, but because a medical professional has proposed a timeline, it's more real than any other time.

So whether you're reading this as the patient, or relative, or friend, you need to get everybody on the same page. Friends and relatives respect and understand what the patient is going through, and the patient (more importantly) needs to respect and understand what the friends and relatives are going through.

The next day more tests were carried out and everything was the same, no improvement, but no difference either. Of course, me being Mr Positive, I grabbed onto the no difference to mean, it's starting to reverse. Yeah, call me mad, I know it doesn't make any sense, but in my mind at the time, it did. I didn't feel any worse than previous days; I was walking about the room, eating, drinking and everything else, so what's with all the doom and gloom?

I will accept that maybe I was a bit muddled with all the drugs, but looking back on it now, I would have made the same decision.

Friday arrived. My last day on earth. Strangely, I felt good. I had a confidence. I wrote it in the diary.

More tests were done, and the results showed a slight improvement (which in my world meant a dramatic and unexpected massive improvement, the like of which the world had never experienced before).

The consultant and doctors were telling me not to get too excited as it was just a minor fluctuation, but in my mind, it was a tectonic shift.

The next day I woke up and thought, Yes, I haven't died. Where's my fuckin' penny?

Once again, tests were done, and yet another improvement was evident. I was told dialysis was no longer on the table.

Two steps forward, one step back. I didn't need dialysis, but now the cancer had spread to my colon. Still, one step at a time, and always forward.

So, I'll bet you're wondering how it all ended. Yeah, I never got the penny. Bummer. But… I'm alive.

IVE (I've) beat it

Okay, so it was a play on words, but both are correct anyway. (IVE - the treatment and I've - I have)

My 9th July 2004 PET scan showed the cancer had returned and the only treatment available (IVE) would be palliative care which would not beat it, just try and control it; but that's not how things played out.

My IVE Chemotherapy Regimen consisted of:

I Ifosphamide

V Etoposide

E Epirubicin

The IVE regimen is high-dose therapy used on patients with relapsed lymphoma.

I took the treatment offered, but it had to be stopped around October time as the side effects were annoying everybody due to my compromised immune system. I was getting treatment week one, going into hospital on week two with an infection, and coming out just in time to start it all again. It was decided to give me a break until January 2005 when I would have one more treatment which would be followed by another PET Scan.

Surprisingly, this time I didn't end up in hospital. Things went better than ever, and I was going around telling everyone that this treatment (January) would be my last as I was finally cured. I don't know where this came from, but I felt it very strongly, so I suppose I believed it.

My next PET scan was scheduled for 11th March 2005, and when the results were available, they showed nothing, nada, zip, zero, zilch, nothing, not even a pin head, not even something smaller than a pin head - no cancer anywhere to be found in my body. Am I being clear enough?

CANCEROLOGY

Lawrence Wray's NHL cancer

Start date: 3rd May 2002

End date: 11th March 2005

Four visits in total from Non-Hodgkin Lymphoma.

Various Estimated Date of Demise deadlines given and ignored.

2 years, 10 months, 8 days.

1043 days in total from official diagnosis to all clear.

What a trip.

I don't know what to believe. I had attacked it head on with a change of diet (nothing radical, just basic healthy eating), daily visualisations, IVE treatment and an extremely positive mental attitude, so I assume that one or all of them worked in some way to rid my body of my little annoyance.

Fast forward to June and I felt great, my hair was growing again, I was eating well (too well), and I was able to exercise.

So, what this means is that if you have cancer or know someone who has, you can take hope from this. There are no guarantees, and that means impending death or expected survival are just ideas. Everything and anything can happen. People who are expected to die, survive (me), and people who are expected to live, die.

Way back on 29th July 2004 I was given my results by my haematologist and told the future was very bleak, and after taking everything offered to me, and doing everything I was told to do and more, I beat the odds, and I beat the cancer, so I guess the advice has to be... Don't give up, and be as positive as it's possible to be.

You have to participate in your own cure.

You have to fight.

You have to believe in yourself, and you have to believe the impossible is possible.

At the very worst, it'll make you feel like you're doing something, which will make you feel better, and at the best… it could make all the difference in the world.

You can look at a cancer diagnosis as the biggest challenge of your life, or you can look at it like something that was probably going to happen as 1 in 2 people are going to be diagnosed anyway.

It's a blip.

A pain? Yes.

Scary? Yes.

Inevitable death? NO

Winners and losers

Are there really winners and losers with cancer? Yes.

But just because someone dies, it doesn't make them a loser.

My brother was a loser. He gave up the day he was diagnosed.

With cancer there are winners and there are losers, and if you haven't been through the process, you'll probably assume the winners are those who don't die, but that's not true.

There are those who fight throughout the process and push themselves every step of the way; some survive and are winners, and some don't make it, but… they are also winners and should be admired. They grabbed cancer by the throat and fought like hell. It's just a horrible fact that not everyone survives.

There also are those who complain about everything, don't push themselves and constantly moan about how life isn't fair. They rely on the medicine and don't participate in their own cure. Irrespective of the outcome, they are losers. Some live and proclaim, 'I'm a winner'. Sorry, nope. You can't be a winner if you didn't try.

There is more chance of surviving if you fight, and some people have said that the word 'fight' in the title of this book suggests the body can overcome the cancer cells, and that isn't true, but there is a fight through the treatment. There is a constant mind battle with yourself, a battle against exercise, eating, drinking, motivating yourself to even go outside.

Be a winner.

"My cancer scare changed my life. I'm grateful for every new, healthy day I have. It has helped me prioritize my life." – Olivia Newton John

Newton's third law

The mental state in patients who survived cancer can be impacted by their journey through treatment.

Think of the attitude knowing you had cancer and survived because the doctors cured you, compared to the attitude knowing you survived because you fought.

If you survived because of medical intervention, your attitude afterwards isn't going to be that of a winner. 'It was awful. It was a horrible process. I was sick. It's the worst thing in the world.'

Now compare that to someone who fought all the way through their cancer. They fought to force themselves to eat; they fought to force themselves to exercise; they fought to force themselves to read books on cancer that they had really no interest in but needed to read to understand and fight their disease. They forced themselves to sleep when they didn't want to sleep; forced themselves to meditate, forced themselves to visualise, and then it happened: they beat cancer.

I survived cancer is good, but I beat cancer is better.

When someone beats cancer as a result of fighting, their attitude towards life is permanently changed for the better. They didn't survive cancer; they beat cancer.

But... wasn't it because of the medicine? Yes, of course it was, but I have to insert a big 'and their attitude' as well. Medicine and a positive attitude are an extremely powerful combination.

When you beat cancer and eventually go back to work, you find that problems that were previously mountains are now just minor inconveniences. If someone asks, "Do you think you might be able to do whatever?" your response is, "Are you kidding me? I beat cancer; I can fly to the moon without a rocket, dude."

There is an inner strength as a result of your ordeal; a reward if you will.

You come out the other side a much stronger, more confident person. Yes, don't get me wrong, you're still going to panic and think every little health hiccup is cancer returning, but you've also got the knowledge that you beat it.

I've spoken to three people who have had at least two recurrences of their cancer, and they all basically said the same thing. "If it came back, I'd just beat it again."

Just beat it again; think about that.

Worry, of course, but it's like a muscle memory, you do it once, you can do it again.

Compare that attitude with someone diagnosed for the first time. There is a strength knowing you participated in your own cure, but unfortunately, for those diagnosed for the first time with no experience, it's the worst thing to ever happen to them. It's understandable and it's a pity; and that's where talking to others can help so much.

Beating cancer is a strength, a power that (thankfully) ordinary people don't possess, but if the doctors cured you, and you didn't participate in your own cure and cancer revisits, you have nothing to fall back on as you relied entirely on others, and that's nowhere near as powerful.

The hope of the patient who didn't participate in their own cure is in sharp contrast to somebody who says, "I beat it before, I'll beat it again." The idea of hoping for a good outcome isn't present.

Cancer is the most hateful disease in our world, yet it can change you for the better, depending on how you tackle it.

I'm not suggesting cancer is a thing everyone should try to be a better person, but it's seldom you get something that doesn't have a positive as well as a negative. Newton's third law states that for every action, there is an equal and opposite reaction, and when you think about it, it really works in relation to a cancer journey.

If you look back at cancer being the worst thing you've ever experienced, it's going to have a negative impact on your outlook; but if you ask, 'What did that teach me? What can I learn from the problems I overcame?" you change your outcome, you change your psychology, you change your mindset, you change your outlook for the rest of your life...and it's power. It's a weird son of a bitch.

Depends how you look at it

When strangers find out I've had cancer seventeen times and survived, most say, 'You must be really unlucky to have had it that many times.'

I suppose there is two ways of looking at it, but for me, I think I'm the luckiest guy alive. Seventeen times, and I've beaten it every time?

How the hell is that unlucky?

You've read my Twenty Three section and know that people have died throughout my journey, so, for me, I'm the lucky one.

Not my circus, not my monkeys

Late 2005, after having had Non-Hodgkin Lymphoma four times and been given the all clear, I was asked to give a talk at one of the groups I attended; tell them my story, explain how I felt, tell them about my stem cell transplant, and give encouragement. I started with the attitude needed and progressed to; you have to participate in your own cure. (Yes, even way back then I was promoting this phrase) At this stage, one of the guys put his hand up and asked me to explain what I meant as it was the doctor's job to cure him and not his. I explained that although this was correct, the doctor couldn't be with him at home and that due to the chemotherapy he might not feel like eating, drinking, or exercising, so he had to look after himself, take responsibility, and participate in his own cure. He immediately stood up and asked if I had any idea how long he had worked and how much he had paid into the health service by way of taxes and National Insurance Contributions.

This was the first time I had ever spoken in public, so I looked at the organisers for help, but I was on my own.

I said I had no idea, but the fact that he had paid, meant he was getting the best treatment possible, and not only that, he was getting it free of charge.

He then said that as he had worked so hard and paid so much, if it was essential to his treatment that he should be eating, drinking, and exercising, the hospital should either provide him with a nurse full time, or admit him to hospital for the duration of his treatment, after all, that's what he paid for.

Someone at his beck and call 24/7 to make sure he did everything he was supposed to do. I don't think that's a nurse, I think it's a servant.

Another patient started to clap, then they all joined in.

What the hell?

I thought about sitting down, but no, typical me, I started to argue back, after all, A) I knew what I was talking about as I had watched others and B) would he rather die. (Yeah, I'm blunt.)

Eventually, one of the organisers came to the front and said that irrespective of whether or not they agreed with me, I was right.

The guy then walked out, followed by two others.

I didn't offer to speak in public for a long time after that.

Thinking about it afterwards, if he had been offered a full-time nurse, he wouldn't have wanted her fussing around at his home, and if he had been admitted to hospital for three months to receive treatment, he wouldn't have wanted that either.

Irrespective of how much you've paid into a system, or how good your health insurance is, or what your views are on the standard of care you receive, you are the one that needs to take responsibility for doing everything the doctors advise and participate in your own cure. Nobody can force you to do something you don't want to do, that's where the fight comes into the equation. You have to make yourself do it. Argue all you like if you don't agree with me, but ultimately, it's your life and if you don't value it and prefer to waste time arguing, that's up to you.

You only get one chance to get it right, so it's common sense to do everything in your power to survive.

What if it all goes to shit?

Hopefully, it doesn't, and yes, I'm talking about death or a prognosis so severe, it has to be acted on (having said that, any cancer diagnosis has to be acted on immediately anyway).

Well… the first thing to remember is that I was given three days to live while on palliative care with cancer number four, I went into renal failure and against the odds, I didn't die. That's not to say it will or won't happen to you (getting an Estimated

Date of Demise that is), and I hope you never have to go through it.

But peace of mind, calms the mind. Being organised (in my case, for the first time in my life) is calming.

We all know from an early age and from experience that we are going to die; it's just a matter of when. The how? Really? Is that important? It might be in our sleep, or we might step out in front of a bus, car, van, lorry, train, or a house might fall on top of us, or we might drown, or a plane might fall out of the sky on us, or we might trip and bang our head, or… Jeez, it goes on and on and on and the possibilities are endless, yet it is certain, and the best we can hope for is a quick painless death, unlike the passengers in my dad's taxi when he fell asleep at the wheel. Nah, just jokin' ya.

From the minute we're born, we are dying. It's just a matter of when.

So don't just sit there, get organised. Irrespective of your condition this is something you should already have done.

Make a will

People who wait until the eleventh hour to make a will, usually die at ten-fifty-five.

The first thing I need to point out is that a lot of places now offer a free will making service, and in most cases, it's not a good idea. On one hand you save the normal fee (which usually isn't much anyway considering the knowledge required to protect assets) but the catch is they appoint themselves as executor of the will—so when you die and expect everything to be left to your nearest and dearest—they (as executor) charge a fee for estate administration, whereas, if you appoint the executor, there is no charge.

There's no such thing as a free lunch, and anything concerning legal matters rarely comes cheap.

But how high can the fees be? Obviously, they're reasonable? Yeah, cuz everybody is honest. How about 10% of your estate? That means you have a house valued at say 100,000; your FREE will just cost your family 10,000, and if your estate is worth more, then the fee goes up. If that's free, I'm a banana.

Q: What do you call 100 solicitors/lawyers at the bottom of the sea? A: A good start.

There's a reason for a lot of jokes.

The culprits are solicitors, lawyers, banks, charities, estate agents, insurance companies, and even car sales companies, etc. Always ask about what happens when you die, and if there is a fee to execute the will, walk away.

There is no such thing as a 'free' service.

And what about afterwards?

Well, if you've made a mark, you'll be remembered for that, and if you haven't there's always family, but if there are kids?

We live in interesting times where we carry a small device capable of wonderous things in our pocket, like recording a video.

If you have a solicitor/lawyer/legal advisor/friend you can rely on, you could look at the possibility of recording videos for the anniversary of your death (wow, morbid or what?) and having them distribute a recording of you saying something. Something? What, specifically? Well, you'll have to work that one out for yourself and it will depend on your demeanour, your family and your circumstances, but for someone like me who doesn't take life—let alone death—seriously, I'd be saying something like: "So, a year? Honestly, time flies and I didn't even notice. What have I missed? How are you all doing?" etc. I'd be jolly and messing about. Why change the habit of a lifetime?

Be careful naming people who might just be where you are now. Yeah, I didn't say it would be easy. It takes a lot of thought to get right.

Obviously, this isn't going to suit everybody, or even most, but it might tickle a few, and as you're reading this and maybe thinking, gosh darn it, that is a strangely weird but good idea, you can throw on a thinking cap and write your own script.

Birthdays and Christmas or other major celebrations where there are potentially going to be lots of people present might not be ideal, but then again, if you're weird and they sorta expect it, where's the harm?

As I said, it's not going to be for everyone, but you already know best what might or might not work, so if you do decide to do it, set a timeframe and plan for special events like births, birthdays, graduations, engagements and weddings you're not going to be around for. You can even record something to allow for something bad happening where you can give comfort from the grave. Gran, Grandfather, Mum or Dad dying, or divorce, or… Yeah, I did mention the word morbid already. But think of it this way, when you last had a major event in your life like a birth or a death or divorce, would you have liked to have been congratulated or comforted by a loved one who has gone before?

Look, I have these ideas and I throw them out there, and if you like them or hate them, at least I've presented something you probably haven't given much consideration to…and I suspect that's because most people are sane and haven't been given an estimated date of demise. It makes you think, both in a good way and in a weird way, but how's that a bad thing?

My funeral

It's just my opinion, but funerals are for the living. They are a way to say goodbye to loved ones and gain some sort of closure and are usually an excuse for a good booze-up afterwards. The problem is they are expensive. You'll need a fancy coffin with all the bells and whistles (to rot in the ground or be burnt), a ceremony, a hearse and a couple of limousines for the nearest and dearest, and then a humungous bar bill afterwards, followed by the cost of a headstone and engraving.

Some people look on it as a celebration of life, but for me, I want the quickest simplest funeral available, after my body is used for medical research/training. Although I am a registered donor, nothing can be used for transplant due to cancer, but they may be able to cut me up (dissect, for those purists) and find something of relevance that could potentially illuminate the who, what, why, where, and when the cancer got me. Who knows, but as I won't be there, I wish them well.

My ideal departure would be a plastic bag (with me in it, obviously), thrown in the back of a van (no need for a hearse), then off to the crematorium. No celebration of life, no order of service, no attendees, no singing, no nothing. That's it. I'm gone. Who? The guy who wrote the book about his cancer. Can't remember his name but he's dead. That's that.

If you have the opportunity to plan your own funeral (which, if you're reading this, you do), give it some thought. Sure, it's morbid, but then again, it's pragmatic. Make your wishes known. Have it done your way, and not the way some might assume you wanted it.

My way won't be right for most people, but for me it seems the quickest and easiest way to finish.

"*Knowledge is of no value unless you put it into practice.*" ~
Anton Chekov

You're takin' the piss

Fast forward to Wednesday, 23rd November 2011 when I went for a pee (as you do) and was mid-stream when I heard something hit the porcelain. I looked down and there was a little lump at the bottom of the bowl, then another popped out. I finished, but instead of flushing, I used the toilet brush to retrieve the little pieces of whatever had decided to appear. It looked like dried blood.

For the ladies reading this, you won't have the same experience as a guy standing to wee, so it would be a good idea to see if anything has popped out if you have the sensation of something other than liquid coming down the pipe.

I immediately rang my doctor, and he made an appointment for the afternoon and instructed me to bring the samples. At the surgery he said, "Don't worry, it's not cancer." But I knew from reading everything I had been given regarding my chemotherapy drugs, that Cyclophosphamide (Cytoxan®) was known to have a potential side effect of secondary cancer, and in particular, bladder cancer. When I brought this up, he was unaware of this possibility—which is understandable as it's a very specialised drug, and it would be unreasonable to expect a general practitioner to have knowledge of every drug used in every chemo treatment. He decided to refer me to hospital for a cystoscopy (camera up the waterworks and into the bladder), but again advised that it was, "Probably nothing to worry about."

As usual, I wasn't worried, but I wanted it sorted as soon as.

The appointment was a week later (probably as a result of my history), and if the thought of this procedure makes your eyes water, don't worry, it's not as bad as it seems.

Cystoscopy

Friday 2nd December 2011 (9 days later)

A cystoscopy is similar to the endoscopy test as they use a camera to view your insides, but this one is inserted up your water pipe. Yeah, I did mention your eyes would probably water.

They can, if you insist, give you something to make you sleep through the procedure; otherwise, they simply freeze the entrance with a local anaesthetic. In all the times I've had it carried out I've only ever had the local anaesthetic, as once they explain there is virtually no feeling inside, it's not a problem, but—there's always a but—you will feel uncomfortable when they pass the camera through the sphincter muscle that stops urine leaking. The first time it's a bit of a shock, but honestly, it's nothing to worry about and doesn't even last a second. You won't jump or shout out, but you will be aware.

Once inside, the consultant will be able to have a look around for any potential problems, and during this time you will feel nothing. Depending on the equipment used, you may be able to see what the doctor sees on a flat screen, although I've had it done in two different hospitals where one had the screen and one didn't. It's not for everybody and you don't have to look, but I found it fascinating (no surprise there).

There are two types of cystoscopes: a flexible cystoscopy camera is about the width of a thin pencil and can be moved inside the bladder to view everything, and a rigid cystoscopy camera doesn't bend and is used while you are anaesthetised, the latter mostly being used to remove any tumours found.

On screen I was shown where the cancer cells were. Colourful little buggers that looked like tiny mushrooms swaying gently in the water they pump into you to fill the bladder. I was told they were superficial and not to worry, although I would need an operation to remove them.

That's it. The whole thing takes less than ten minutes and is not a problem.

However, the first pee afterwards can sting a bit and sometimes blood appears for a couple of days, but it's not something to worry about, just keep drinking and everything returns to normal after the third or fourth day. The first pee I have after a cystoscopy always has me tensing and standing on my tip toes, but once it starts, I'm left wondering what all the fuss was about.

I've now had it done at least twenty times, give or take, as I've lost count. I have no fear of having it done again and as bladder cancer requires a check-up every three months, it's gonna happen anyway.

I wouldn't be qualified to do the procedure, but the thought of inserting the camera myself and guiding it into the bladder wouldn't be something I would worry about. It's that easy.

Pain rating is only ½/10. (if even) Nothing to worry about.

Problems afterwards? Slight nip with the first pee, but once the flow starts it's not a problem. There is also the possibility of infection (which I've had numerous times), so if you start running to the loo every 10-15 minutes and wondering why you bothered as nothing worthwhile comes out, you should contact your doctor and get antibiotics.

Thursday 15th December 2011 (13 days later)

Just under two weeks later I had the tumours removed. At this stage I'm going to just throw everything into the mix about my bladder cancer as although I've now had it twelve times, it's a case of the same thing repeated over and over and over…

TURBT

The first stage in treating bladder cancer is a Trans Urethral Removal of Bladder Tumour (TURBT).

A scope is inserted up the urethra and the tumours are either burnt away with a laser or cut out. Afterwards you may notice blood in your urine for up to five days.

I've had twelve TURBTs in total with no real problems other than detailed below. It's a scary thing when they tell you tumours are going to be removed and I've seen lots of questions on the Facebook forums from people in a panic about their impending appointment, but I've never had a problem.

They anaesthetise you using one of the methods described below and get on with it. You don't feel anything during the procedure, and afterwards the potential problems are a stinging/burning sensation for the first couple of urinations, and the possibility of infection. There are other things that can happen such as excessive bleeding (which I've never experienced), but these will be taken care of before you are allowed home.

Epidural TURBT

For my first of many bladder operations, I had an epidural, which is where they inject anaesthetic into your spine which freezes everything from the waist down.

The benefit is you are awake throughout the procedure and feel nothing. I remember touching my legs and they felt like they belonged to someone else. Weird.

The initial injection and operation were not a problem, but afterwards in the recovery room I started to shiver; however, this is expected, and not only did they wrap me in metallic blankets, but they put a plastic blanket over me which was connected to a hot air blower, so the blanket inflated and the hot air started to come out the little holes at the bottom and warm me up. Bliss.

The benefit of an epidural is that you can drive away afterwards, which you can't do with a general anaesthetic, the drawback is pins and needles as the effects wore off. I didn't like it. It drove me crazy and that was my one and only epidural.

Other patients seem to like it and have no problems, but given the option, I always took something else.

Pain rating is only ½/10. (if even) Nothing to worry about.

The pins and needles and shivering afterwards get a frustration rating of 9/10. Not painful, but bloody annoying.

Problems afterwards? None for the procedure, but… that first wee. That's something entirely different.

Local Anaesthetic TURBT

I only had a procedure performed once under local anaesthetic as they normally use a rigid cystoscopy camera which requires a general, but when given the option, I jumped at it. The opportunity to watch surgery being carried out while I was awake was something I couldn't miss.

Initially, it's the same as a normal cystoscopy test; the cream is applied to the opening of the urethra and the scope slid in and up past the sphincter, then off we go.

For this operation the tumours were embryonic, and laser surgery was being used. I watched everything on the screen and just before he lasered the first tumour, I was told to expect an unusual mild pain. Unusual? Okay, not painful, as such, but weird, like nothing I'd ever felt before. A nip might describe the pain element, but there was a tingling sort of sensation. I can't do it justice here and I've never felt anything like it again as local was used only once, but I'd recommend it if it's offered as an option. The surgeon simply aligned the laser up and tapped on a foot pedal to initiate the blast.

On screen it was like watching a galactic battle in Star Wars as the tumours exploded in all directions, yet (apart from the tingling which lasted less than a second on each tumour) I felt nothing.

Pain rating is only ½-1/10. Nothing to worry about and you get to see the little buggers being burnt and explode.

Problems afterwards? None, apart from the first pee stinging a little.

General Anaesthetic TURBT

A canula in the arm, a countdown, and it's all over. You awake in recovery and they give you tea and toast. The only problem is you can't drive after receiving a general anaesthetic, so you will need to organise a lift home. You may be kept in overnight and I've mostly been allowed out same day and kept overnight on occasion.

Same problems afterwards with the first pee, although one time it was mega. I went out for tea after escaping and had to use the men's room, I was apprehensive as usual but started anyway, then screamed. I had previously heard it described as peeing razor blades and laughed at the very idea as I (super dude that I am) had never experienced it, but just when you thought it was safe… it wasn't. Now, I've painted a bad picture here and throughout all my other operations I've never had it since; however, it only lasted for the first few seconds then went back to normal, but it really did make my eyes water. Next pee I was very uptight, but it didn't repeat. I think it might have been caused by a combination of internal bleeding and a chemo flush that is normally given after the operation.

But, then there was pee number two after another TURBT. A good one this time. Again, I was out having a meal, but when I went into the men's room there were four other guys peeing into one of those trough things where all the pee flows to the end and down a drain. For me, it was urgent as I'd just been released from hospital, so as the only slot free was at the top, I raced in and started. Then… the room went silent. I was staring either at the ceiling or wall and was just glad to be emptying, but when everything went quiet, I looked around. Everyone was looking at me. What?? I looked down and followed the flow of my blood down the trough.

Yes, I did explain, but honestly, it looked like somebody had been slaughtered. I laughed, but for some reason, everybody continued to look at me like I had two heads. Fun or what?

So, out of 12 TURBTs so far, one produced a painful pee. A couple produced blood, but most were event free.

Pain rating is only ½/10. Nothing to worry about.

Problems afterwards? Unless you experience my one-time problem, there is nothing to worry about, just a little sting and burn that decreases after you start. But… as with all general anaesthetics, there is a strong possibility of constipation afterwards, so as with the chemo advice previously, ask about the possibility and plan ahead. I've learnt the hard way and I always take a laxative on the morning of surgery, and if I'm kept overnight, I get another after the operation.

Catheter

A catheter is something you may have to get used to if the doctors are working on your water works. It's simply a soft thin tube inserted up your water pipe and into the bladder, where a small balloon is inflated to stop the catheter falling out, and the other end is usually connected to a bag which can be on a stand, or attached to a bed, or strapped to your leg.

I've had one inserted on four occasions (once for fourteen days), and although it's uncomfortable, it's tolerable, but take it easy when you have one; don't go jogging and you won't have any problems, but—and this one is just for the guys—don't get excited with a catheter in. No, really. If you wake up with a *morning glory*, you're gonna regret it. Get out of bed and go for a walk. Having a hard-on with a catheter in isn't funny, it's painful, and not in a good way, so if it happens, get yourself out of bed and distract yourself. Take a cold shower or wet a towel with cold water and use that. You'd be amazed just how quickly things return to normal when everything is hit with cold.

For the girls, I can't see this being a problem, but for the guys, it's a hard one (See what I did there?).

If you find that it's painful, you should contact your doctor for advice, but the main problem I had was friction when moving, as the dry tube rubs against the dry skin in what is a very sensitive area. The solution is to use a lubricant to stop the friction, but the easiest way is to just lie about the house and avoid walking, after all, it's not like you have to run to the loo for a pee.

Pain rating is only ½/10. Nothing to worry about.

Problems afterwards? Irritation and potential for urinary tract infections which have to be treated with antibiotics. In fairness, I've only had one infection, so shouldn't be a problem for most people.

Kidney Cancer

I'm not going to go into great depths about my kidney cancer for the simple reason that out of all the cancers I have had, it was the easiest to deal with.

It was caught early during a routine cystoscopy check-up, investigated further, and the decision was made to remove it as soon as possible. (12 days later)

On the day of surgery (Tuesday, 25th October, 2016 The day I turned 56), I turned up early after having fasted the night before. They did the standard basic checks followed by loads of questions, which another nurse double-checked.

Then a nurse inserted a cannula in my arm (which I didn't feel because I used the distraction methods), then transfer from bed to trolly and away we went.

Just outside the theatre, there were loads more questions confirming the questions already answered, then the syringe with the white liquid appeared and all I had to do was a count from ten down to one.

The one thing I do remember is when the drug was administered, I had a kaleidoscope of colours before my eyes. It was a most wonderful feeling.

I found out later there was fentanyl in the mix, which I suspect I've had before but never experienced the multi-coloured waking dream stage.

Then I awoke in bed, and that was that.

One minute you're tripping on colours floating across a ceiling; the next, you're on a bed with a nurse asking, "How are you feeling?"

Before the operation, I was told that—depending on the complexity of the procedure—I might need a significant incision to remove the kidney, but in the end, it was done with laparoscopic (Keyhole) surgery.

I have three scars to the left of my belly button, the biggest being around 2½ inches/6.5cm/65mm and the other two around ½inch/1.2cm/12mm each. Did I have any hassle? No

I was discharged the following afternoon and told to take things easy for the next couple of weeks.

All through this book I've been advising you to exercise, and I live by that because it's always been my method and it has served me well. I go out walking on chemo and I'm the only one on the planet exercising in that area with cancer and being on chemo. It gives me a lift, so, I arrived home, went to bed, got up the next day, drove to a car park and went for a walk.

I parked in the middle and made it as far as the edge of the carpark, which—having measured it for this book—turned out to be 41 feet, and that was as far as I could manage. I had to sit down gently because of the stitches, rest, then manoeuvre myself back to the car and then sit resting for a good 20 minutes thinking, *you dickhead...* but the next day I went up to the same car park, and I managed from the middle of the car park to the edge and back in one go. No rest required.

The third day, I did half a lap of the car park. I was able to walk from the middle to the edge then do a semi-circle and then walk back to my car and rest.

The next day I did a full complete circle of the park, and I felt great.

The next day—like an idiot—I did a slow jog.

I was wearing a light grey tracksuit and was running around without a care in the world when a girl came into the park with her dog. As I approached, I waved, then... watched her face change, then she let out a little whimper and pointed.

It was like something out of a massacre movie. My top looked like I'd been shot in the belly and the trousers all down one leg was glistening red blood. Oops.

It turns out a couple of the stitches thought jogging was a bit silly, so they didn't try as hard as they might to keep everything neat and tidy.

I knew it was nowhere near as bad as it looked, so I threw some newspapers on the seat of the car and drove to my surgery. Funny enough, when I entered, I didn't have to queue, they took one look at me and threw me in a wheelchair then straight to a doctor to get patched up.

All in all, not too bad, and yes, the next day I did a slow walk around the park (no jogging). It was probably about a month before I attempted a slow jog again.

So overall, the operation was easy. Recovery was easy. Even the burst stitches were easy. I really had no problem with it. It was the easiest of all my cancers. Sorry, I keep using the word 'easy' repeatedly because it's the most appropriate word. There was no problem at all (other than having to ditch my tracksuit).

I have a check-up every six months, and have Chronic Kidney Disease (CKD) with the remaining kidney operating at around 27-29%, but I live with it without incident or problem. It is no hindrance whatsoever.

There was no chemo needed or suggested as the cancer was contained in the kidney and hadn't spread, and they had caught it early, so whip it out, and that was it.

Some of you may—quite rightly—be thinking that I'm not giving enough importance to kidney cancer, and that is, in a way right, because it is based on my experience with other cancers that were caught late and had spread.

Any type of cancer is extremely serious, and people die as a result of having kidney cancer, so I hope you understand where I'm coming from.

Ultimately, a cancer diagnosis is a scary and life-threatening thing, irrespective of the type, spread, stage or grade.

Laparoscopic surgery

Laparoscopic surgery, otherwise known as keyhole surgery, is a procedure where small incisions are made in the skin instead of one big one.

The surgeon uses an instrument called a laparoscope, which is similar to an endoscope or a cystoscope in that it's a small tube with a light source and a camera at the end which sends the information back to television monitors so the surgeon can see inside.

The advantages over this technique include:

A much shorter hospital stay.

Less scarring.

Less pain.

Less bleeding after the operation.

Laparoscopy is performed under general anaesthetic.

The surgeon will make one or more incisions—in my case it was three—and then a tube pumps gas into the abdomen to keep it inflated, so the surgeon has room to look around.

After the procedure, the gas is let out, then the incisions are closed using stitches, and you're usually kept in overnight.

A recent development in laparoscopy is robotic-assisted laparoscopic surgery, where the surgeon uses a console located outside the theatre and does everything by controlling robotic arms.

Pain rating is 0/10.

Problems afterwards? Not really, but you already know what happened.

"*Knowledge is only power if you use it. If you know what you should do and don't do it, you're an idiot.*" ~ Lawrence Wray

Long term side effects from treatment

I've already covered chemo-brain, which does get better with time and is not only something you can live with, but a small price to pay; but there are others.

The wall of sleep

Sometimes, I have no energy. It happens about once/twice a month without warning and even after a good night's sleep. I get up, have breakfast and get ready for the day ahead, then it strikes. I describe it to friends as walking into a wall of sleep.

The only way to deal with it is to go with the flow and go back to bed or lie on a couch. If it happens when you're driving (and yes, it does happen and it's sudden) don't try to drive through it; opening windows and forcing yourself to stay awake doesn't work, so find a safe place to pull over and have a nap. I suspect it's the body's way of telling you it's had enough for now and rest isn't optional, but irrespective of whether or not you do go back to bed, from experience, it's not a good idea to get behind the wheel of a car or do anything remotely dangerous, such as operating machinery.

You won't know until it hits you, so it might be an idea to let your employer know in advance that on occasion you may not be at work and explain that it's a long-term side effect of chemotherapy. You can always make up the lost time afterwards when you'll be able to work better anyway.

Peripheral neuropathy

The other wonderful visitor is peripheral neuropathy, and no, it's not brain related.

Some drugs such as vincristine, cisplatin, paclitaxel, etoposide, tenoposide, thalidomide, interferon, and others, can damage the peripheral (extremities) nerves which results in a numbness, burning sensation, or tingling of hands or feet, loss of sensation to touch, loss of positional sense (knowing where parts of your body are without having to look), and cramping or pain in the hands and feet.

The good news is that for some, they never suffer any symptoms at all, but for others, the symptoms peak 3-5 months after the final treatment and should disappear completely months later. The bad news is that sometimes the problem remains with you permanently.

For me, I never experienced numbness or any burning sensation, but I do suffer from loss of touch and I drop a lot of things. I can burn my fingers if I'm not careful and I only know about it when I notice a blister, of course, once I do notice it, the feeling returns just when you don't want it. Occasionally, I get intense pins and needles and irrespective of the time of day, the only way to alleviate the problem is movement. Flex the fingers if it's in the hands and wiggle the toes or go for a walk if it's in the feet.

Cold Agglutinin Disease

This is a rare side effect and, of course, I've got it. Cold Agglutinin Disease can be a side effect of any autoimmune disease such as lupus, leukaemia, Non-Hodgkin lymphoma, etc. Normally your immune system makes antibodies that attack bacteria and viruses, but when you have Cold Agglutinin Disease, the body's immune system mistakenly attacks and destroys its own red blood cells. Red blood cells are made in the bone marrow inside your bones and have a life span of about 120 days. The word 'cold' in Cold Agglutinin Disease is very relevant as it's usually only in cold temperatures that problems arise, but living in Northern Ireland means it's with me most of the year.

Cold Agglutinin Disease destroys red blood cells faster than the bone marrow can make new ones, which means they are killed off after only a few days.

Symptoms include an increased heartbeat, chills, pale skin, shortness of breath, chest pain, dark urine, an enlarged spleen, weakness and fatigue.

For me it seems to work in conjunction with peripheral neuropathy, with extreme coldness and pain in my feet and hands.

I initially found out I had it when dark patches of skin appeared on the heel of both feet. Not only was it sore to walk, but pressing on the affected areas felt as if there was a hole below the skin.

I was sent to a local hospital and had both a visual inspection and a blood test carried out.

When I was diagnosed, it involved a blood test that had to be transported immediately from the hospital to a laboratory in a taxi to ensure it arrived in time to carry out the tests. The presence of cold agglutinin is evaluated by measuring the red cell agglutinating antibody activity at different temperatures. The test measures the number of red blood cells, white blood cells, and platelets, as well as the size, how much protein the cells contain, and how much space they take up in the blood. They also look for evidence of blood cell destruction and the level of bilirubin, which is a strong indicator of Cold Agglutinin Disease as it increases when blood cells are destroyed.

The primary treatment is to avoid being in low temperatures and other than that. there is no realistic treatment available.

For me, Cold Agglutinin Disease means my hands and feet can't retain heat, and even during the summer months my hands are like touching ice while the rest of me is comfortable. I've learned to accept it and it's not unusual for me to wear two pairs of woollen socks or a pair of stretch gloves with the tips of the fingers cut off when I'm typing. I frequently wash my hands just to get them under hot water.

Exercise does work wonders sometimes, but it's a short-term solution to a long-term problem. Anything that produces sweat such as star jumps or jogging on the spot will usually alleviate the problem for at least an hour, but after that, you have to do it all over again.

Blurry vision

Some chemotherapy drugs can cause cataracts, and although I've been tested and given the all clear, I do suffer from blurry vision at times. It's usually first thing in the morning and clears up as the day progresses, but sometimes it's an all-day thing. Eye drops do help, but in my case the effects diminish after around ten minutes and the blur returns. It's not a biggie, and if you plan for it, you can do everything as normal.

Dry eyes

Dry eyes are a common short-term side effect as some chemotherapy drugs can affect the inside of the eyelid. Eye drops are the obvious solution but talk to your consultant if it appears and get appropriate treatment. Occasionally, years later, I awake to find I have dry eyes, but I always keep a bottle of drops beside the bed which sorts the problem. It can be painful, so avoid rubbing as it makes matters worse. If you don't have eye drops handy, find some water.

Other problems

Lots of survivors have few or no lasting/late side effects after treatment ends, but there are exceptions depending on the aggressiveness of the treatment necessary to achieve a cure. Most are nothing more than an inconvenience; however, still better to have long-term side effects than no term at all.

Late side effects of surgery

Depending on the area of the body the surgery was performed, and whether a tumour may have had an effect on healthy tissue, or the amount of normal tissue removed as a caution, there are a number of side effects that may present.

Scarring on the skin, problems fighting infection, swelling of arms or legs, nutritional problems, cognitive problems, changes in sexual function, reduction or loss of fertility, moderate to severe pain, difficulty with speech, difficulty swallowing, emotional side effects such as body image after surgery.

Most of these are easily dealt with, and if you experience any of the above, you should seek professional help at the first signs.

Late side effects of chemotherapy

Chemotherapy kills cancer cells, but it also affects normal healthy cells, which is why short-term side effects appear such as changes to fingernails, skin, and hair loss.

Organs that have been affected by cancer can cause problems well after treatment has ended due to the damage from both the cancer and the treatment.

You may experience fatigue, chemo-brain, early menopause, heart problems, infertility, reduced lung capacity, kidney and urinary problems, nerve problems (Peripheral Neuropathy/Cold Agglutinin Disease), bone and joint problems, muscle weakness, and secondary cancers. Cyclophosphamide (used in my Non-Hodgkin Lymphoma treatment) is thought to be responsible for my bladder cancer, as it's a known potential side effect, however, nobody can say for definite whether or not it is actually responsible. Again, on the bladder cancer forums, some people are in the same position as me and attribute their bladder cancer to previous treatment, with the inevitable comment that if they had known then what they know now, they would have refused treatment. Of course, this would have worked if only they had known and could have easily avoided bladder cancer by refusing treatment and dying. Great idea. Duhhh.

Late side effects of radiation therapy

Radiation therapy is constantly getting better with more targeted treatment, but by necessity, it also has an effect on healthy tissue to make certain that all the cancer in the area is treated.

Potential problems include cataracts, fatigue, dry mouth, permanent hair loss, problems with thyroid or adrenal glands, infertility, slowed or halted bone development, decreased range of motion in the area treated, skin sensitivity to sun exposure, and secondary cancers.

Before treatment, your consultant will discuss any potentials with you, and although the list above is intimidating, you have to bear in mind that the area being treated may (or may not) trigger a side effect.

A weird one for you

Technically, this is a side effect, but it's indirect, and it's the association you have with vomiting and your chemo nurse, but it's a good example of how your mind puts things together and how powerful the mind can be.

I've never experienced this one myself as I only read about it, until I met another survivor at a check-up years later and we got to talking. In between check-ups he had been out shopping with his wife when he came face-to-face with his chemo nurse. In his words: "I seen her, I smiled, she smiled, I threw up."

It's classical conditioning as in Pavlov's dogs where he rang a bell every time he fed the dogs, which meant that any time he rang the bell, the dogs started salivating with expectation. If every time a cancer patient is sick on chemo and makes the link to the chemo nurse, the nurse becomes the bell.

My opinion on late side effects

Yeah, you knew I would have an opinion.

They can be a pain; but you only get them if you've survived cancer, so as you ain't dead, what's to complain about?

I don't think there is any medicine that doesn't come with a warning about side effects, and it would be unreasonable to expect your consultant to point out every potential long term side effect that may never develop, yet I see lots of Facebook groups complaining about the fact they were never notified about the possibility of future problems prior to treatment. The fact is the information leaflets supplied before the treatment starts lists all potential problems, but as you need the drug to survive, you're probably not going to be too concerned about what might happen later.

Realistically, when you've just been diagnosed, the last thing you want to hear about is the possibility of problems after you've beaten your cancer. It's a one-step-at-a-time approach. Let's get the cancer out of the way before we start worrying about problems that may never materialise.

I have asked other survivors about problems they experienced as a result of treatment, and without exception, they all concluded they were just glad to be alive and could cope with anything after having survived cancer.

One of the nice side effects is just knowing you've survived. It gives you a special strength. Some cancer survivors have a swager, or a glow, or a confidence that comes with surviving that which has tried its hardest to kill. Ultimately, it's not all bad. It's only bad if you allow it to be bad.

You've beaten something that kills a lot of people and you're a survivor, a winner, a warrior; one who can tackle anything life throws at them because… well, because you're alive.

Chemotherapy can kill and give you cancer

This is one of the main arguments used by the alternative medicine fraternity, and they talk about it like it's a secret only they know. They ask how something used as medicine can kill, then bash you over the head with facts about how their treatment is gentle; but it's never been a secret, it's a fact. The other problem is using treatments that are so gentle they have no effect, means just that, they don't do anything and that's not a good idea when you have cancer. You need something tough and effective to kill what's trying to kill you. Sorry, that's just the way it works. No use throwing water down a germ-infested toilet and crossing your fingers, you have to use something that is going to kill the germs, so in a crude way, chemotherapy can be thought of as bleach for cancer cells. Now, don't go off on one after the covid debacle and say I'm suggesting an alternative way of curing cancer with bleach. You know better than that.

Chemotherapy can give you cancer is another secret only they know. Well, Cyclophosphamide was one of the drugs I was on which is known to have the potential to develop bladder cancer, which I've had twelve times now. Given the choice between the extra years I've been alive and not developing bladder cancer, would I have refused the drug in the first place? Nope. Not even a possibility. Sure, it's not nice developing another cancer, but it's better to be alive, fighting, than right and dead. One battle at a time.

Chemotherapy kills healthy cells, not just cancer cells. One of the big problems is when it wipes out your immune system leaving you unprotected against infection, and if an infection does take hold that is hard to target with antibiotics, it can end badly. Research is being done to develop treatment that only targets cancer cells, and although we're not there yet, I suspect it won't be too long before it's mainstream.

Useful Websites

Here are just some of the websites worldwide that I have found to be useful in my research.

American Cancer Society (USA) https://www.cancer.org

Canadian Cancer Society (Canada) http://www.cancer.ca

Cancer Australia (Australia) https://canceraustralia.gov.au/

Cancer Research (UK) https://www.cancerresearchuk.org

Irish Cancer Society (Ireland) https://www.cancer.ie/

Lymphoma Action (UK) https://lymphoma-action.org.uk/

Macmillan Cancer Support (UK) https://www.macmillan.org.uk

Marie Curie (UK) https://www.mariecurie.org.uk/

National Cancer Institute (USA) https://www.cancer.gov

The NHS (UK) https://www.nhs.uk/

There are other sites specialising in specific types of cancer, but I think it's fair to say that any information required can be obtained from the sites shown above.

Facebook Support Groups

I have found these groups to be useful; however, if you find a post that recommends you do something, check it out with your doctor first.

As I have had Non-Hodgkin Lymphoma, stem-cell transplant, bladder cancer, and kidney cancer, I can only list the ones relevant to my own diseases, but there are support groups for virtually any disease you can think of.

When choosing one, it's a good idea to look at how many members it has, and also if it allows anyone to post what they like, or if the posts have a moderator. The groups that have a moderator tend to be the best, as there is someone to police the posts, so if somebody tries to post something that is known to be dubious, it won't be posted.

Bladder Cancer Awareness/Support Group
https://www.facebook.com/groups/bladdercancerawareness/

Bladder Cancer Support And Social Group
https://www.facebook.com/groups/558442744366025/

Fight Bladder Cancer: Support
https://www.facebook.com/groups/bladdercanceruk/

Bone Marrow & Stem Cell Transplant Patient Support
https://www.facebook.com/groups/bonemarrowstemcelltransplant

Cold Agglutinin Disease (CAD) CAgD
https://www.facebook.com/groups/CADdisease/

The Depression and Mental Health Support Group
https://www.facebook.com/groups/1590995357823281/

Leukemia Survivors
https://www.facebook.com/groups/2205054913/

Living with CML...Chronic Myelogenous Leukemia
https://www.facebook.com/groups/158621161622/

Lymphoma Support Group
https://www.facebook.com/groups/113903748651959/

Hodgkin's Disease Refractory & Relapsed
https://www.facebook.com/groups/24106758410

Non-Hodgkins Lymphoma Christian Support Group
https://www.facebook.com/groups/480873928746286/

Hodgkin's Lymphoma Cancer Support
https://www.facebook.com/groups/374235959440861/

Hodgkin's Lymphoma Support Group 40796
https://www.facebook.com/groups/320871991340796/

Hodgkin's Non-Hodgkin's Lymphoma Support Group
https://www.facebook.com/groups/LymphomaHodgkins/

U.K Non-Hodgkin's Lymphoma
https://www.facebook.com/UKNHL

Non-Hodgkins Lymphoma Support
https://www.facebook.com/groups/61093336773/

UK Non-Hodgkin's Lymphoma support group
https://www.facebook.com/groups/1412013712343588/

Marginal Zone Non-Hodgkin's Lymphoma Support Group
https://www.facebook.com/groups/1734968436810226

UK NHL Social Network
https://www.facebook.com/groups/785923508115150/

Non-Hodgkin's Lymphoma (NHL)
https://www.facebook.com/groups/18306569192/

Kidney Cancer Help! Kidney Cancer.org
https://www.facebook.com/groups/kcahelps/

Kidney Cancer UK Support Group
https://www.facebook.com/groups/kcuksupportgroup/

Celebrities and cancer

Steve Jobs (died 5th October 2011)

The boss of Apple had the resources to use the best medical facilities in the world but choose to put his trust in alternative therapies before realising they weren't working. For nine months he tried acupuncture, coffee enemas, fruit juices, spiritualists and treatments found on the internet. When he eventually reverted to conventional medicine, the cancer had spread to the surrounding tissue and there was nothing that could be done. He spent $100,000 to have his DNA sequenced and threw more money at any potential solution, but it was too late. It has been speculated that if Jobs had started conventional treatment from the start, the outcome may well have been different: hell, if he had lived the world may well have been different. His biographer disclosed he (Jobs) regretted spending so long trying alternative medicine and should have taken the advice of the medical professionals.

Farrah Fawcett (died 25th June 2009)

The Charlie's Angels actress was diagnosed in 2006 with anal cancer. She opted for aggressive radiation treatment and chemotherapy, which cured the cancer within five months; however, during a routine check-up months later, a malignant polyp was found. Even though conventional treatment had provided a cure the first time, she decided to fly to Germany for alternative treatment that wasn't approved in the United States. She tried chemoablation, which is injecting chemicals directly into the affected organs, laser ablation which heats the tumour to 100 degrees Fahrenheit to try and fry the cancer cells, and immune boosting vitamins. When she returned to the United States, she experienced a blood clot in her abdomen muscles due to the repeated injections she had in Germany. In her documentary 'Farah's Story', she stated she was disillusioned with the German clinic when it used treatment more suitable for palliative care rather than cure. Traditional treatment would have removed the anus and rectum, which would have meant using a colostomy for the rest of her life, but she put her trust in alternative treatment instead, with unsurprising results.

She died on the same day Michael Jackson died which meant media coverage all but ignored her passing.

Olivia Newton-John (alive)

When she was diagnosed with breast cancer in 1992, the singer started chemotherapy and complementary treatments that included herbal supplements, meditation, visualisation and acupuncture, but had initially considered using homeopathic treatments and acupuncture instead of conventional treatment. In an interview with CNN she said: eventually, common sense prevailed and that maintaining a positive mindset throughout the experience also helped her heal.

Steve McQueen (died 7th November 1980)

When diagnosed with mesothelioma in 1989 (A type of cancer that develops in the thin tissue that covers many of the internal organs; the most common being the lining of the lungs and chest wall. The main cause is exposure to asbestos.), he shunned conventional medicine and decided to visit a doctor in Mexico who was a dentist that had been blacklisted by the American Cancer Society. He started a regime of daily vitamins and minerals, psychotherapy, coffee enemas, healing and prayer sessions (healing and prayer sessions are as useful as shouting at the waves of the sea), injections derived from sheep and cattle foetuses, laetrile (Vitamin B17, which isn't a vitamin), and apricot kernel injections (cyanide). Although he claimed he had recovered, he died shortly after completing treatment following surgery to remove tumours from his abdomen and neck.

Stephen Fry (alive)

During the writing of this book, I contacted Stephen Fry to see if he would allow me to use one of his quotations. He replied very quickly, gave me his blessing to use the quotation and wished me well.

What I didn't know at the time was he was going through his own cancer treatment.

It was kept very quiet and only made public around mid-February 2018.

He had been diagnosed with prostate cancer during a routine health check two months previously and needed immediate treatment. At age 60 he confessed it had taken him some time to come to terms with his diagnosis and said, "It's all pretty undignified and unfortunate."

Thankfully, his doctor caught it at the early stages, and after having the prostate and eleven lymph nodes removed (by robotic surgery, no less), he is now back at work.

It makes it all the more appreciated that during his journey through treatment, he took the time to contribute, and I'm in his debt.

Prince Charles (alive)

The problem, when someone who is famous or respected makes a comment, is it is broadly assumed knowledge that isn't available to mere mortals is being made public, when in reality, it's only an opinion; and that was a problem for Prince Charles in 2004 when he mentioned he knew a lady that had terminal cancer and she was cured using the Gerson Method.

As one of the main methods touted as a cure in the Gerson treatment is coffee enema, it didn't go down well with mainstream conventional medicine practitioners. (shoving coffee up your bum isn't something anyone normal would even consider, and especially as a cure for cancer)

At the time, Prince Charles was publicly attacked for recommending the treatment, when, in fact, he only suggested it merited more investigation to see whether it might work.

Again, the problem is when someone of his stature mentions a potential cure, it can be misconstrued as a recommendation.

Still, (and it's only my opinion) he should have either explained it better or not mentioned it in the first place.

…and Prince Charles is mentioned again later in the book, so that's something to look forward to.

Hall of Shame

…and then there are these opportunistic fucktards.

Cancer is a terrible disease, and everyone has a dark respect that means they treat it seriously and don't abuse it. Really? Well, not these people.

Help me, I'm sick.

In 2009, Belle Gibson experienced memory loss, walking difficulties and problems with her vision. She was only twenty years old and not long afterwards had a stroke and was admitted to hospital where they discovered she had terminal brain cancer and was given only four months to live.

She started a regime of chemotherapy and radiotherapy, but after two months, she decided to stop all treatment and explore the world of alternative medicine.

Around the same time, Instagram was launched, and she started posting as a cancer sufferer who was intent on healing herself with nutrition, holistic medicine, colonics, vitamins and oxygen therapy. As the treatment was obviously working, she amassed tens of thousands of followers, all wishing her well and paying attention to the treatment in case they were ever in the same position.

Her Instagram account was: Healing Bell. Belle Gibson. Game changer with brain cancer and a food obsession. She claimed what she was doing was raw and authentic.

Followers increased from tens of thousands to hundreds of thousands, and before long she wrote a book and developed an app called, The Whole Pantry, which went straight to the number one spot in the Apple App Store on launch.

Penguin books gave her an advance of A$132,500 (Australian dollars, approx £70,000 $91,000) which sold 16,000 copies in two months.

She went on a book tour, bought a new BMW, had her teeth straightened, hired a personal trainer and moved to a rented A$1m beach house.

Then it all went wrong.

In 2014 she had a forty-minute seizure at her son's birthday party, but no ambulance was required, as—although this was the worst seizure so far—she was used to them and assured everyone everything would be all right. Later, on Facebook she posted: 'I have seizures often as a result of my brain cancer, but nothing ever this long or intense.'

Within three weeks she was diagnosed with two more cancers, one secondary and one primary. She posted, 'I have cancer in my blood, spleen, brain, uterus, and liver. I am hurting.' Thankfully, she also remembered to promote her book that had made her over half a million dollars so far.

Questions were eventually asked about her lifestyle and how well she looked and how she could still exercise so much when she was so ill.

When the media started to take an interest in her, she finally admitted in 2015 she never had cancer.

In September 2017 she was fined A$410,000 (approx £217,000 $283,000). The judge said, "If there is one theme or pattern which emerges through her conduct, it is her relentless obsession with herself and what best serves her interests."

The book and app were withdrawn and her company 'Injkerman Road Nominees' was liquidated.

I'll miss my kids.

In 2014, Jennifer Flynn Cataldo was diagnosed with terminal cancer and all she wanted to do was take her kids to Disneyland.

She said it all started when dirty instruments were used to perform a biopsy, which resulted in sepsis (blood poisoning) that later turned to cancer. She had three tumours in her brain, twelve in her abdomen, and had to have one of her kidneys removed, even though both had cancer, they removed the one with the least disease.

She sued and was awarded $17 million in damages, but due to a mix-up in the court, the funds were paid out to the wrong person. Thankfully, the recipient understood and promised to forward it to the correct account, but three years later it was still outstanding.

Her father had given her nearly $500,000 to cover medical expenses while waiting for the claim to be paid, and she had received over $38,000 from two GoFundMe campaigns that people had donated to. In total, through social media, she received over $200,000 in donations.

When she was eventually caught, she confessed to making the whole thing up and was sentenced to twenty-five months in prison and ordered to pay $81,270 in restitution.

She addressed the court saying, “I am overcome with sorrow. They trusted me, they loved me. I was deceitful and I lied. I’m sorry. I don’t know a better word than sorry.”

It’s in my family.

Lacy Elizabeth Johnson was diagnosed with untreatable lung cancer, which was the same cancer her mum had died from. Only months later, it had metastasised to the brain and the only help available was in Mexico.

Lacy’s godmother Dorinda Gardner donated $28,000 from her retirement savings, and as Lacy was an active member of her church, they gave thousands to help as well.

Her ex-fiancé claimed that she used his personal details to obtain three credit cards in his name and ran him into more than $40,000 of debt.

After discovering that it was all a scam, Lacy was arrested, but even after that, she continued with a fundraising campaign to help her dad who was suffering from a non-existent skin cancer.

The court sentenced her to 180 days and five years on probation, and ordered that she pay $127,000 in restitution.

In a horrible twist, her grandmother did get cancer and issued the following statement. "Lacy, now I have lung cancer. Eight tumours to be exact, that are not responsive to conventional treatment. The money you stole from me is no longer available to help me in my time of need."

The one that got away.

In May 2014, a nursing assistant called Jenifer Gaskin was diagnosed with medullary thyroid cancer and the disease was terminal. She tackled it head on with a pre-chemo party, but later claimed her doctor recommended stopping chemotherapy and advised her to 'just enjoy the time you have left.'

A close friend started a GoFundMe page to help with medical expenses which raised over $10,000, but instead, Hanns used it to buy her daughter a second-hand car and get her son braces. When her friend suspected everything was not as it seemed, she contacted the police.

On investigation it was found she had faked her illness and never received treatment at any of the hospitals she had mentioned, and even though she was bald as a result of the chemotherapy she never had, it was discovered she had shaved her head in an attempt to convince friends and family of her illness.

GoFundMe took the decision to reimburse all of the donors who contributed, but authorities declined to prosecute Gaskin due to the expense involved in bringing so many witnesses—who donated between $20 and $50—to a trial.

Statistics, interesting stuff, Top 10 lists and a bit of cancer fun

Interesting cancer facts

The ancient Egyptians were the first civilisation to describe cancer. The earliest description was found in the Edwin Smith Papyrus which dates back to 1600BC. Although it describes breast tumours being removed by a tool called a Fire Drill, it also states there is no treatment.

The word cancer originates from the Latin for crab, just like the zodiac sign. When describing certain tumours which had veins or extensions from the main body, doctors originally called them crab-like, or cancerous.

Indoor tanning causes more cases of skin cancer than smoking causes lung cancer. A recent study concluded that there are over 419,000 new cases of skin cancer each year due to tanning in the US alone.

Men who have never married are up to 35% more likely to die from cancer than those who are married. In terms of surviving cancer, women also benefited from being married, but to a lesser extent.

The only known animal that is immune to cancer is the naked mole rat, which is due to a substance called hyaluronan that stops cancers growing.

It is more common to have breast cancer, kidney cancer, and melanoma on the left-hand-side. When I had my kidney cancer, it was on the left-hand side.

Currently there are over 43.8 million cancer survivors worldwide, and you need to be one of them.

CANCEROLOGY

Only 5-20% of cancers are hereditary.

Over fifty million people have died in the last decade due to tobacco.

Cancer is responsible for more deaths than AIDS, tuberculosis, and malaria combined.

Skin cancer is the most common form of cancer in the U.S., with over 2 million cases diagnosed every year. Many cases could be prevented by protecting the skin from overexposure to the sun and avoiding indoor tanning.

Less than six hours sleep a night puts you at risk of developing colon cancer.

One in every eight deaths worldwide are due to cancer.

Over 26,000 people die every day from cancer.

Cancer patients have twice the risk of suicide than the general population. Men are more likely to kill themselves immediately after a diagnosis.

The most common cancer that women suffer from is breast cancer. In 2018 25.4% of women diagnosed with cancer had breast cancer. The top three for women were: breast, colorectal, and lung cancer which contributed 43.9% of the total (excluding non-melanoma skin cancer).

African Americans are more likely than any other racial group to develop and die from cancer.

Asian Americans and Pacific Islanders have the lowest overall cancer rates.

Cancer is not just one disease; rather it is a set of diseases. Different agents cause each type of cancer.

The most common cancer that men suffer is lung cancer which contributed 15.5% of the total worldwide in 2018. The top three are lung, prostate, and colorectal cancer making up 44.4% of all cancers (excluding non-melanoma skin cancer).

It is estimated that 90% of lung cancer is caused by smoking.

Poor dental health can lead to systemic inflammation, which, in turn, increases the likelihood of developing cancer.

Women who have no children or who have their first pregnancy after the age of 30 have a slightly higher risk of developing breast cancer than those who become pregnant while they are younger. Breast-feeding may also reduce the risk of breast cancer slightly.

The lifetime risk of a man in the United States of developing an invasive cancer is 47%.

Breast cancer is considered a taboo in many Middle Eastern countries, and many women will not get tested because they fear being examined by male doctors.

During a 13.5-hour surgery in Texas, physicians were able to pull out a malignant brain tumour through an 11-year-old girl's nose.

Scientists claim that the nuclear disaster at Chernobyl produced the largest group of cancers in history from a single incident.

An alternative medical dictionary

Artery - The study of paintings.
Bacteria - Back door to cafeteria.
Barium - What doctors do when patients die.
Benign - What you be, after you be eight.
Caesarean Section - A neighbourhood in Rome.
Cat scan - Searching for kitty.
Cauterize - Make eye contact with her.
Colic - A sheep dog.
Coma - A punctuation mark.
Dilate - To not die early.
Enema - Not a friend.
Fester - Quicker than someone else.
Fibula - A small lie.
Impotent - Distinguished or well known.
Labour Pain - Getting hurt at work.
Medical Staff - A doctor's cane that may or may not have magic powers.
Morbid - Another higher offer.
Nitrates - Higher than day rates.
Node - I knew it.
Outpatient - A patient who has fainted.
Pelvis - Second cousin to Elvis.
Postoperative - A letter carrier.
Recovery Room - Where upholstery is done.
Rectum - Nearly killed him.
Secretion - Hiding something.
Seizure - Roman Emperor.
Tablet – Similar to a computer, but no keyboard.
Terminal Illness - Getting sick at the airport.
Tumour – Add another two.
Urine - Opposite of you're out.
Varicose - Near/close by.

The Top Ten Lists

10 Good things about having cancer

1) You can usually get to the front of any queue and get a seat in any waiting room. Walk unsteadily as you approach and explain you're dying of cancer. Cough in their general direction. (Okay, so this was written before Covid19 and I'm not changing it in the expectation/hope it's gonna be over soon, but you get the drift and you can still cough with a mask on if covid is still a pain when you read this.)

2) You can lose your inhibitions. What's the point of being embarrassed at this stage? Karaoke, speeches, dancing, whatever you were scared of is now just silly.

3) You'll find out who your real friends are. Some will be there for you whatever, and some just vanish like they never knew you.

4) You can laugh at other people who are less sick than you. They say, 'I've got a really bad cold I can't shift,' and you reply, 'Wanna swap? I'll see your silly cold and raise you terminal cancer.'

5) If you get caught speeding or double parked and somebody starts to write you a ticket, ask them the timescale to appear in court, and then tell them you'll be dead from your cancer before then. They usually stop writing at this stage.

6) You don't have to get up for work as a) they won't want you there and b) you're not strong enough anyway.

7) You can park anywhere with your disabled badge, and you can shout at people who take disabled spots and haven't got a badge.

8) If you're on holiday you don't have to leave the room early as it's your last holiday EVER. Who's gonna throw you out? All you have to say is that social media will love their attitude.

9) You can fart anywhere and blame it on the chemo.

10) You can use cancer as an excuse. 'I've got cancer,' is your phrase to get away with virtually anything.

And one last quick one for the ladies. You don't have to shave your legs anytime soon.

10 bad things about having cancer

1) You might die.

2) Your treatment could kill you.

3) They'll replace you at work.

4) Your relationship could change.

5) Your treatment will make you feel ill.

6) Your hair will probably fall out.

7) You'll have no energy.

8) You can't sleep when you want to.

9) You can't stay awake when you want to.

10) You might die.

See? The list of good things about cancer outweighs the list of bad, and you can have some fun at the same time.

10 Motivational Songs for Cancer

1) 'Always Look On The Bright Side Of Life' by Eric Idle.
You can't beat this one first thing in the morning.

2) 'Bring Me Sunshine' by Morcambe and Wise.
If this doesn't bring a smile to your face, nothing will.

3) 'Don't Stop Thinking About Tomorrow' by Fleetwood Mac.
This one works for my 'tomorrow will be better' mantra.

4) 'One Shot' by Eminem.

Yes, it's about a rapper, but still someone facing and overcoming fear.

5) 'I'm Still Standing' by Elton John and Bernie Taupin.
It just screams, never give up.

6) 'It's My Life' by Bon Jovi.
'It's my life, and it's now or never.' What more do you need?

7) 'I'm a survivor' by Destiny's Child.
I think the title says more than I ever could.

8) 'I Will Survive' by Gloria Gaynor.
Say goodbye to your cancer by changing some of the lyrics.

9) 'Don't Stop Believing' by Journey.
Believe it's going to be okay, treatment works.

10) 'Eye of the Tiger' by Survivor.
Sing this one during chemo sessions and get everyone to join in.

Finally, a sing-a-long song for the ward. 'We Are the Champions' by Queen
'I consider it a challenge before the whole human race, and I never lose.' It's all in the chorus.

10 Ways to Know You are a Cancer Survivor

1: Your alarm clock goes off at 6 a.m. and you're glad to hear it.

2: Your mother-in-law invites you to lunch and you just say, 'No.'

3: You're back in the family rotation to take out the garbage.

4: When you no longer have an urge to choke the person who says, 'All you need to beat cancer is the right attitude.'

5: When your dental floss runs out and you buy 1000 yards.

6: When you use your toothbrush to brush your teeth instead of your hair.

7: You have a chance to buy additional life insurance, but you buy a new convertible instead.

8: Your doctor tells you to lose weight and do something about your cholesterol, and you actually listen.

9: When your biggest annual celebration is again your birthday, and not the day you were diagnosed.

10: When you use your Visa card more than your hospital parking pass.

The best things to say to someone with cancer.

I don't really know what to say.
Honest and straight to the point.

You look good.
Even when you know it's a lie, it still makes you feel better.

How can I help?
Something that can be appreciated.

I'm sorry this has happened to you.
Genuine feelings.

If you ever feel like talking, I'm here to listen.
You need someone like this.

I care about you.
This statement always gives a little lift.

I'm thinking about you.
Always nice to know.

If you need a lift or need groceries or help with the housework, just call and I'll organise everything.
Really appreciated.

I'm sorry you're going through this.
Genuine sympathy.

I'll remember you in my prayers.

Whether you believe or not, it's a nice thing to hear.

And again, the best one last.

I'm really sorry and I know it's tough, but I had the same thing so ask me anything.
Just the fact they've beat it gives you a lift and confirms that it can be beat.

Things you should never say to someone with cancer.

Everybody means well, and sometimes it's a case of not knowing the right thing to say at the time and just blurting out the first thing that comes to mind. Understand and forgive when it happens to you.

A friend of mine who is suffering from Non-Hodgkin Lymphoma stage 4 was told that it was a good cancer to have, when in fact the old way of thinking was that Hodgkin Lymphoma was the best out of the two as it has the Reed Steenberg cell that can be better targeted by chemotherapy, but things have now changed with treatment and both are treated equal.

My friend had done her research and knew about the new thinking, but her friend was mixing the two up, and although trying to be helpful, was just an annoyance.

The main problem, is when someone who has never had cancer, knows better than the sufferer what it's like.

When something is said that frustrates, just realise it comes from a good place, thank them, and move on.

Common phrases include:

"You're are so brave."
"I don't have a choice, do I? It's here and I'm dealing with it."

"Have you thought about trying XYZ, it worked for my friend?"
"Gee, I'll have to tell the doctors they've got it wrong, as you (you idiot) know better."

"That's a good cancer to have."
"Really? Ya think? Lucky me. It's only trying to kill me."

"Cancer treatment isn't as hard as it used to be."
"And you would know this how? All treatment is hard when you're going through it."

"If anyone can beat this, you can."
"Yeah, you're right, I can, which means that the others who died didn't fight hard enough."

"What caused your cancer?"
"Nobody knows exactly what causes cancer, but you think I should know?"

"Have you tried praying?"
"Did that before and my lottery numbers never came up, but I hear it's what all the hospitals recommend now."

"I've always wanted to shave my head."
"Great, all my friends are doing it on Saturday to show their support, here, let me get you the name of the hairdresser."

"God never gives you anything you can't deal with."
"I must remember to thank him."

"Remember, there's always someone worse off than you."
"Yeah, like you. Born without a brain."

"You got this."
"Yeah, cancer. I got cancer. It's not like I'm good at it?"

"I didn't think you'd be up for chemo."
"Wow, is that because the alternative is so much better?"

"You'll be fine."
"And you know this how?"

“At least you don’t have to work.”
“Which is great, as the cancer fairy left a suitcase full of cash under the bed.”

“I know how you feel.”
“No, you don’t. You haven’t a clue unless you’ve been through it.”

“My advice is, you shouldn’t mope around and get up and do something.”
“Great, now I know what to do with all this excess energy I don’t have.”

“I suppose you’re scared of dying?”
“No, it’s something I’m really looking forward to, how about you?”

“My friend died from that.”
“Thanks for that. Have you thought about taking up motivational speaking?”

I saved the best till last, and yes, I’ve had this said to me so many times.

“Look at you, I thought you were dead.”
“How was my funeral? Were there many there?”

Sometimes, in trying to help someone feel better, we end up invalidating their feelings.

Statements like “you shouldn’t feel that way”, or “it could be worse”, although well-meaning, can be quite damaging. They deny that person’s perspective and make them feel worse.

You can validate a person’s emotional experience without necessarily agreeing with it. Try to understand why they feel that way. Just be willing to listen, and withhold judgment.

Avoid offering unsolicited advice or forcing positivity on them. Create a safe space for the other person to feel their feelings.

Cancer statistics

WorldwidePopulation 7.67 billion

Estimated number of new cases each year is 18.1 million (49,589 per day/2066 per hour/34 per minute) Just think about that, more than one new case every two seconds?

By 2030 it is forecast the figure will rise to 23.6 million each year.

Estimated number of deaths from cancer each year is 9.6 million (26,300 per day/1098 per hour/18 per minute) Just under four seconds and cancer has murdered someone else.

United States of America

Population 328.2 million

Estimated number of new cases each year is 1,762,450 (4,828 per day)

Estimated number of deaths from cancer each year is 609,640 (1,670 per day)

United Kingdom

Population 66.65 million

Estimated number of new cases each year is 367,000 (1005 per day)

Estimated number of deaths from cancer each year is 165,000 (452 per day)

Canada

Population 37.59 million

Estimated number of new cases each year is 220,400 (603 per day)

Estimated number of deaths from cancer each year is 82,100 (224 per day)

Australia

Population 25.36 million

Estimated number of new cases each year is 145,000 (397 per day)

Estimated number of deaths from cancer each year is 50,000 (136 per day)

Ireland

Population 4.90 million

Estimated number of new cases each year is over 40,000 (109 per day)

Estimated number of deaths from cancer each year is over 9,000 (24 per day)

The figures were taken from government and major charity websites in the relevant countries and are mostly 2019/20 figures. By the time they're published they're already out of date, but for the purposes of illustrating how serious the problem is, they will suffice.

Frequency of cancer by country

Age-standardised rate for all cancers (excluding non-melanoma skin cancer) ordered by the countries with the 50 highest rates at the time of going to print.

1. Denmark
338.1 per 100,000

2. France
324.6 per 100,000

3. Australia
323.0 per 100,000

4. Belgium
321.1 per 100,000

5. Norway
318.3 per 100,000

6. United States
318.0 per 100,000

7. Ireland
307.9 per 100,000

8. South Korea
307.8 per 100,000

9. The Netherlands
304.8 per 100,000

10. New Caledonia
297.9 per 100,000

11. Slovenia
296.3 per 100,000

12. Canada
295.7 per 100,000

13. New Zealand
295.0 per 100,000

14. Czech Republic
293.8 per 100,000

15. Switzerland
287.0 per 100,000

16. Hungary
285.4 per 100,000

17. Iceland
284.3 per 100,000

18. Germany
283.8 per 100,000

19. Israel
283. per 100,000

20. Luxembourg
280.3 per 100,000

21. Italy
278.6 per 100,000

22. Slovakia
276.9 per 100,000

23. United Kingdom
272.9 per 100,000

24. Sweden
270.0 per 100,000

25. Serbia
269.7 per 100,000

26. Croatia
266.9 per 100,000

27. Barbados
263.1 per 100,000

28. Armenia
257.0 per 100,000

29. Finland
256.8 per 100,000

30. French Polynesia
255.0 per 100,000

31. Austria
254.1 per 100,000

32. Lithuania
251.9 per 100,000

33. Uruguay
251.0 per 100,000

34. Spain
249.0 per 100,000

35. Latvia
246.8 per 100,000

36. Portugal
246.2 per 100,000

37. France, Martinique
245 per 100,000

38. Malta
242.9 per 100,000

39. Estonia
242.8 per 100,000

40. Macedonia
239.3 per 100,000

41. Montenegro
238.3 per 100,000

42. Kazakhstan
236.5 per 100,000

43. Bulgaria
234.8 per 100,000

44. Poland
229.6 per 100,000

45. Romania
224.2 per 100,000

46. Belarus
218.7 per 100,000

47. Cuba
218.0 per 100,000

48. Japan
217.1 per 100,000

49. Argentina
216.7 per 100,000

50. Puerto Rico
211.1 per 100,000

Let's find some humour in your tumour

Yes folks, we got cancer jokes.
This section isn't meant to offend, but it's a humorous look at cancer.
People have asked how I can joke about something so serious, but having had it so many times, if I can't laugh at it, nobody can. It's a coping mechanism and I do have a mischievous sense of humour as friends on my Facebook page can confirm, so you've been warned.
If you feel it's inappropriate to joke about the subject or too early in your journey, then please skip this section and accept my apologies.

I went to see my doctor, he said, "Tell me, what's your star sign?"
"Cancer," I replied.
"Oh, what a coincidence."

I started smoking to impress this girl who liked people who were into cancer.
Turns out she was talking about the star sign. Anyway, I've three months to live.

Q: What's the difference between God and a Surgeon?
A: God doesn't think he's a surgeon.

A man isn't feeling well, so he goes to see his doctor.
The doctor examines him, then asks to speak with his wife. He tells her that her husband has cancer.
The wife asks, "Can he be cured?"
The doctor replies, "There's a chance we can cure him with chemotherapy, but you will need to take care of him every day for the next year—cooking all the meals, cleaning up the vomit, changing the bed pan, driving him to the hospital for daily treatments, and so on."
When the wife comes out to the waiting room, the husband asks her what the doctor said.
The wife answers, "He said you're going to die."

Q: How can nurses stand to work in busy hospitals?
A: They have lots of patients.

Q: What do you call a doctor who is always on the telephone?
A: An ON-CALLogist.

Q: What do you call bugs with cancer?
A: MalignANT and BEEnign.

A patient visited his urologist for testicular cancer and expressed concern about being able to perform after the operation. The patient was also worried about the chemotherapy.
The doctor said, “I too had testicular cancer a few years ago. Ten days after the operation I made passionate love with my wife and forgot all my worries. Try it and see for yourself.”
Three weeks later the patient returns and thanks the doctor effusively.
The doctor says, “I’m glad my advice helped.”
The patient thanks him again, and as he’s leaving says, “By the way, Doc, you have a really beautiful house.”

Cancer cures smoking, eventually.

Dark humour is like a child with cancer. It never gets old.

When I told a friend that I have cancer, he replied, “I thought you were a Scorpio.”

A man hears from his doctor that he has cancer and has six months to live. The doctor recommends he marry an accountant and move to a posh neighbourhood.
The man asks, “Will this cure my cancer?”
“No,” said the doctor, “but the six months will seem a hell of a lot longer.”

Doctor: “I’ve got your test results and I have some bad news. You have Cancer and Alzheimer’s.”
Patient: “Wow, that’s lucky, I was afraid I had cancer.”

CANCEROLOGY

Q: What do you call a person who has a compulsion to get lymphoma over and over again?
A: A Lymphomaniac.

Smoking causes cancer, but it cures salmon.

On a flight, the pilot announced, "That thump you heard was our last engine conking out. I'm really sorry to tell you this, but we are going to crash into the ocean."
In the stunned silence that followed, an angry voice spoke out. "Dammit. That stupid doctor of mine said I was going to die of cancer."

Q: Why did the cancer victim cross the road?
A: He was hoping to get hit by a truck.

Did you hear about the clown who couldn't stop laughing about his cancer?
Yeah, he had a weird sense of tumour.

Mary was walking through Tesco when she ran into Harry, who she hadn't seen in a couple of years. They got to talking and eventually Harry enquired after her husband.
"Oh, haven't you heard? He's no longer with us."
"He's dead?"
"Yes."
"I'm sorry to hear that. If it's not too intrusive, can I enquire what he died of?"
"The big C got him."
"Oh my God," he replied. "Cancer is so common nowadays."
"It wasn't cancer, he fell overboard the Belfast to Liverpool ferry, and drowned in the big sea."

An Irishman named Mike O'Leary went to his doctor after a long illness. The doctor, after a lengthy examination, sighed, looked Mike in the eye and said, "I've some bad news for you . . . you have a cancer known as Galloping Leukaemia and it can't be cured. I give you two weeks to a month at best."

Mike, who was shocked and saddened by the news, managed to compose himself and walk from the doctor's office into the waiting room. There he saw his son and said, "Son, we Irish celebrate when things are good, and we celebrate when things don't go so well. In this case, things aren't so well. I have cancer and I've been given a short time to live. Let's head for the pub and have a few pints."

After three or four pints, the two were feeling a little less sombre. There were some laughs, some tears, and more beers. They were eventually approached by some of Mike's old friends who asked what the two were celebrating. Mike told them that the Irish celebrate the good and the bad. He went on to tell them that they were drinking to his impending end. He told his friends, "I've only got a few weeks to live as I have been diagnosed with AIDS." The friends gave O'Leary their condolences and they all had a few more beers.

After his friends left, Mike's son leaned over and whispered in confusion, "Dad, I thought you said you were dying from cancer. You just told your friends you were dying from AIDS."

Mike replied, "I am dying from cancer, Son. I just don't want any of them sleeping with your mother after I'm gone."

Doctor: It's a very serious cancer.
Patient: Just tell me how long I've got, Doc.
Doctor: Ten—
Patient: Ten years, Ten months?
Doctor: Nine, eight, seven…

CANCEROLOGY

Three guys were talking about death and dying. One asked, "When you're in your casket and friends and family are mourning, what would you like to hear them say?"
The first guy says, "I would like to hear them say I was a great doctor of my time and a great family man."
The second man says, "I would like to hear I was a wonderful husband and schoolteacher who made a huge difference in our children of tomorrow."
The last guy says, "I would like to hear them say, *look, he's moving*."

Q: How many cancer patients does it take to screw in a light bulb?
A: Just one, but it takes a support group to cheer him on, and there's a lot of grieving afterwards.

Q: What's the difference between an oral and a rectal thermometer?
A: The taste.

Real Doctor's Notes

1. Patient has two teenage children, but no other abnormalities.
2. Patient has chest pain if she lies on her left side for over a year.
3. On the second day, the knee was better, and then on the third day it disappeared.
4. The patient is tearful and crying constantly. She also appears to be depressed.
5. Discharge status: Alive, but without my permission.
6. Healthy-appearing decrepit, 69-year-old male, mentally alert but forgetful.
7. The patient refused autopsy.
8. The patient has no previous history of successful suicides.
9. Patient has left his white blood cells at another hospital.
10. Patient's medical history has been remarkably insignificant with only a 40-pound weight gain in the last three days.
11. She is numb from her toes down.

12. Occasional, constant, infrequent headaches.
13. I saw your patient today, who is still under our car [sic] for physical therapy.
14. Skin: somewhat pale but present.
15. The patient has been depressed since she began seeing me.

Q: What's the difference between a skinhead and a cancer victim?
A: The skinhead's not going to die from a horrible, incurable disease.

Q: What's the difference between a cancer victim and someone with AIDS?
A: You won't get sick from shagging a cancer victim.

Q: How many cancer victims does it take to change a light bulb?
A: None: they're too weak to climb the ladder.

Q: What does chemotherapy have in common with its patients?
A: They both have half-lives. (a little chemistry joke there)

Q: You know what's so great about cancer?
A: Nothing.

"Hey, Doctor, those suppository things you prescribed taste horrible and stick to my teeth."
"What? You didn't swallow them, did you?"
"What else was I supposed to do with them? Shove them up my ass?"

Did you hear they finally found a cure for cancer? It's called Death.

I don't get why cancer is so hard to beat. I'm already on stage 4.

What do you call a kid with cancer walking through the airport?
Terminal

CANCEROLOGY

A rich Arab oil sheikh discovers he has a rare form of blood cancer, so he scours the world looking for a match for his blood type, which is also rare. He discovers a Scottish man as a match and the Scottish man agrees to donate blood to him.
The sheikh rewards him with lavish gifts, fancy cars, a mansion, and the finest luxury clothes.
Two years later, the sheikh discovers his cancer has returned. He reaches out again to the Scottish man, who once again agrees to donate blood.
The sheikh rewards the Scottish man with a coupon for a small coffee at a local cafe.
The Scottish man says "Well, thank you for that, but you were a bit more generous last time."
The Sheikh replies, "Well yes, but… that was before I had Scottish blood in me."

The leading cause of cancers is having sex in October.

Cancer sucks at first... But it grows on you over time.

Q: How would you best describe prostate cancer?
A: It is somewhere between a dick and an asshole.

My friend's mother always has a positive attitude. When she learned of her daughter's cancer diagnosis she said, "Well honey, at least you'll lose some weight."

Q: What do you call a movie that has kids with cancer?
A: Finding Chemo.

A woman visits her doctor as she has some stomach pains and suspects she may be pregnant. After her examination, the doctor says, "I hope you like changing nappies."
She replies: "Oh my god, so I'm pregnant?"
The doctor shakes his head. "No, you've got bowel cancer."

Q: What's the most expensive haircut in the world?
A: Chemotherapy.

Q: What's long and bald and moves slowly?
A: The conga line in the cancer ward.

A woman goes to the doctor and says, "I think I have cancer."
The doctor checks her and says, "It's all in your head."
"Phew," she says.
"Yes," the doctor says, "one big tumour, right in the middle."

The unlucky Lord.
When the Lord of the Manor comes back from vacation, he meets his gardener at the gates of his park looking a bit shifty.
Lord: "Has something happened while I was gone?"
Gardener: "Nothing much, I just broke a shovel while I was burying your dog."
Lord: "My dog died?"
Gardener: "Yes, it choked on the smoke when your mansion burnt down."
Lord: "My mansion? Burnt down? How?"
Gardener: "Well, your wife was distraught and dropped a candle on the curtains."
Lord: "Why was she distraught?"
Gardener: "She received the news of your daughter being kidnapped."
Lord: My daughter, kidnapped? Don't you have any positive news for me?"
Gardener: "Oh right, nearly forgot. Your cancer test results came back."

Doctor: "You're as healthy as a horse, Jimmy."
Jimmy: "That's great."
Doctor: "Yeah, A horse with cancer."

Alternative medicine

"Alternative medicine people call themselves "holistic" and say it's the "whole" approach. Well, if it's the whole approach, let it be the mind as well. Use logic, use sense, use the incredible five wits you were given by creation." ~ Stephen Fry

The cancer bandwagon

Once upon a time, before Twitter, Facebook, Snapchat, TikTok and Instagram; cancer was (and still is, to a lesser extent) a taboo subject. Nobody wanted it, and people talked about it in hushed voices. There was a dark fear of it and anyone who was going through treatment was also treated with respect. It wasn't something to be taken lightly. But all that changed when social media opened both the world and the con artists to the benefits of an easy scam.

Snake oil salesmen climbed on board promising a quick and complete cure for any type of cancer, as long as you were stupid enough and had the cash to buy the new super snake oil cures they were now peddling.

YouTube introduced the world to doctors (who may, or may not have been worthy of the honorific) who extolled the benefits of the new products and everything was tickety-boo; except the con men kept getting richer, and the cancer sufferers? Well, as the snake oil didn't work, they just died. Still, there was a money-back guarantee, but nobody was around to avail of it.

Let me, for a minute, give you a ridiculous example.

You have a severe headache, and you mention it to your doctor.

"Not to worry," he says, "we'll make some coffee."

"I just drink the coffee and it cures my headache?"

"No, we have to wait until it cools down a bit, then we pour it into this bag."

You look at the bag and notice the long tube at the bottom. "Then I drink it?"

"No," he replies, "then we stick this tube up your bum and squirt in the coffee."

"Are you nuts?" you scream, making sure to give the door a loud bang on the way out.

Now, the question is: is this a realistic scenario in the circumstances?

For most people, the answer is yes. Why would anyone think putting coffee up your bum would cure a headache? Yet for cancer sufferers, this is the suggested protocol the quacks recommend, and their patients accept it without question in an attempt to beat their cancer. (Steve McQueen/Steve Jobs)

Nobody would consider it for a headache, yet cancer?

Coffee enemas are one of the most popular alternative cures for cancer, yet they don't work; but people watch the videos, read the blurb, and convince themselves.

The con men have you where they want you. Vulnerable and open to suggestions, no matter how foolish they may seem.

I found a site over a year ago (which is no longer there) that had a convincing video of a guy who had the same cancer as me, and after using a new and revolutionary magnetic therapy treatment (which doesn't work) had a complete remission in only six weeks. The doctor had initially told him he needed chemotherapy and radiation, but he did his research and discovered magnetic therapy and it was a miracle, hallelujah. The doctors couldn't believe it, etc. I knew it was rubbish but as the video was so convincing, I bookmarked it and forgot about it. Then later, as a result of having my heart checked and discovering my rhythm was odd, I did a bit of research and discovered the same guy in another video. This time he was scheduled for triple bypass surgery, but after checking the web and discovering magnetic therapy, blah, blah, blah.

The company concerned had obviously hired an actor and used him to promote both cancer and heart cures using a magnetic pulse machine. Same background, same graphics, same machine, and he was even wearing the same trousers and shirt. They didn't even think it necessary to use a different actor as people will believe anything. I bookmarked it too and wrote a whole piece on it, but as the site has now either been removed or the owners made so much money they didn't need it anymore, it's gone. I often wonder how many people fell for the $3000+ scam and how many relied on it and died as a result.

The Magic Cure

Everyone, including me, wants to believe there is a magic cure for cancer, and while I have no doubt research will eventually find one, I doubt one of the numerous bogus sites on the internet will develop it. Think about it for a minute; if the cure is found by someone outside conventional research, they would become overnight bazillionaires, but not by trying to sell one or two at a time at inflated prices on the internet. Worldwide recognition and untold wealth await anyone who finds it, yet the claim is made every day on social media and nobody thinks to question why it's not all over the real news. The reason is—it doesn't work. It's a scam. Someone gets rich and someone dies. That's life.

The beliefs of those who want to believe without questioning the validity of the claims made, is a type of ostrich syndrome, where they're not just sticking their head in the sand, but up their own backside.

While it is true that all of the scam cures that don't have any effect can trigger the placebo effect, they offer no real treatment, although some that can have an effect—such as apricot kernels—can actually kill (cyanide poisoning, thank you very much).

There is a reason the cons work, and that is, they play on our fears and offer a magic solution. We want to believe, and we need to believe, so we believe, irrespective of overwhelming evidence it's just a con, and when it doesn't work, we explain it away with the excuse that conventional medicine sometimes fails as well.

The only thing I can think of that is worse than offering a cure that doesn't work, is someone who commits murder, but, in effect, that's what these people are doing anyway. Don't use conventional methods, buy from us instead. Just die, we don't care.

Why would anyone listen? Why would anyone believe? But they do.

So-Called Alternative Medicine

Let's just call it SCAM for short, because that's what it is.

Q: "You know what they call alternative medicine that's been proved to work? A: Medicine." ~ Tim Minchin

There are people on this world that claim to have a cure for cancer. Only they have it, and for a fee, you can have it too.

They claim their cures are not available in hospitals as Big Pharma won't let the hospitals use it as it would cost them billions.

The people who peddle this crap are liars, thieves, cheats, con-artists, and ultimately, murderers. They have no qualms about the outcome as long as their bank balance benefits. And yes, murderer is the right word as their treatment does nothing towards achieving a cure. It's a scam to cheat sufferers out of their money with a cure that doesn't exist—simple as that.

Anyone who preys on cancer sufferers (or victims of any other illness for that matter) with the sole aim of getting rich by empty promises, should be dealt with in the same manner as other murderers.

Anyway, rant over. Just my opinion.

Magical Mexico

Mexico is a beautiful country, famous for its food, sombreros, fabulous beaches, and the Mexican Wave that's used at sporting events to celebrate victories. It's when people stand up at different times, throw their arms in the air then sit again, and it creates a ripple effect across a crowd; it's wonderful, and it's very popular.

But did you know there are two Mexican Waves? The second one is where someone with cancer goes to an alternative treatment centre in Mexico for a magic cure and waves goodbye not only to their money—usually around £20-£50,000—but also their life, as the treatments are usually bogus and do not cure cancer.

The world centre for alternative, emotionally driven cancer cures—or to put it another way, treatments that don't work—is Mexico. It is becoming a top medical tourism destination for patients from around the world, and over one million people are expected to travel to Mexico this year for affordable alternative medical procedures. The reason they're affordable is they do nothing. They don't work. But, hey, they're profitable.

Many of these people hail from the United States where healthcare costs keep rising; however, people from all parts of the globe visit in the hope of a miracle cure. Basically, if someone doesn't like the sound of surgery, chemo, or radiation, some conman will offer a cure (that doesn't work) that is easier to tolerate—until, that is, you die.

Part of the attraction is its unconventional cancer treatments, which are either too expensive to access in patients' home countries or not approved in general (because they don't do anything).

They sell hope—false hope, to cancer sufferers. They even include the word 'hope' in some of the hospital names?

Mexico's medical tourism industry generates over three billion US dollars a year, with new clinics and alternative health facilities always under construction.

Diego Ballesteros Pino, the Director of Oncology at the Baja California Health Authority, is a conventional cancer specialist in Mexico. He says: "They (the clinics) are definitely predatory, and they're making a profit from people's lives."

Dr Kurt W Donsbach DC ND PhD was one of the major players, until the FBI arrested him. He ran the Hospital Santa Monica, which was subsequently renamed The Alpha Medical Clinic and moved to new premises after his arrest. He didn't have any qualifications and was selling a product called Poly-MVA under the brand name Quercetin Plus that he had modified with synthetic estrogen/oestrogen, which, when taken without blood thinners, causes severe blood clots and can lead to death.

His big mistake was when he stepped over the border into the US for a radio show where he promised a 99% cure for prostate cancer in his broadcast, without having anything to back it up. "Come to my hospital in Mexico and bring $23,000 (cash-up-front, of course) and I'll cure you," he said.

Over 400,000 pages of evidence were presented at his trial, and it was discovered that over an eighteen-month period, he had accumulated over $32m from his fake cancer cures. Thirty-Two Million Dollars? He was sentenced to one year in prison but ended up with six months of house arrest after coming to a deal to testify in another court case.

In an undercover video interview with his replacement, Dr Humberto Barboza (who took over running the clinic under the new name) stated, "Mexican law is not too tight, like in the US," and "if you want to cut your life, do chemotherapy." He then went on to bargain with, "how much will you pay for your life, it's only $21,000."

For treatment that doesn't work? It's emotional blackmail at its best, and—let's not beat around the bush—at its worst, it's murder, plain and simple.

Some may ask why Mexico allow these clinics to operate, but the surprising fact is they are not registered as hospitals but rather palliative care centres, which means they deal with end-of-life patients. I suppose a 'what's the harm, they're gonna die anyway' attitude could apply. The problem is, palliative care is used to make the patient comfortable, whereas the clinics are unashamedly offering a cure for cancer—which is not the intended use.

Still, as long as they can refuel their Lear Jets and buy the girlfriend a new Bentley occasionally, who really gets hurt?

They sell hope to patients who can't afford conventional treatment, or who have no other alternatives, and with the cost of extended medical care in, say, America, a miracle cure that is capped at only $30,000 in Mexico seems like a bargain, only they forget to mention that in addition to the payment it could cost you your life.

The fact these alternative doctors operating in Mexico aren't even recognised as doctors anywhere else in the civilised world should start alarm bells ringing, although, to be fair, if you believe putting liquid coffee up your bum is a cure for cancer, you're in trouble anyway.

You would think given the success rate being non-existent would give those so-called doctors a clue their cure isn't working, but as it's all about the money, it doesn't matter.

Before he retired, Edzard Ernst was a Professor of Complementary Medicine at Exeter University. He describes some of the cures offered in Mexico as irresponsible and criminal as the claims are not supported by evidence and are illegal. He says: "As the internet is uncontrollable, the sites offering bogus cures can offer any therapies they wish without fear of prosecution." He goes on to say: "There is no alternative cancer cure, full stop, and there never will be one."

One of the examples Ernst gives is Ozonated Hyperthermia Treatment which the Mexican clinics recommend. The theory revolves around the fact that cell death occurs when a temperature of 42°C/107.6°F is achieved, so raising the core body temperature will kill cancer cells. At the temperature required, not only do cells die, but the person does as well. The Mexican clinics counter this argument by saying a normal sauna is well in excess of this temperature, and although this is true, the body temperature of a healthy person is automatically maintained to within 1-2^{0}C/2-4°F of normal—which means, it could never work anyway.

The fact is the practises allowed in Mexico are not allowed anywhere else in the civilised world.

I have a question for the government of Mexico which authorises and regulates these clinics. If a clinic in Mexico offers a bogus cure, that everyone—including their own qualified cancer specialists—knows doesn't work, and someone dies as a result, why isn't anyone charged with the murder of that person?

It seems to me that as long as this bogus and distasteful practice keeps bringing investment to Mexico, the government isn't concerned with the outcome for the patients and turns a blind eye.

Alternative Treatment

There have been a multitude of cases worldwide where an alternative practitioner has diagnosed someone with cancer and then offered them the lifesaving treatment that only they provide. Unfortunately, a lot of people that have had the cancer treatment, never had cancer in the first place, so when they're cured of the cancer they didn't have—it's a miracle. Praise the Lord and throw your hands in the air.

If you feel unwell, your first point of contact should be with a real doctor. Once tests such as blood work, biopsy, CT scan, etc., have been done, then a diagnosis can be arrived at, but when somebody asks you to place your palm on a metal plate and hold a metal rod, then they hit a few buttons and say you have brain cancer—but not to worry because they can cure you with eight treatments on their cutting-edge machine—you need to take a step back and wonder why real hospitals aren't using this wondrous technology. The answer is real hospitals don't use it as it doesn't work. No, not even a little-itty bit. Nothing. Nada. It's nothing more than a con. (Bioresonance is the practice I'm talking about, but there are loads of other interesting machines that do nothing as well)

Some of you will be reading this and wondering why anyone would be so easily taken in, but right back at the start of this book I pointed out that the brain will do everything in a frantic scramble to obtain a cure, and this also includes suspension of disbelief. You will sacrifice realism and logic in an attempt to beat your cancer.

In fairness, the charlatans are extremely convincing, and even use actors to give them glorious praise in their promotional videos; but then most con artists are experts at deception, by definition.

What you read on the internet will be plausible

A lot of the supposedly scientific experiments quoted are based on the principle of cell destruction in a petri dish; the theory being that if something kills the cancer cells, then it must be good for you; which could be construed as a logical conclusion but for the fact that acid and bleach also kill cells in a dish, so would it be a good idea to drink acid or bleach, or inject it?

The complexity of the body means that just because something works in a dish, it won't necessarily work when introduced into the human body.

The throw everything at it approach

It's worth pointing out that a lot of alternative medicine practitioners suggest any number of treatments for the disease in the hope something will stick. Enemas, nuts, diet, praying, voodoo, etc.

Unlike conventional medicine where they weigh you and prescribe a treatment plan in a strictly monitored order, the alternative treatments include anything and everything currently in vogue in an attempt to separate you from your money.

I would ask that if the treatment actually works, why is it not a standard regime for every patient based on quantifiable medical parameters?

Why does every alternative treatment practitioner recommend different regimes for the same condition?

Trust me, I'm a doctor.

How valid is your doctor? Are they what they claim to be?

If you are considering alternative treatment, get advice first and research it thoroughly.

A lot of treatment centres have their own websites and they use Doctors to validate their claims (in one case, the doctor turned out to be a vet).

In a huge amount of cases, it was doctors who had completed an online course. Courses not recognised by any genuine medical establishment anywhere in the world, and they usually have no relevant medical training to treat cancer patients.

Did you know you can call yourself a Cancer Coach by simply logging on to beatcancer.org/services/cancer-certification, pay $500 and do an online course? At the time of writing the course has an advertised value of $15,474, but they're offering a discount of $14,974. I have to confess, the discount alone made me wonder how much anything offered is actually worth. If you went to buy a new car at $15K and the salesman instantly dropped the price to $500, I think you would wonder if the car was worth buying in the first place.

If someone told me they were a cancer coach, I would assume they had both medical training and experience working in a hospital, but no, apparently, it's not a requirement.

Even more worrying is the fact you can do an online course and call yourself a Doctor of Natural Medicine or a Doctor of Integrative Medicine from as little as $2500 and doing forty hours study, which, of course, anyone can do on your behalf if you're too busy. There are no checks and balances and you're a qualified Doctor. The question is: qualified for what?

Some don't even bother with any type of course and just make the claim of being a doctor as they know nobody will check.

Real doctors spend a huge amount of time studying and doing practical exams before even being allowed on a ward, let alone treat a patient.

If you put your life in the hands of one of these bogus doctors—because that's what you're doing—and it doesn't turn out well, will it really be a surprise?

Be very wary of anything you see online promising a quick cure in exchange for money.

If it's in Latin, it's believable

Sometimes—like the legal profession—the sellers of various treatments intentionally confuse with words like in-vitro or in-vivo and we look at them and think, that must mean something scientific. Sounds impressive, so it must be real.

In-vitro means something is done in a test tube, petri dish, culture dish, or a container outside the human body. When the alternative community say in-vitro testing has been done and 100% of cancer cells were eradicated; it's the same as saying, we put cancer cells in a dish and poured bleach/whiskey/vodka on them and they died. Yeah, that's what happens; but killing something isolated in a dish isn't the same as killing it in the human body with the complexities of other cells and tissue.

That's why chemo is so hard on the body as it can't differentiate the good cells from the bad; it kills them all

In-vivo is when something is done within a living organism such as the human body and isn't something the alternative medicine fraternity normally mention.

When meeting a client for the first time, lawyers/solicitors like to say, 'you have a prima facie case here', and you think, 'wow, I have a prima facie case, so that's like, good, isn't it? Not just an ordinary case but a prima facie case—I can't lose.' What it really means is, on the first impression, you may have a case. Translated it means, I'll take your money and let's see what happens. Prima facie only means that based on what you've told the lawyer/solicitor, it sounds like you have a good case, but that's before the other side dispute what you say and it all goes tits up. In-vitro basically means the same thing. First impression is this works in a dish, but that ultimately means nothing until it's tested in-vivo.

Caveat emptor

Yes, now I'm showing off; it's something I learnt when I was in business and my solicitor told me about it when I bought something that turned out to be not as described.

Caveat emptor is a Latin phrase favoured by the legal profession. Its translation is, 'Let the buyer beware', and it's a good phrase to remember when buying something claiming to cure or help in the battle against cancer on the internet, or anywhere else for that matter.

Well before the internet was even thought of, my mum always insisted that pen and paper refuse nothing. The same claim can be made for the internet, and it's an unfortunate fact that anyone can upload a website and sell just about anything, make any claims they like, and provided they're clever in how they go about it, they can sail off into the sunset, pockets bulging and not a care in the world; you, on the other hand?

Marketing is a priority to attract new customers and some sites employ actors to pose as individuals who have allegedly beaten cancer with whatever new and exciting method they are selling, and they invite you to view their blog through cancer forums, again acting as sufferers who endorse the product. Once you click on the link, you will find information on how they cured themselves using product ABC123Plus, which, by sheer coincidence, they can sell you.

The cliché, 'if it seems too good to be true, it probably is', is very relevant to the miracle cures offered online. When you're looking for something to help you beat cancer, you're in a vulnerable state where you will try anything, and this can be taken advantage of.

I have found some scams on the internet where a product is given numerous glowing reviews and is guaranteed to beat cancer. This is usually accompanied with a case study where someone claims they have been cured, and you see their before and after pictures and they explain their journey. Everything seems wonderful, so you assume it's legitimate and decide to purchase the product. Thankfully, there is a handy link, but this is the clever part—when you click on the link, it takes you to a different website that offers the product; only on this site—and only if you look carefully—you will find a disclaimer in the small print that advises the product offered has no medical qualities and no claims are made in relation to any potential cure for any disease. In effect, you have purchased something you wanted, and they have merely supplied just that. They haven't claimed anything they can't stand over, so if they say it has Omega oil, then it will contain just that, but the fact you've been told it cures cancer is irrelevant as it hasn't been claimed by the seller.

We've all clicked to accept terms and conditions of trading for multiple websites without bothering to read them, but a simple phrase releases the seller of any responsibility for claims made elsewhere.

You buy it, and it doesn't work. Caveat emptor.

Nice and easy, no harm done. But if it doesn't work as a cure for cancer, it's not like a broken radio—it's life and death we're dealing with. You die, and they fly—first class, thanks for your donation.

My first death threat

To let you know just how serious people take this source of income (as in scamming people that have cancer), I was on Facebook and in contact with a guy who was selling a cure that was nothing but fakery. A machine made in Russia that he claimed was able to scan your brain and tell what diseases you had already had, what you currently have and what you are going to get in the future.

What you had, currently have, and what you're going to get? Wow.

I asked him if it could tell me next week's lottery numbers, which seemed to annoy him somewhat, then I called him out on it and we had a very long conversation during which time I found the manufacture's website, which, categorically stated their machine is not designed to detect or diagnose cancer, yet here was a guy using it for that specific purpose.

Now at this juncture, any reasonable person would assume he would leave the conversation with his tail firmly between his legs, but no, he asked me where I lived, then proceeded to issue a very detailed death threat. Yeah, that's how dumb some of these guys are. Not only do they threaten you, but they do it on the most public forum on the planet in written form. Not a hint or a suggestion about what might happen, but a detailed threat to end your life with the use of a hammer. They (allegedly) have the intelligence to use one of these specialised machines, and not only diagnose cancer, but treat it as well, then they put death threats in writing that can be traced right back to them. I think it's a minimum requirement that someone treating cancer would at least have some common sense in addition to the qualifications they don't have.

I reported the whole conversation to Facebook, who immediately removed him from the site, both his business page and his private page. I suppose I could have taken it further, but what was the point? He was over 3000 miles away. However, it does illustrate the lengths these guys will go to protect their revenue stream. That's how lucrative fake cancer cures can be.

The manufacturers state the machine is designed for the complex scanning and treatment of the human body and operates on bio-resonance impetus principles (whatever they are).

The device in question is the Seneitive Imago, and if you check their promotional video, it looks like you sit in front of a monitor, wear some sort of headset, place one hand on a plate and hold a metal rod with the other. You are then analysed by computer.

It does a full body scan? With you sitting down? That's like me admiring the view beyond a brick wall, while only looking at the wall. How does it do it? Is it magic?

It also analyses your Biorhythms and can re-align them. This intrigued me as I had no idea what a Biorhythm was, so I looked it up: a recurring cycle in the physiology or functioning of an organism, such as the daily cycle of sleeping and waking. A cyclic pattern of physical, emotional or mental activity believed to occur in a person's life. To be honest, even having read the definition, I'm still unsure if it's a thing or just a pattern, either way, I don't see it having any effect on cancer.

The machines are certified as Class 2 medical equipment in the EU, which operators use as a selling point to make it more credible, but although it has the certification, it only means it's safe to use in a hospital environment. If you propose to use a hairdryer in a hospital as part of the equipment, it has to pass the same test, and like the BioResonance machine, it's only tested for safety and not to see if it will actually dry your hair, so the certificate in no way lends any credibility as to the effectiveness of the machine. Plug it in and it won't electrocute you or give off radiation or magnetic fields that may interfere with other equipment, that's about it. Users of the machine keep throwing this certification in our face as if it makes the machine more credible due to the testing involved, when, in fact, it means nothing like that.

The only relevant fact about this machine is that for the diagnosis or treatment of cancer, it don't work.

Sorry, guys, I'm not convinced. Not even a little bit.

This next section came about as a result of people asking for my opinion on recommendations made on websites, or programmes offered, or YouTube videos. I've put the most popular first, but all of them have convinced people that they have the answer to cancer, and conventional treatment is bad.

The biggest problem I had was that although people asked for my opinion, they had already convinced themselves everything made sense and these guys had the cure for cancer Big Pharma wouldn't allow because it would reduce profits.

Local newspapers ran an article about a guy with cancer (who had asked my opinion and ignored it) who was trying to raise money for treatment in Mexico the health service wouldn't provide, and the newspapers bought into it as well and asked for donations. Thankfully, this was before fundraising pages on the internet and he had to rely on conventional treatment, which, cured him anyway without the need to travel 5148 miles.

Some people have asked why I'm always so hard to convince, and it's because I've been self-employed since I turned 20, and during the 80s and 90s I had a string of companies that—let's say—bent the rules somewhat. I didn't break them, but I came close. A friend describes me as a poacher turned gamekeeper, and I quite like that. I tend to see things without looking; words like probably, could, potentially, may… they always jump out

It has been said that conventional therapy doesn't guarantee a cure either, but the difference is where a site claims Wee Willie Winkey was cured of a cancer growth on his nose, therefore their cure works, versus multiple clinical trials with published results. While this is a light-hearted example, it's based on the experience of Dr David Jockers (as recommended by The Truth About Cancer). I have a video of him telling how he had a growth on his nose and—as his grandfather had the same type of growth and died of skin cancer—he just knew it was cancer, so he changed his diet, slowed down, rested a lot, prayed a lot, and it went away. Hallelujah.

Don't get me wrong, I'm glad he didn't die, but… he just knew it was cancer? There was no biopsy, no scans, no consultations with a doctor; he just knew.

Could it have been… a pimple? A wart? A sting? A rash?

Is there the slightest possibility it wasn't cancer in the first place?

We'll never know, but:

Dr. David Jockers is a natural health doctor, functional nutritionist, corrective care chiropractor, exercise physiologist and certified strength & conditioning specialist. (Yeah, I lifted it from his bio.)

…so it follows that someone as qualified as that knows what they're talking about.

Sounds like moo-cow-poo and probably smells like it as well.

Anyway, in comparison to conventional therapy, they don't point to Wee Willie Winkey and hope you'll be convinced, no, they have numerous validated studies to show that 61.7% or 89.6% (or whatever figure they quote) managed to achieve remission based on this specific protocol for this specific cancer out of 500+ patients, not one.

When alternative therapies don't work, they say it's because you didn't believe it would work. It's your fault.

When conventional therapy doesn't work, they find something else. Move on to the next level. If they say your hair will fall out, it doesn't matter whether you believe or not, your hair will fall out.

In fairness, all the sites are slick and believable, until you do just the tiniest bit of digging. No deep searching required, just type in the person or website, add the word 'quack' or 'fraud' or 'scam' at the end and hit search.

I'm not convinced ~ Ty Bollinger / The Truth About Cancer

The best name for a cancer site anywhere. The truth…the whole truth… and nothing but the truth…about cancer.

But… it all depends how you define truth.

One of the glitziest sites on the web. Host to once-a-year medical extravaganzas with lots of doctors (who aren't really doctors) claiming their method is the magic cure; which begs the question, if every treatment is different, who's right?

If there is just one cure, how come there are so many being offered? Praying, Gerson Therapy, Essential Oils, dancing around a pole naked at midnight chanting 'cure me, cure me,' etc. (Okay, I made that last one up.)

Ty Bollinger. He's a likeable guy who loves the Lord and makes a point of telling you as much as possible, because if you love the Lord, you just can't be a bad guy, can you?

It seems to be a theme with alternative therapy sites as Chris Wark (below) is also a God fearin' guy who throws God at you at every opportunity.

Ty and Charlene Bollinger are always centre stage and always going on about how they don't make money and Big Pharma is trying to shut them down, and the internet is censoring them, and their daffodils didn't bloom this year… Honestly, I almost feel sorry for them.

Doesn't take a lot of digging to find sites that suggest they do make money from promoting doctors who aren't doctors and cures that don't work. (Although I would never suggest that.)

But they do seem to promote a lot of discredited "doctors" who have qualified through internet courses. They do seem to promote a lot of "doctors" who have been involved in court cases. The do seem to promote a lot of stuff they don't sell but can recommend a site where you can purchase it, but… they don't make any money.

If it walks like a duck and it quacks like a duck…

They're currently running their 'Quest for the Cures [FINAL CHAPTER]' video series which you can watch for free for a limited time, or purchase for only $97, which is the 50% off bronze package, or go for the gold package at 60% off which is at the unbelievable price of only… wait for it… $197. Yeah, they don't make money?

In a recent email they said: Please remember, we're not Big Pharma (with deep pockets) and we don't have advertisers. Much like PBS (Public Broadcasting Service), we need your support to continue broadcasting free information to the world and continue saving lives.

According to Wickipedia the Bollingers claim to have paid $12 million to partner groups. Yes, you did read that right. They claim to not make money but claim to have paid $12 million. Bet you wish you were that broke as well.

They didn't convince me they were telling the truth about cancer, but they did convince me they make a lot of money and live a fantastic lifestyle because of people willing to believe (or hope) their connections have the answer.

I'm not convinced ~ www.chrisbeatcancer.com

The one big selling point on the ChrisBeatCancer website is diet. Yes folks, by changing your diet you can cure yourself of cancer.

Just by way of illustrating a point, let's say you are out shopping when someone picks your pocket and steals your keys, but as you're unaware of the theft you visit a coffee shop and treat yourself to a fancy coffee you've never tried before, but when you go back to your car your keys are missing, so you immediately equate drinking a fancy coffee means your keys vanish. Would you consider this to be a reasonable assumption?

I think everyone would agree the coffee had nothing to do with the loss of the keys, so if someone has a tumour and it is subsequently removed by a surgeon, is it reasonable to assume that just because they changed their diet after the operation, the diet is responsible for the cure?

You may think the website ChrisBeatCancer.com means what it says: that a person called, Chris, beat a disease called cancer. You may even go as far as to think he did this all on his own, without surgery, or chemo, or radiation, or any kind of treatment, but you would be wrong.

It would be wonderful if Chris were one of those guys who was diagnosed and subsequently changed his life through nutrition and hey-presto the cancer vanished, but unfortunately, that's not what happened. At the time of his original diagnosis, it was recommended the tumour be removed with surgery, which they did. Chris then decided (once the cancer had been surgically removed) to decline adjuvant chemotherapy and proceed to cure himself by diet. Hallelujah, praise the dude in the sky, etc.

At this stage, it should be made clear that adjuvant chemotherapy is a bit like someone brushing a yard (surgery) then going over everything with a power washer (adjuvant chemotherapy) to get the little pieces that have been missed by the brush. In this case, the doctors were taking no risks with his treatment in recommending adjuvant therapy to make sure the surgery had removed all the cancer. It's simply a common-sense approach, but he refused, which makes his claim—I refused chemotherapy and still beat cancer—true, but not true, if you get my meaning.

I posted a question on the ChrisBeatCancer website and asked him: If you hadn't had the operation in the first place, would your recommendations on diet and lifestyle have cured the cancer?

Unfortunately, he didn't reply, so I don't know what he thinks.

I sent him numerous emails and asked: If you hadn't had surgery to remove your tumour, would your methods still have beaten the cancer?

I eventually received an answer to an email I sent on 12th January 2018. The reply on 14th January from Julie Johnson stated: Unfortunately, I've never heard Chris speak about that subject, I'm so sorry. She did give me a list of YouTube and website links where Chris talks about his journey, but the question was never answered.

I have no doubt Chris is a good guy who is trying to do the best he can for cancer patients, and some of the recommendations he makes are well thought out and very helpful in regard to nutrition, but for me, his claims about how to cure cancer through nutrition or supplements or smoothies, simply don't add up or make sense.

Let me put it another way; the doctors cured his cancer with surgery and his change of diet did not cure his cancer; unless him eating healthy had an effect on the bit they cut out of him that was cancerous and the hospital held onto it to see what happened. (nope, don't think so)

He has some interesting videos where he interviews cancer doctors (some of whom have no qualifications whatsoever to confirm their status as doctors) and some survivors that followed his protocols; however, some of the patients who had their cancer cured were never actually diagnosed by real doctors, which begs the question; did they have cancer in the first place? It's not hard to cure something that wasn't there to cure.

At the end of one of his promotional videos, he states, "Sometimes, things get worse before they get better and if this happens, just stick with it." Sometimes? Really? That would infer that *sometimes*, they just continue to get worse, but, hey, don't worry yourself, have some trust in the process.

If you're having conventional treatment and things get worse, the doctor will investigate further. Do you honestly think that when someone with cancer gets worse you should just 'stick with it', or 'give it time', or 'die'? If you decide to go alternative, you're on your own. You can't consult the seller as they're mostly in it for the money. No medical qualifications that mean anything. At the very least, the statement: "sometimes, things get worse before they get better," doesn't inspire confidence.

It seems at first glance Chris is only providing a service, as although he recommends various sites that products can be purchased from, you can't make a purchase on his site, but, as with everything, money does raise its head, and at the end, he will invite you to purchase his video course, which, of course, has helped numerous people beat cancer through diet, which, as any idiot knows, has no effect on existing cancer cells.

I'm not convinced ~ Dr Leonard Coldwell

Mr Cancer himself. Jeez, this guy is good. He can cure any cancer (yes, any cancer) in two to six weeks.

Yeah, you read that right, any cancer cured in weeks.

No messing about with success rates or percentages, it's a guaranteed 100% cure. Any cancer.

He has many videos on the web and—as I'm on his email list—I know he can cure a multitude of problems in addition to mere cancer.

Leonard Coldwell was born in 1958, but not as Leonard Coldwell; he was allegedly born as Bernd Klein and changed his name when he moved to America.

He first discovered his ability to cure people of cancer at the age of 12 when his mother was diagnosed with final stage liver cancer that was terminal and was given six months to live, but at only 12 and with no medical training, he cured her when doctors couldn't. Wow, what a guy. Sounds almost too good to be true.

In fairness, he seems to be a clever guy, and extremely modest. He says, "In the opinion of most experts that I have ever spoken to, I have the highest cancer cure rate in the world."

His qualifications are impressive:

ND – Naturopathic Doctor.

CNHP – Certified Natural Health Professional.

DIP.PHC – Diploma in Primary Health Care.

DNM – Doctor of Naturopathic Medicine.

LCHC – Legally Certified Healthcare Constructor.

PhD – Doctor of Philosophy.

D.Hum – Doctor of Humanities. (Honorary).

…and Four Doctor Degrees. (No idea what these might be).

But all his qualifications have proved hard to confirm as genuine. He does have a doctorate in psychology from Columbia State University, which sounds good until you find out the University sold diplomas and was closed by court order. Not that impressive then.

In 2011, he claimed to have cured 35,000 cancer patients. Wow.

I'm just going to give you some of his comments from one of his videos (6m 55s long) followed by my comments and you can make up your own mind.

In his most popular video, he says, "The viewer needs to understand that cancer is the easiest condition to cure. If you have cancer, be happy that you don't have anything more serious or something that might be harder to fix. Because cancer is nothing more than a symptom."

So there you have it, folks, nothing to worry about.

"There are over 400 natural cancer cures out there. So don't worry." Well, that's reassuring.

"In my experience, every cancer can be cured in two to 16 weeks. Some cancers can be cured in minutes."

"The second you alkaline, the cancer already stops. It can take a couple of days, a couple of weeks, but it stops." This is so wrong it's hard to comprehend. You can't change your pH level, and if you could, you would die, but then again, so would the cancer, so maybe he has a point.

He recommends altering your pH level, eating a raw diet, drinking a gallon of water a day with half a teaspoon of sea salt, a vegan diet, oxygen therapy, vitamin C injections, etc. I have to wonder how he cured his mum way back, when all the things he now recommends weren't even things.

"In my personal experience, the tumours of the cancerous growth was basically gone within a couple of days." Impressive. Two days to cure cancer.

He then discusses salt, which he says is made up of salt, sand, and glass (one third each), which, when you ingest it, the glass cuts the insides of your veins? He must be working on different bodies to the rest of us because if you swallow grains of sand or glass, it comes out with your poo. There's no way it can enter your veins.

The video was uploaded to YouTube on 28th November 2011, and if I'm being totally honest, if I had seen it when first diagnosed, I would have believed this guy, and with nearly eight million views (WTF? He's like a rock star.), eighty-five thousand likes and only six thousand thumbs down, how could he not be the real thing? The viewing figures and likes confirm he's legit.

Selling is easy, especially when it's a cure for a life-threatening disease.

Tell people what they want to hear and tell them it's true because you've tested it and you've got qualifications to prove you know what you're talking about. Tell them they were right all along, and they believe; that's it. Why would they check? You've just confirmed what they already knew/hoped. You're on the internet. You're plausible. You look professional, and you sound professional, especially in Dr Caldwell's case because he has that little squeaky moustache, fancy accent, and always dresses well with his little pocket square. So, your brain says okeydokey, sounds tickety-boo. Let's go with that.

Sadly, he's a fruitcake at best or someone who has cost people their lives at worst, but either way, he's believable.

You can watch the original video at www.cancerology.co/2to6 and I have also made a video with comments about Dr Coldwell on the same page.

I'm not convinced ~ David Sereda's Light Stream Wand

The main problem with new inventions on the internet, is the quacks seem to be winning over a substantial proportion of people.

I'm on Facebook daily, and when something new pops up, I watch the comments. Some ask questions about effectiveness or price, but most seem to believe without questioning. The surprising thing is the number of people who tag another person to see the post, probably because they think it might work or be of interest.

I recently followed a post from David Sereda who is offering a resonance wand that cures almost every disease known. Reading the post and watching the video, it seems there is nothing this magic wand can't cure.

The intro states: Learn how stage 4 cancer patients who had only six months to live were able to virtually eliminate cancer markers in six weeks without chemotherapy, radiation or surgery (I love it when they use words like virtually or probably. Always lends credibility),

It then goes on to display the gizmo that looks just like a torch and which it is claimed can accelerate health and vitality, improve flexibility, raise your energy, give you inner peace, improve your sleep, restructure your water and food, enhance brain waves, etc.

On the pdf information sheet, it states the wand generates a vortex electromagnetic energy field about 5-10 feet in diameter and you just need to be within 6 feet of the wand for it to work.

He has separate posts detailing what the wand can do for heart disease, type 2 diabetes, abdominal inflammation, gallbladder diseases and gallstones, pain relief, hernia, foot disease, facelifts, migraine, prostate, candida, liver disease, lyme disease, nerve pain, benign tumours, swelling, herniated disk, interverbal disk displacement, periodontal disease, bacterial infections, parasites, haemorrhoids, human papilloma virus, cysts, irritable bowel, skin regeneration(?), gastritis, tinnitus, brain hemisphere synchronisation(?), hair regeneration, glaucoma, eyesight improvement, itchy skin, abscesses, headache, staph and strep, high blood pressure, phobia, pelvic floor muscles strength, restless leg syndrome, muscle spasms, removal of eye bags, erectile dysfunction, impotence, threadworms, knee joint pain, sciatica, constipation, cataracts, anti-aging, memory improvement, weight loss, muscle growth, immune system boost, sinusitis, intestinal healing, colds and flu, male enlargement, tooth regeneration(?), circulation. Honestly, I have to stop here; otherwise, I'd be writing another book. Is there anything this bloody thing can't cure?

But I saved the best till last as usual: Brain tumour (seriously, I kid you not).

Surely anyone reading this would question the validity of such claims? Seems a lot don't.

I did some research on Mr Sereda and discovered he has previously had other miracle cures for cancer including healing crystals, which begs the question, if they worked, why has he now moved on?

The wand has seven rubies, 33 tourmalines, and a quartz crystal, which make it look nice, but he's using them as a qualifying sales aid, when, in fact, they do nothing.

He suggests the ancient Egyptians used a wand or transmitting device to activate(?) the stones of the pyramids and for human DNA upgrade activation, and he helpfully includes a picture showing just this.

Interestingly, even though I posted all kinds of questions and linked to other sites that prove the theory doesn't work, he didn't answer personally, but those who were interested defended him vigorously.

It must be great to know you're selling something bogus and have others defend your product, even though they haven't used it themselves.

The sales video and accompanying literature is impressive, and I'm sure it cost a lot of money and time to produce, but even claims made in the video contradict those in the literature, and still, they defend him. Go figure.

The video shows metal balls spinning on plates due to the magnetic pulses emitted from the device, but in what world is this useful in the fight against cancer?

He claims cancer cells have specific frequencies and his wand can target them, and while this is true in an isolated test with singular cancer cells being subjected to frequency, we're back to bleach killing cells in a petri dish, but you wouldn't drink it; although I suspect if he recommended it, someone would be stupid enough to try it.

The disclaimer specifically states the device is harmless and has no effect on human cells, which would seem to contradict his sales pitch that it kills cancer cells. Which one is it?

The problem is people have a desire to believe, and especially if mainstream medicine says there is nothing more to be done, so I suppose a 'what's the harm' mentality comes to the fore, but the fact is the only thing you are doing is lining his pockets.

There is a picture of a nurse who has used the wand to cure patients, but the picture is a clip art depiction of a nurse and not an actual person. Surely, she would benefit from the advertising and would want to appear. Why are the cured not shown to endorse the product?

The nurse (who we don't see) says: "I had three cancer clients who were at stage 4 cancer with less than six months to live. After their Light Stream Wand treatments, their tumour markers dropped dramatically, and the doctors couldn't believe what happened..." - Cheryl. 37-year veteran nurse.

The list of problems with this device are numerous, yet almost all the comments are positive or enquiring about the price. One even said they would sell their car to purchase a wand.

The price? A snip at $2,121 for the entry level wand and $7,171 for the Quartz wand, and he invented them himself. Wow, how does he do it so cheap and make a profit?

I'm not convinced ~ Homeopathy

Homoeopathy was invented by a German physician by the name of Samuel Hahnemann in 1796.

The main idea behind it is that 'like cures like', so if you're allergic to peanuts, you should rub them on your skin until you're not allergic anymore; and we all know that doesn't work.

The second idea is that diluting with a large quantity of water increases potency. I looked up the word dilute, and it's defined as 'to make a liquid thinner or weaker by adding water or another solvent to it.' But, in the world of homoeopathy the definition is, 'the more something is diluted, the stronger it becomes.' So the next time you come home from work and think, 'I would love a gin and tonic,' just put the tiniest little drop of gin in the tonic and you're good to go, because homoeopathy says so.

Or could it be the other way around? If you go out for a night on the town and get completely hammered and wake up with the hangover from hell, then the teeniest drop of whatever alcohol you were drinking in a glass of water will fix you right up. I don't think so.

I think we could stop talking about homoeopathy at this point but there is more.

The third idea is that water has memory. Bet you didn't know that did you?

The overall theory sounds similar to a vaccine in that it infects you with a tiny dose of what's troubling you, and your body then builds up a resistance because 'like cures like', but there is one very major problem, and that is the ingredients used. If 'like cures like', you would assume they use something from the common cold to cure the common cold, but no, they use flowers, berries, roots, red onions, herbs, Belladonna, poison ivy, nettles, and even crushed bees, yes, those little things that fly around; homeopathists grab them and crush them to make medicine. Wow.

Another convincing thing homoeopathic remedies have in their favour is that most of them look very like Latin, which of course means that it sounds like something you've never heard before, so it's specialised and esoteric and probably the real thing, because quidquid latine dictum sit altum videtur (Anything said in Latin sounds profound).

The dilution process is one drop of the 'cure' into 99/100 drops of water (some say 99% some say 100%), mix well, then remove 1 drop and put that into 99 drops of water, mix well, then... and you do that 30 times (30C), which is the most popular ratio.

Fact: In a 13C dilution, there will not be a single molecule of the active ingredient present.

Bear in mind that 30C is a standard, but they do go up to 1000C and I have no idea how many zeros would be at the end of that.

I found it hard to get my head around the 30C figure, so rather than try to explain it in detail with equations, I'll just give you the number.

1:1,000,000,000,000,000,000,000,000,000,000,000,000,000,000,000,000,000,000,000,000,000.

The dilution is 1 in What???, no idea how you'd even go about saying this number. It's got 60 zeros. I Googled it and it's called a Novemdecillion.

Now, being of sound mind, could anyone really think any of the original drop is left? Irrespective of how good a memory the water has.

That got me thinking, is it normal tap water they use or is this the same water that Jack watered the beanstalk beans with? Is it magic water?

If this idea was put forward at a school science class, the kids would ask you if you were a head case.

A 2015 report from the Australian Government, the National Health and Medical Research Council (NHMRC) concluded that after reviewing around 200 studies on homoeopathy; the remedies were no better than the sugar pills used to put the dilution into.

And if that's not enough to convince you, there are homoeopathic asthma inhalers being sold that have no active ingredient, they do nothing. Completely useless. If you have an attack and use one, you better pray someone can let you use their real one.

Another thing homoeopaths tend to say, "you will not get any side effects with our medicine. It will not do any harm to your body whatsoever." Well, if you have cancer, you kinda want the cancer cells to be given a bit of a kicking. You want to do damage to them. So if homoeopathy doesn't do any damage at all, whatsoever, in any way; it doesn't do anything.

The other thing they say is that homoeopathy is not medicine, which is a great get-out clause. They say it promotes the body's natural response, helping the body make itself better. They can't explain how it does this. But that's what happens. You just got to trust that water has memory and they know what they're talking about.

Still not convinced. Okay, I can go one better. You're going to love this. They have made a homoeopathic treatment in order to alleviate the effects of depression from the bricks of the Berlin Wall.

Wait what? Like as in a brick? Concrete stuff?

Yes, the bricks of the Berlin Wall have absorbed something over the years that when diluted properly (30C with magic water), treats depression.

I think I've said enough about homeopathy.

But, as it's homeopathy, once again, Prince Charles is in the frame.

One would think that after being caught up in the last, "Oh yes, I recommend the Gerson method," nonsense. He would learn to, you know, just stay in the background slightly and not put his head on the chopping block, but he has now volunteered to be the patron of the Faculty of Homeopathy. Now, don't get me wrong, I do not have any problem with the royal family in any way, and in fact, I met the good man himself at the Royal Victoria Hospital in Belfast, quite by accident.

Funny story. I was going in for a PET scan and—unbeknown to me—he was there opening the new wing. I remember walking in that morning thinking, wow, there are an awful lot of police here, what's going on? But nobody bothered me. Bald guy, obvious cancer patient, not a threat. I walked through the main doors, and he was the lead man coming out. He said, "Oh," and nodded. There was a load of people behind him, who, oddly enough, rushed forward to me and asked stupid questions like, "What are you doing here?" To which I replied, "It's a hospital. I've got cancer, duhhh."

I think the royals are great and I do support them, but when you've got a member of the royal family who is not a doctor putting his recommendation behind something that has no scientific proof behind it, you've got to wonder.

I'm not convinced ~ CBD oil

CBD oil is made from hemp, which is a variety of the cannabis sativa plant and has a lot less THC than marijuana.

Cannabidiol (CBD) is one of the chemicals found in cannabis, but it doesn't have the psychoactive or mind-altering effects that cannabis has because it does not contain tetrahydrocannabinol (THC) which is what gives you the high if you use cannabis on its own.

CBD oil should not have any THC in it, as it would then be classified as a drug.

Primarily used with a dropper under the tongue, it can also be applied to the skin and even used for vaping.

Just for the fun of it, and because I'm a fun guy, I went to a shopping centre where there was a CBD shop, went in and said I had cancer and asked if CBD oil was any good for treating cancer or preventing it or curing it or what did it do? The assistant said, "I'll get my manager as he knows more than me."

The manager came out and started to ramble on about how he had several customers with advanced cancers that came to him regularly, and it was a miracle drug as one of them had gone into complete remission after doctors told her she had less than three months to live, and I should start using it immediately.

He didn't ask what type of cancer I had or what stage it was, which would have been irrelevant anyway as I didn't have cancer.

I said, "That's amazing. How much is it?"

He discussed prices and recommended I should sign up for a payment plan and buy it monthly. He said I should be on it now, then told me how hospitals won't allow you to take it because it's a cure that doesn't cost as much as chemotherapy, so they don't make any money out of it (which is an irrelevant argument in the UK where healthcare is free).

It was at this stage I produced a dictation machine, pointed to the microphone attached to my lapel, and said, "I'm writing an article on CBD and cancer. Can I have your name?"

For some reason, his face changed from the cheerful, helpful guy he had been and started to push me out of the shop.

I said, "If you assault a guy with cancer, you will be arrested. You cannot assault somebody who has cancer."

He backed down, but he did call the shopping centre security to ask me to leave.

I picked up some leaflets and thought I would ring the head office, but when I called, he answered. It was a one shop chain and he was the owner. When I introduced myself, he hung up.

One of the manufacturer's leaflets stated CBD oil should not be used to treat cancer. I think that says everything.

Weeks later, I did the same thing in another shop in Belfast, and the experience was identical. CBD oil cures cancer. It can make the blind see again. You can walk on water if you use it, and you can fly without wings. Whatever you want to hear, they will tell you to get a sale.

In 2019, The Centre for Medical Cannabis tested thirty products advertising themselves as CBD oil bought on the high street and online.

After testing, it was found that 45% had levels of THC that made them technically illegal in the UK as they have the potential to give you a high, just like cannabis.

Seven of the products tested had the solvent Dichloromethane which causes shortness of breath and wheezing. Unsurprisingly—to me anyway—they also found that one sample bought from a high street chain had no CBD in it at all, and it sold for £53.00.

Of all the products tested, only 30% had levels of CBD within 10% of the amount advertised.

The problem is there's no legal requirement for CBD oil to be tested because it's not a medicine; it doesn't claim to be a cure. The manufacturers/suppliers can't say anything about it treating anything because if they did, the product would have to be tested to confirm.

They rely on social media, and people saying they used CBD oil and it cured them. After that, word of mouth and sharing does the rest.

In fairness, some medically approved products are authorised to treat seizures, but it does nothing for cancer.

In another study in 2019, CBD oil was tested on mice, and it was discovered the mice that received high doses experienced severe liver damage within one day.

Some good news is that in another study in 2016, CBD oil inhibited the growth of many types of tumour cells in a test tube.

Bad news is it wasn't done on people, so it doesn't really have any relevance—you're back to the old bleach kills cancer cells in a petri dish scenario.

They also found that some types of cannabinoids suppress the immune system allowing tumours to grow unchecked, which is not a good thing.

The other red flag for cancer patients is that CBD oil can interfere with how your body processes cancer drugs. Using CBD oil while on chemotherapy can (depending on the chemotherapy used) make the treatment more toxic or make it less effective.

Bottom line is, if you're thinking of using CBD oil, talk to your oncologist. My recommendation—based on research by Queens University, Belfast, and a lot of online sources—is you shouldn't use it as it has not been proved in any way to treat cancer.

A lot of companies have added CBD oil to coffee, soap, soft drinks, gummies, etc., and they claim to have a calming effect and blah, blah, blah, but when they've been tested, there is so little CBD in them, there is no possibility of any sort of biological effect.

It's funny that the only sites on the web that recommend CBD oil as a cure for cancer are those that sell CBD oil as a cure for cancer.

I'm not convinced ~ Rick Simpson oil (RSO)

Rick Simpson oil is basically like CBD oil, except it is made from cannabis and not hemp, which means it contains tetrahydrocannabinol (THC) which will give you a high the same as ordinary cannabis, so irrespective of whether it cures you, you'll be happy.

Tetrahydrocannabinol (THC) comes with its own range of psychological symptoms, such as:
Anxiety.
Depression.
Disorientation.
Hallucinations.
Irritability.
Paranoia.

It can also have physical side effects, such as:
Bloodshot eyes.
Dizziness.
Impaired memory.
Impaired motor control and reaction time.
Low blood pressure.
Sleeping issues.
Slow digestion.

However, the physical side effects do not pose any significant risk and usually only last a couple of hours.

Driving or operating machinery while using RSO should be avoided until the high wears off.

In addition to cancer, the oil can also treat:
Arthritis.
Asthma.
Depression.
High blood pressure.
Infections.
Inflammation.
Insomnia.
Multiple sclerosis.
Tinnitus.

Now, call me jaded, but doesn't snake oil also claim to cure anything and everything. Which is it? Is it a cure for cancer or a cure for every illness known? If it sounds too good to be true…

It's interesting to note that one of the side effects of THC is depression, which, if I'm understanding this properly, the oil can treat. Seems like a contradiction to me.

The claim is that Mr Simpson had skin cancer on his face, and after having it surgically removed (the cancer, not his face), it returned. He then tried his marijuana oil directly on the skin cancers, and a few days later, they had completely disappeared, according to Rick.

The poor old cancers were probably high and just lost their balance and fell off.

His mum had psoriasis, which is a skin condition, and after a few weeks, her sores had also disappeared.

The first red flag is he can cure cancer quicker than psoriasis, which, for me, is kinda hard to believe, but I'll give him the benefit of the doubt.

It was used on a patient with glaucoma, and it reduced the pressure on the eye and improved vision.

Diabetic patients were completely healed with a 60-gram dose.

The second red flag is, I can understand the oil having some effect on the skin cancers as it was applied directly, but how does that work when it's an internal cancer? Its not like you can unzip your belly and rub some on you colon, and I've no idea how it would work for brain cancer, but if Rick says it does…

Mr Simpson was arrested by the police in Canada and sent to jail. Now, don't get me wrong, that doesn't mean the oil doesn't work, but the evidence above has me convinced, as well as all the research facilities that tested it and found no benefit to cancer patients.

I'm not convinced ~ Dog dewormer

Joe Tippens is the man who allegedly cured his cancer with a dog dewormer. Yes, you read that right.

In 2016, Joe was diagnosed with small cell lung cancer and was told, “what you have, can’t be cured.”

He received chemotherapy and radiation; then he got the old good-news- bad-news. Good news was the treatment had worked, and his left lung was completely clear. Bad news was a pet scan showed cancer in his right lung, neck, stomach, bladder, pancreas, liver, and tailbone. He had dozens of tumours, and the prognosis was less than 1% survivability, and he wasn’t expected to last any more than three months.

His oncologist mentioned a clinical trial and managed to get Joe included, but even then, the best outcome might only extend his life for a year.

Joe went on the internet and found a post that said, ‘if you have cancer or know someone who does, give me a shout.’

The guy was a veterinarian in Western Oklahoma who told Joe that a scientist at Merck animal health had done some cancer research on mice and had come across a product that was batting 1000 and killing cancer. The scientist had been diagnosed with stage four brain cancer and given three months to live. Joe decided. ‘what the heck’ and started taking dog dewormer which contained Fenbendazole (FenBen). (Panacur and Safe-Guard canine dewormer are two popular sources)

In January 2017—when he was on the clinical trial—he also started using bio-available curcumin 600 milligrams per day, and 25 milligrams a day of CBD oil.

Straightaway, we have a bit of a complicated regime. Dog dewormer, and a clinical trial, and now CBD oil, and Curcumin. How did we get here? If the dog dewormer works, why were the other two added?

Joe says he doesn’t give medical advice, but on his website, he has details of the protocol that cured him, except he’s updated it after he was cured.

Initially, it was take the dewormer for three days then skip four days, but now (well after he has been cured and still isn't medically qualified), he states, 'I now believe that seven days per week is now prudent for virtually everyone, and there is no longer believed to be a need to take four days off per week.

He believes?

Virtually? Damn, that's so exact. Must be true.

No longer believed? What does that even mean?

Just take it every day as it does no harm anyway. Which begs the question, if it does no harm, what does it do?

He has a note saying, 'Because cancer is notorious for recurrences, I plan on taking this regime the rest of my life.' And then he has "Why not?"

People ask him whether or not it can be taken while on chemotherapy, radiation or immunotherapy, and he says yes to all three. And again, we have another "Why not? followed by "My recommendation is do just that."

Based on what? He doesn't give medical advice, but... kinda looks like he does.

He then states, 'about 80% of the people who have followed my lead have been transparent with their oncologists, and of those, about 80% of the oncologists have been supportive.' I find that hard to believe. Had I gone to my consultant and said, "Look, I know you're doing your best, and you're giving me the best possible treatment, but I've decided to munch some dog deworming tablets because I think they're probably going to be better." I have a fair idea what might have been their reply. If I was a haematologist or oncologist, I know what I'd be saying, and I wouldn't be okay with it.

This following statement from Joe is so good, I'm going to include it verbatim; "In my regular quarterly PET scan in the first week of May 2017, my Tuesday week meeting was my first sign that the positive thinking, the prayer posse, the humour, the supplements and yes, the canine dewormer all combined, might just be working."

So, dog dewormer cures cancer; but you have to also take curcumin. and CBD oil, oh, and let's not forget the clinical trial, and the prayer posse, and the humour, and the positive thinking, and...

Turns out his oncologist was 'literally stupefied'.

Three months prior, there was cancer all over his body that left 99% of its victims dead within three months, and now, Joe was completely clear.

It is funny he doesn't mention what clinical trial he was on or what treatment he received, which niggles, and I'll tell you why; when I had my fourth cancer, they said three months at best; then I got the all-clear. Was I on anything else outside? Nope. The chemo worked. That's it.

Could it be possible that Joe was cured because he was on the clinical trial? Why does he not mention the treatment? I searched everywhere but couldn't find any details.

Once cured, he told his doctor about the dewormer and the doctor said, "We have known for decades that these anthelmintic drugs (which is the term used to describe a drug to treat animals for parasitic worms) could have possible efficacy against cancer and in fact, in the 80s and 90s, there was a drug called Levamisole that was used on colon cancer and it's an anthelmintic drug."

I'm not saying the guy didn't say that but... It's hard to believe a qualified oncologist would basically say, 'yeah, I know dog medicine is better, but what the hell? I thought I'd try ineffective conventional treatment.' Why would someone admit that?

In fairness, Joe does say that there is no way to prove that it was the deworming drug that vanished his cancer. But it was, only it wasn't, but use it anyway as it works, or doesn't, definitely, maybe, who knows?

The next bit is boring

This next section is about alternative treatments, and if you're not considering alternative treatment, there really is no need to read it because, putting it bluntly, it's boring. It lists all the alternative medicines and what they claim, and why they don't work.

Where it might be helpful is when (not if) someone suggests a treatment for your cancer they have heard of or found; you can look it up and see if it's there and what I've said about it.

For me, having researched it, I found it really interesting what some people are trying to sell as medicine, and what some people are willing to believe.

So ultimately, I will leave it up to you to decide what you do next, but you have been warned.

You could also just skip to 'And finally' which is the next section.

Alternative therapies debunked

126–F

126–F is a liquid formula containing inositol, nitric acid, sodium sulphite, potassium hydroxide, sulfuric acid, and catechol, that it is claimed cures Alzheimer's disease, multiple sclerosis, diabetes, AIDS, and cancer.
The claim is the mixture can lower the voltage of cells, causing them to digest themselves; a claim that was found to be false.
The ingredients were tested by the National Cancer Institute and found to have no effect on cancer in humans, either separately or combined.

714-X

714-X or Trimethylbicyclonitramineoheptane chloride, is a mixture of chemicals marketed as a cure for cancer and other serious diseases.

It was developed by Gaston Naessens from France and is made using camphor in a chemical reaction with ammonia and sodium chloride.
Banned in the US by the Food and Drug Administration, it has been tested and found to have no effect on cancer.
The main ingredient in the potion is water.
In 1989 Naessens was arrested and charged with murder after a patient using 714-X died after refusing conventional treatment, but although arrested, he never went to trial and was acquitted.

Actaea racemosa
Actaea racemose is a flowering plant that is claimed to have health-giving properties. According to Cancer Research UK, there is no evidence to support any claims that it treats or prevents cancer.

Alkaline Diet
The alkaline diet is a restrictive regime of non-acid foods, such as that proposed by Edgar Cayce (1877–1945), which is based on the claim this will affect the pH of the body generally, so reducing the risk of heart disease and cancer.
The alternative practitioners claim that cancer cells can't survive in a non-acidic environment and lowering the pH level will kill the cells, and although the claim has some merit in so far that cancer cells in a petri dish die, the level required to kill the cancer cells will also kill all the other cells necessary to survive, so if you could lower your pH to the required level, you would die anyway.

Aloe (See also T-UP)
Aloe is made of plants from Africa and is mainly used to treat minor skin problems, but some alternative practitioners recommend injecting it into the veins or directly into the tumour, as well as adding it to shakes or ingesting it in other ways.
Several deaths have been caused by injections of aloe, and in America the practice and claims are illegal.

There is no evidence to show it having any effect on cancer and it can cause severe side-effects and death when used as a cancer treatment.

Ambrotose

Glyconutrients is a type of sugar which is extracted from plants.
A company called Mannatech repackaged this sugar and marketed it under the brand name Ambrotose, which, it is claimed, promotes cellular health and boosts the immune system.
It's surprising a company is promoting sugar to cure cancer when others are saying sugar feeds cancer cells, but as it doesn't work, it's redundant anyway.
The Memorial Sloan Kettering Cancer Center says there is no evidence of glyconutrients having any effect on cancer.

Amygdalin/Amygdalina

Amygdalin is obtained from the pits or seeds of apricots, apples, peaches, red cherries, plums, and other fruits as well as bitter almonds.
It was first patented in the 1950s and was known as Laetrile.
Touted as an alternative cancer treatment in the 60s and 70s, it is banned by the Federal Drugs and Administration due to the fact that when your intestines break it down, it converts into cyanide.
The idea is that cyanide kills the cancer cells, but the reality is that numerous deaths have been attributed to its use.
It was then repackaged as Vitamin B17 in an effort to get around regulations for drugs, but it isn't a vitamin and doesn't act like a vitamin.
There is no vitamin that reduces blood pressure to dangerous levels and induces a coma.
As little as 50 grams of amygdalin, or whatever name they choose to call it, can kill you.
Unsurprisingly, clinics in Mexico still promote its use, but after analysis by the Food and Drug Administration, some samples were found to have excessive levels of bacteria, and samples had been bulked out with other harmful substances.

Amygdalin has been independently tested on up to 20 animal tumours and found to have no benefit either alone or together with other substances.
In a clinical trial in 1982 by the Mayo Clinic and three other cancer centres, it was administered as recommended to advanced cancer patients for which there was no other treatment available. Out of 178 patients, there was no improvement, but in those still alive after seven months, their tumours had increased, and several patients experienced symptoms of cyanide poisoning and had to stop treatment.
In a US Supreme Court ruling in 1979, it was determined that the general public deserve protection from amygdalin and called it a fraudulent cure.

American Coneflower Therapy
American coneflower therapy (also known as echinacea) is a herbal supplement derived from plants in the daisy family.
It is marketed primarily to prevent and lessen the symptoms of cold and flu.
Others sell it as a cure for cancer, but there is no evidence of this anywhere other than in their sales pitch.
In addition, some products have been found to be contaminated with arsenic, lead, and selenium.
According to Cancer Research UK, there is no scientific evidence to show that echinacea can help treat, prevent, or cure cancer in any way.

Andrographis Paniculata
Andrographis paniculata is promoted as a dietary supplement and also a cure for cancer.
It is a herb plant with a bitter taste and is one of the ingredients used in Ayurvedic medicine.
The Memorial Sloan-Kettering Cancer Center has stated that there is no evidence that it helps prevent or cure cancer.

CANCEROLOGY

Antineoplaston therapy
Antineoplaston therapy was invented by Stanislaw R. Burzynski MD in the 70s. It is a name invented by him to describe substances extracted from urine or synthesized in a laboratory.
It is claimed to be a form of chemotherapy; however, it doesn't work. In 1995, a federal grand jury indicted Burzynski for marketing an unapproved drug.
Patients treated with this protocol died, and there is no evidence of it having any effect on cancer as it was simply a scam to make money, but it is still practised in Mexico.

Apitherapy
Apitherapy is products such as honey and bee venom which is claimed to have an anti-cancer effect.
Tests have shown it to have no effect on cancer.

Aveloz
Aveloz is a shrub from Africa or South America. The sap is promoted as a cancer treatment/cure, but studies have found that it can suppress the immune system, promote the growth of a tumour and lead to cancer.
Around 1880 a Brazilian physician called Pamfilio is credited with the introduction of aveloz to conventional medicine, then around 1980 it was promoted as a cure for cancer.
It is claimed that: One drop of aveloz sap, diluted in a glass of distilled water and taken by the tablespoonful every hour, eliminates cancerous growths in one week.
The fact: It irritates the skin and mucous membranes, causes conjunctivitis of the eyes, burning in the mouth and throat, diarrhoea, and gastroenteritis.
The chemicals contained in the sap act as tumour promotors that suppress the immune system, promote tumour growth, and lead to the development of cancer.
All things considered, it's probably one of the worst things you could try.

Ayurvedic Medicine

Ayurvedic medicine is a 5000-year-old system of traditional medicine which originated on the Indian subcontinent.

Unfortunately, it has been tested to substantiate the claims made and the conclusion is that there is no scientific evidence to prove that Ayurvedic medicine can treat or cure cancer or any other disease.

The biggest problem is that—depending on the practitioner—no two treatments are formulated in the same way. It's simply a matter of throwing a number of secret ingredients into the mix and hoping for the best.

When it doesn't work, other experts claim that the mix was wrong, and you should have come to them in the first place. Not exactly confidence inspiring.

B17

B17 is another name for Amygdalin, which is obtained from the pits or seeds of apricots, apples, peaches, red cherries, plums, and other fruits as well as bitter almonds.

It was first patented in the 1950s and was known as Laetrile. Touted as an alternative cancer treatment in the 60s and 70s, it is banned by the Federal Drugs and Administration due to the fact that when your intestines break it down, it converts into cyanide. The idea is that cyanide kills the cancer cells, but the reality is that numerous deaths have been attributed to its use.

It was then repackaged as Vitamin B17 in an effort to get around regulations for drugs, but it isn't a vitamin and doesn't act like a vitamin.

There is no vitamin that reduces blood pressure to dangerous levels and induces a coma.

As little as 50 grams of amygdalin, or whatever name they choose to call it, can kill you.

Unsurprisingly, clinics in Mexico still promote its use, but after analysis by the Food and Drug Administration, some samples were found to have excessive levels of bacteria, and samples had been bulked out with other harmful substances.

Amygdalin has been independently tested on up to 20 animal tumours and found to have no benefit either alone or together with other substances.
In a clinical trial in 1982 by the Mayo Clinic and three other cancer centres, it was administered as recommended to advanced cancer patients for which there was no other treatment available. Out of 178 patients there was no improvement, but in those still alive after seven months, their tumours had increased, and several patients experienced symptoms of cyanide poisoning and had to stop treatment.
In a US Supreme Court ruling in 1979, it was determined that the general public deserve protection from amygdalin and called it a fraudulent cure.

Bach Flower Remedies
Based on preparations invented by Edward Bach in the 1920s in which tiny amounts of plant material are diluted in a mixture of water and brandy.
According to Cancer Research UK, this remedy is promoted as having the capability to boost the immune system, but there is no scientific evidence to prove it having any effect over the immune system or any type of cancer.

Baking soda
Baking soda is another name for sodium bicarbonate, which is promoted as a cure for cancer based on the theory that cancer is a fungus and is always white; both of which are wrong.
Treatment is most commonly administered by direct injection into a tumour, which can lead to death.
At its most basic, it's a treatment based on an incorrect assumption, and tests have concluded that the claims are false.

Bee venom
It has been claimed that bee venom has an anti-cancer effect. They take a bee, make it sting you in the area of the cancer and hey-presto, you're cured. Problem is a) it don't work and b) (yeah nice pun there) they can't sting your liver, or your bladder, etc., so

just thinking about it rationally would make you question it anyway. Tests have shown it has no effect on cancer and it hurts.

Biobran

Biobran is made from breaking down rice bran with enzymes from the Shitake mushroom.

It is claimed to increase the number of natural killer (NK) cells in the blood as NK cells are part of the immune system.

As it has been promoted for a cancer cure for at least twelve years, it's surprising the manufacturers haven't conducted any clinical trials to prove its effectiveness.

There is no evidence to confirm it has any effect on NK or cancer cells.

Biologically guided chemotherapy

Biologically guided chemotherapy is another name for Revici's Guided Chemotherapy, which is another cancer cure linked to acidity in the body.

Despite using the word chemotherapy, it doesn't even fulfil the definition, but does lend credibility to the treatment.

It was invented by Emanuel Revici 1896-1997, who in 1993 had his medical licence permanently revoked by New York State.

Administered by either mouth or injection, it is a chemical mixture that includes lipid alcohol, zinc, iron, caffeine, and various metals.

There is no evidence of it having any positive effect on cancer and has serious side effects.

Bioresonance Therapy

Bioresonance therapy is based on the theory that cancer cells emit electromagnetic oscillations that can be found and treated using an electrical device.

In a petri dish with isolated cancer cells, this does work, but targeting specific cells in the human body is—at this stage—impossible.

I've carried out a lot of research on this topic and even the manufactures of the machines go to great lengths to say that the machine cannot detect or treat cancer, yet practitioners still make outrageous claims of their success in cancer treatment.
The Memorial Sloan Kettering Cancer Center says that such claims are not supported by any evidence, which would also seem to confirm the manufacturer's claims, and in addition, the US Food and Drug Administration has prosecuted sellers of such devices.

Black Cohosh
Actaea racemose is a flowering plant that is claimed to have health giving properties. According to Cancer Research UK, there is no evidence to support any claims that it treats or prevents cancer.

Black Salve
Black Salve is a dangerous paste used in alternative medicine to treat tumours near the skin, such as a breast cancer tumour. The paste is spread on the area and left to burn the tumour out. It burns through the skin, destroys skin tissue, leaves a thick scar, and it doesn't work.
The US Food and Drug Administration has listed it as a fake cancer cure that has no effect on cancer.

Black Sampson Therapy
Black Sampson therapy (also known as echinacea) is a herbal supplement derived from plants in the daisy family.
It is marketed primarily to prevent and lessen the symptoms of cold and flu.
Others sell it as a cure for cancer, but there is no evidence of this anywhere other than in their sales pitch.
In addition, some products have been found to be contaminated with arsenic, lead, and selenium.
According to Cancer Research UK, there is no scientific evidence to show that echinacea can help treat, prevent, or cure cancer in any way.

Breuss diet

The breuss diet is a diet based on vegetable juice and tea devised by Rudolf Breuss (1899–1990), who claimed it could cure cancer. It has been proven that cancer diets are simply a marketing ploy to make money, and there is no evidence of a change in diet having any effect on cancer and can actually make matters worse. If you think about it, when fighting cancer, the body needs more energy than normal, so restricting food intake or supplementing it with woo-woo fads just can't make any sense.

Budwig Protocol (Diet)

The Budwig Protocol is an anti-cancer diet developed in the 1950s by Johanna Budwig (1908–2003). The diet is rich in flaxseed oil mixed with cottage cheese, and emphasises meals high in fruits, vegetables, and fibre; it avoids sugar, salad oil, animal fats, meats, butter, and margarine.

It has been proven that cancer diets are simply a marketing ploy to make money, and there is no evidence of a change in diet having any effect on cancer and can actually make matters worse. If you think about it, when fighting cancer, the body needs more energy than normal, so restricting food intake or supplementing it with woo-woo fads just can't make any sense.

Caesium chloride

Caesium chloride is a toxic salt that is promoted as a cancer cure that targets cancer cells

Tests have concluded that the salt has no effect on cancer in the human body, and its use can induce cardiac arrest, hypokalemia, arrythmia, and death.

Cancell

Cancell is a liquid formula containing inositol, nitric acid, sodium sulfite, potassium hydroxide, sulfuric acid, and catechol, that it is claimed cures Alzheimer's disease, multiple sclerosis, diabetes, AIDS, and cancer.

The claim is the mixture can lower the voltage of cells, causing them to digest themselves; a claim that was found to be false.

The ingredients were tested by the National Cancer Institute and found to have no effect on cancer in humans, either separately or combined.

Cannabis

Cannabis or Marijuana is dried buds from varieties of the cannabis sativa plant.

Also known as pot, grass, weed, hemp, hash, ganja and lots of other names.

It seems to kill cancer cells in a dish, but there aren't enough trials to confirm or deny how successful it is on humans, and there are so many strains and variations, it's going to take time. There seems to be potential, but there is no evidence to suggest it cures cancer.

What I can confirm is that when you are on treatment and have no appetite, cannabis will give you the 'munchies', and you'll eat again, and sometimes it makes the food taste way better than normal, which is great if chemo has taken your taste away.

I can also help with sleep, which again, if you're on chemo and can't sleep, is a good thing.

In some countries, you can get it legally, in others you can't, but I don't know of any country where you can't get some somewhere.

I wouldn't recommend smoking joints filled with tobacco, as that sort of defeats the point, but edibles—where no smoke is generated—would probably be okay; but I'm not recommending it. I can't. Then again, I did use it when I was on chemo and for taste and sleeping it was wonderful when I had access to it.

If you do decide to try it, be sensible.

Cantron

Cantron is a liquid formula containing inositol, nitric acid, sodium sulfite, potassium hydroxide, sulfuric acid, and catechol, that it is claimed cures Alzheimer's disease, multiple sclerosis, diabetes, AIDS, and cancer.

The claim is the mixture can lower the voltage of cells, causing them to digest themselves; a claim that was found to be false.

The ingredients were tested by the National Cancer Institute and found to have no effect on cancer in humans, either separately or combined.

Cansema
Cansema is also known as Black Salve, which is a dangerous paste used in alternative medicine to treat tumours near the skin, such as a breast cancer tumour. The paste is spread on the area and left to burn the tumour out. It burns through the skin, destroys skin tissue, leaves a thick scar, and it doesn't work.
The US Food and Drug Administration has listed it as a fake cancer cure that has no effect on cancer.

Capsicum
Capsicum is a product derived from plants in the nightshade family such as hot chilli peppers, cayenne pepper, and jalapeños. It is marketed under various names including capsicum, cayenne and conoids.
It can be administered by various methods including teas and capsules.
Depending on the type of cancer cell, in studies Capsicum has been shown to both promote the growth of cancer cells (particularly skin cancer cells), whilst killing others.
Research is ongoing, but at this time, research trials have not been conducted on humans, so it is not recommended by any recognised institution as a cancer treatment.

Carcalon
Carcalon is another name for Krebiozen, which is a mineral oil-based liquid claimed to cure cancer.
Analysis of the oil has proved that it is nothing more than basic mineral oil with a price tag of $170,000 per gram.
The American Cancer Society say that there is no evidence of it having any effect on cancer, and the US Food and Drug Administration say it has been linked to several dangerous side effects.

Carctol
Carctol is a mixture of eight herbs marketed by Dr Nandlal Tiwari in 1968 and now sold as pills.
The claim is that although none of the herbs have any anti-cancer properties, the mixture makes them special.
Allegedly, the mixture removes acid from your body leaving a low pH environment where cancer cells can't live.
The alternative practitioners claim that cancer cells can't survive in a non-acidic environment and lowering the pH level will kill the cells, and although the claim has some merit in so far that cancer cells in a petri dish die, the level required to kill the cancer cells will also kill all the other cells necessary to survive, so if you could lower your pH to the required level, you would die anyway.
There are a lot of side effects such as stomach cramps, diarrhoea, allergic reactions, irregular heart rhythm, low levels of blood potassium, short term kidney changes, changes in mind function.
Not only does it not work, but if it did you would be dead anyway.

Cassava
Cassava is a woody shrub from South America, rich in carbohydrate, it also produces cyanide to deter animals from eating it.
The idea is to introduce it to the cancer cells with the aim of causing them to commit suicide; unfortunately, it can lead to cyanide poisoning.
Although research has been carried out on rats, there was insufficient evidence to conduct human trials.
It has no effect on cancer cells other than in a petri dish.

Castor Oil Therapy
Castor oil is made from the seeds of the castor oil plant
It is claimed that application to the skin can cure cancer, but even in a petri dish, it has little or no effect on cancer cells, and with that in mind, it has no effect on skin cancer or any other cancer either.

Cat's claw

Cat's claw is another name for uncaria tomentosa, which is a woody vine found in the tropical jungles of South and Central America, which is promoted as a cure for cancer.
It has been tested and found to have no effect on cancer, however, its use does have some serious side effects which include death.

Cayenne Pepper

Cayenne pepper is a product derived from plants in the nightshade family such as hot chilli peppers and jalapeños.
It is marketed under various names including capsicum, cayenne, and conoids.
It can be administered by various methods including teas and capsules.
Depending on the type of cancer cell, in studies Capsicum has been shown to both promote the growth of cancer cells (particularly skin cancer cells), whilst killing others.
Research is ongoing, but at this time, research trials have not been conducted on humans, so it is not recommended by any recognised institution as a cancer treatment.

CD protocol or CDS

CD protocol is another name for Miracle Mineral Supplement, which is a toxic solution of 28% sodium chlorine in citrus juice, promoted for treating cancer, HIV, malaria, common colds, Parkinson's, autism, acne, AIDS, and other ailments.
Its main use is as an industrial bleach.
Side effects include nausea, vomiting, diarrhoea, symptoms of severe dehydration, renal failure, and other life-threatening conditions.
It was invented by Jim Humble, a former scientologist who promoted it in his 2006 book, The Miracle Mineral Solution of the 21st Century.
It is reported that in August 2009, a woman took it as a preventative for malaria and within 15 minutes she was ill, and 12 hours later was dead.

Celandine
Celandine is made from chelidonium majus, a member of the poppy family promoted for its ability to treat cancer.
According to the American Cancer Society, available scientific evidence does not support claims that celandine is effective in treating cancer.

CBD Oil
CBD oil is made from hemp, and some claim it cures everything under the sun.
It has any effect on cancer, and if used in conjunction with other drugs, can have dangerous effects.
Please see article on CBD oil before this section for more details.

Cell therapy or Cellular therapy
Cell therapy involves the use of fresh embryonic cells taken from the corresponding organ of an animal and injected into the patient.
The claim is that the recipient's body transports the animal cells to target the organ and repair the cancerous tissue.
The American Cancer Society says that there is no evidence to suggest that this works, and the practice has caused serious side effects and death.

Chaga tea
Chaga tea is made from the inonotus obliquus (chaga) mushroom
Originally used as a folk remedy in Siberia and Russia since the 16th century, it is now promoted as Chaga Tea, with the claim that it can cure cancer.
It is widely promoted on the internet and is freely available to purchase.
There is no scientific evidence that it has any effect on cancer, and if used in conjunction with other drugs, can have dangerous effects.

Chaparral
Chaparral is made from leaves and twigs from the creosote bush.

Although it contains biologically active molecules that have been successful in blocking cellular division of cancer cells in a petri dish, it had no effect on cancer cells in the human body.
Several patients (not in any trial) who drank chaparral tea regularly developed kidney cysts, kidney cancer and liver damage.
There is no evidence to show it having any effect on cancer cells in the body.

Chelation therapy
Chelation therapy is promoted as a cure for cancer by removing metals from the body. Although it is a legitimate therapy used in cases of heavy metal poisoning, it has no effect on cancer.
It involves the injection of chelating agents that can remove heavy metals, chemical toxins, fatty plaques, and mineral deposits from the body.
Side effects include irregular heartbeat, kidney damage, and death.
It is widely used as a cancer cure in Mexico.

Chelidonium majus
Chelidonium majus is a member of the poppy family promoted for its ability to treat cancer.
According to the American Cancer Society, available scientific evidence does not support claims that celandine is effective in treating cancer.

Chinese yam
Chinese yam is made from the roots of the wild yam and is made into creams and dietary supplements that are claimed to prevent and cure cancer.
Scientific tests have proved that it has no preventative or curative effects on cancer and is completely ineffective.

Chlorella
Chlorella is a type of algae that is promoted to treat cancer. No clinical trials have been carried out to confirm its effectiveness, but when tested in a petri dish, it had no effect on cancer cells.

Chlorine Dioxide Solution
Chlorine Dioxide Solution is another name for Miracle Mineral Supplement, which is a toxic solution of 28% sodium chlorine in citrus juice, promoted for treating cancer, HIV, malaria, common colds, Parkinson's, autism, acne, AIDS, and other ailments.
Its main use is as an industrial bleach.
Side effects include nausea, vomiting, diarrhoea, symptoms of severe dehydration, renal failure, and other life-threatening conditions.
It was invented by Jim Humble, a former scientologist who promoted it in his 2006 book, The Miracle Mineral Solution of the 21st Century.
It is reported that in August 2009, a woman took it as a preventative for malaria and within 15 minutes she was ill, and 12 hours later was dead.

Chromotherapy
The use of different coloured light is used which allegedly corresponds to chakras or different organs in the body.
According to the American Cancer Society, chromotherapy or the use of light boxes have no effect on any type of cancer.

Clark's Cure for All Cancers
A magical cure for cancer invented/concocted by Hulda Clark, Ph.D., ND., 1928-2009, who claimed that all cancers are caused by parasites, toxins and pollutants. With this in mind, she deduced that by killing the parasites and eliminating chemicals, she could cure all cancers. She used black walnut hulls, wormwood and common cloves in her mixture, and in her book, Cure for All Cancers, she cites 103 case histories where her magic cure worked. However, a quick analysis of her reports would suggest

that most of her patients did not have cancer anyway, and those that did, had received conventional treatment in the first place. Her notions have been described as absurd nonsense, and, considering the fact that she died from cancer in 2009, the phrase, physician heal thyself, is somewhat redundant.

Colloidal silver

Colloidal silver is a liquid of silver particles sold as a dietary supplement and claimed to cure cancer

The idea is that it can convert cancerous cells back to normal by killing microbes.

The Memorial Sloan-Kettering Cancer Center says colloidal silver cannot cure cancer, AIDS, or diabetes. Taking too much colloidal silver by mouth can cause skin discoloration, seizures, and kidney damage.

Colon cleansing

Widely promoted as a cure for cancer by introducing coffee or laxatives into the colon.

The idea that putting coffee up your bum has any effect on cancer just mystifies me.

Not unexpectedly, The American Cancer Society say that there is no evidence of this practice having any effect on cancer.

Coneflower Therapy

Coneflower therapy (also known as echinacea) is a herbal supplement derived from plants in the daisy family.

It is marketed primarily to prevent and lessen the symptoms of cold and flu.

Others sell it as a cure for cancer, but there is no evidence of this anywhere other than in their sales pitch.

In addition, some products have been found to be contaminated with arsenic, lead, and selenium.

According to Cancer Research UK, there is no scientific evidence to show that echinacea can help treat, prevent, or cure cancer in any way.

Conoid Therapy

Capsicum (marketed as conoid therapy) is a product derived from plants in the nightshade family such as hot chilli peppers, cayenne pepper, and jalapeños.

It is marketed under various names including capsicum, cayenne and conoids.

It can be administered by various methods including teas and capsules.

Depending on the type of cancer cell, in studies Capsicum has been shown to both promote the growth of cancer cells (particularly skin cancer cells), whilst killing others.

Research is ongoing, but at this time, research trials have not been conducted on humans, so it is not recommended by any recognised institution as a cancer treatment.

Contreras Therapy

What is it? That's a good question. It varies from alternative practice to alternative practice, with no apparent reasoning behind the various treatments thrown into the schedules.

The protocol was designed by Dr Ernesto Contreras, who seems to have thought that by throwing everything into the mix, something might work.

The therapy includes psychology, spiritual guidance, singing and laughter sessions, because as everybody knows, laughter stimulates the immune system and cures cancer. Seriously? Spiritual guidance? Why don't they bring in a witch doctor as well? If your doctor is having to pray for you, I'd be worried. Is it a doctor looking after you or a cleric? In what realm does any of this make sense?

It is primarily offered as an alternative treatment in Mexico and includes the use of amygdalin and metabolic therapy.

The Memorial Sloan-Kettering Cancer Centre says that it demonstrates no evidence of efficacy.

Coral calcium

A dietary supplement made from crushed coral promoted to cure cancer.

The National Center for Complementary and Alternative Medicine says there is no scientific evidence of it having any effect on cancer.

Creatine

Creatine is another name for Krebiozen, which is a mineral oil-based liquid claimed to cure cancer.

Analysis of the oil has proved that it is nothing more than basic mineral oil with a price tag of $170,000 per gram.

The American Cancer Society say that there is no evidence of it having any effect on cancer, and the US Food and Drug Administration say it has been linked to several dangerous side effects.

Crocinic Acid

Crocinic Acid is a liquid formula containing inositol, nitric acid, sodium sulfite, potassium hydroxide, sulfuric acid, and catechol, that it is claimed cures Alzheimer's disease, multiple sclerosis, diabetes, AIDS, and cancer.

The claim is the mixture can lower the voltage of cells, causing them to digest themselves; a claim that was found to be false.

The ingredients were tested by the National Cancer Institute and found to have no effect on cancer in humans, either separately or combined.

Dandelion Root

The root of a dandelion is said to kill 98% of cancer cells in only 48 hours.

This claim is based on a 72-year-old man sent home to die with chronic myelomonocytic leukaemia who—after drinking dandelion tea—was cured within four months.

The fact is that dandelion root has not been shown to treat or prevent cancer.

In a laboratory environment, it can have an effect on cancer cells, but so can bleach. No similar findings have been shown in humans with cancer.

The explanation for the man's cure will never be known, but if he had changed his diet to drinking vinegar, I suspect that it too would be considered a wonder drug.

Di Bella Therapy

Di Bella Therapy was devised by Luigi di Bella 1912-2003 and is a mixture of drugs, vitamins, and hormones.
Side effects include vomiting, increased blood sugar levels, low blood pressure, vomiting, diarrhoea, and neurological symptoms.
The American Cancer Society say there is no evidence to showing it having any effect on cancer and can be extremely dangerous.

Dimethyl sulfoxide

Dimethyl sulfoxide is an organosulfur compound (organic material that contains sulfur) promoted since the 60s as a cure for cancer.
It has been tested and found to have no effect on cancer.

DMSO

DMSO is another name for Dimethyl sulfoxide which is an organosulfur compound (organic material that contains sulfur) promoted since the 60s as a cure for cancer.
It has been tested and found to have no effect on cancer.

Drug X

Drug X is another name for Krebiozen, which is a mineral oil-based liquid claimed to cure cancer.
Analysis of the oil has proved that it is nothing more than basic mineral oil with a price tag of $170,000 per gram.
The American Cancer Society say that there is no evidence of it having any effect on cancer, and the US Food and Drug Administration say it has been linked to several dangerous side effects.

Echinacea

Echinacea is a herbal supplement derived from plants in the daisy family. It is marketed primarily to prevent and lessen the symptoms of cold and flu.

Others sell it as a cure for cancer, but there is no evidence of this anywhere other than in their sales pitch.

In addition, some products have been found to be contaminated with arsenic, lead, and selenium.

According to Cancer Research UK, there is no scientific evidence to show that echinacea can help treat, prevent, or cure cancer in any way.

Electro Physiological Feedback Xrroid (EPFX)

Electro Physiological Feedback Xrroid (EPFX) is an energy machine which reads the body's reaction to frequencies and makes changes.

It is a Quantum Xrroid device (??) that claims to balance bio-energetic forces that have never been found in any scientific study.

Mainly, it reflects the skin's resistance to low-voltage electric currents, which, of course, has no effect on any known cancer.

As a result of using this therapy, there have been deaths reported, and the machine is banned in the USA.

Electrohomeopathy

Electrohomeopathy or the Mattei cancer cure is a treatment devised by Count Cesare Mattei (1809–1896), who suggested that different colours of electricity could be used to treat cancer.

I'm struggling to understand just what colours of electricity are available, but although this cure was popular in the late nineteenth century, it has been described as idiotic by those who actually know about the effect electricity has on the human body, and specifically cancer cells.

Ellagic Acid

Ellagic acid is found in strawberries, raspberries, blackberries, and walnuts.

Although it may bind to chemicals that cause cancer and prevent growth in laboratories, it has no quantifiable effect on cancer in humans.
Companies selling it as a cancer cure in America have received warning letters from the Food and Drug Administration.

Emu oil
Emu oil is derived from the adipose tissue (body fat) of the emu. It is claimed to cure a wide range of diseases including cancer. The US Food and Drug Administration have said it's a prime example of a rip-off, as it does nothing.

Entelev
Entelev is a liquid formula containing inositol, nitric acid, sodium sulfite, potassium hydroxide, sulfuric acid, and catechol, that it is claimed cures Alzheimer's disease, multiple sclerosis, diabetes, AIDS, and cancer.
The claim is the mixture can lower the voltage of cells, causing them to digest themselves; a claim that was found to be false. The ingredients were tested by the National Cancer Institute and found to have no effect on cancer in humans, either separately or combined.

Essiac Tea
Invented in the 20s by Rene Caisse (Essiac is the surname reversed), it was originally a recipe from an Ojibwa medicine man. (Lot of credibility and cutting-edge technology there.)
It is a type of tea made from five different types of roots, which are believed to be burdock, sorrel, Indian rhubarb, and slippery elm, as well as other undisclosed ingredients.
Rene Cassie had a cancer clinic for terminal cancer patients from 1935-1941. Shortly before her death in 1978, she provided the secret formula to The Resperin Corporation, who provided it on the Canadian market.
Several animal tests have been carried out and no evidence found of it having any effect on cancer cells. In addition, a review of 86

cancer patients who voluntarily used it, found no evidence of any beneficial effect.
It is on a Food and Drug Administration list of fake cancer cures. Of course, it is still recommended and available on the internet, and people still buy it in the mistaken belief that it can provide the magic cancer cure.

Faith healing
Faith healing is an attempt to wish your cancer away.
Although there may be a placebo effect depending on how strong your belief in the process is, there is (unsurprisingly) no medical evidence to prove effectiveness.
It's interesting to note that faith healing is only ever practised in places of worship and never in a medical environment where it could be checked. The internet is full of videos of people coming under the spell, dancing, fainting, spinning around, etc., but only in places of worship. Makes you wonder, though, doesn't it?

Fasting
Fasting has been claimed by some alternative medicine practitioners to help fight cancer, perhaps by starving tumours. The clue as to its effectiveness is in the word perhaps.
If you starve the tumours, you starve yourself of the energy needed to live and fight, and patients who try this while on chemotherapy can reduce the effects of treatment and (without medical intervention) ultimately die.

Fenbendazole or FenBen
Fenbendazole or FenBen is the main ingredient in dog deworming treatment.
Please see article on dog dewormer before this section for more details.

Gc-MAF
Around 2008 Gc-MAF (Gc protein-derived macrophage activating factor) was first promoted as a cure for cancer.

In 2015 the UK Medicines and Healthcare Products Regulatory Agency (MHRA) closed a factory in Cambridgeshire that was marketing GcMAF as a cancer cure.
According to Cancer Research UK there is no scientific evidence to show that the treatment is safe or effective.

German New Medicine
German New Medicine is a medical system invented by Ryke Geerd Hamer 1935-2017, on the theory that disease comes from emotional shock. He also thought mainstream medicine is a conspiracy by Jews to kill non-Jews.
Hammer had his medical licence revoked for malpractice in 1986.
It is based on five laws:
1) Cold disease presents with cold skin, stress, weight loss and skin disorders.
2) Rheumatic fever, infections and allergies.
3) Disease is controlled by the brain
4) Microbes heal the body, but modern medicine stops them working.
5) Disease doesn't exist, what we call disease is a special meaningful program of nature.
Several patients have died or deteriorated so badly that government intervention was necessary to save their lives.
There is no evidence of it being able to cure cancer and it has killed patients.

Germanium
Germanium is a metalloid sold as a dietary supplement with the claim that it cures cancer.
It can be found in garlic, ginseng, aloe, and comfrey, and is also a by-product of coal combustion and zinc ore processing.
The water in Lourde's, France, has a high concentration and it is recommended that you bathe in it, drink it and a magic cure appears for AIDS, cancer, asthma, HIV, arthritis, etc.
Serious side effects include kidney, lung, and nerve damage.

The Memorial Sloan Kettering Cancer Center states that it has no effect on cancer and can lead to chronic kidney failure and death.

Gerson Therapy

Mostly diet based, it limits salt, protein and other foods, while recommending a large quantity of fruits, vegetables, and raw calf's liver, that are juiced and drunk, one gallon per day. Oh, and coffee enemas.

The theory is that by juicing fruits and vegetables, it eliminates toxins from the body and augments the intake of potassium and iodine.

The practice also includes liver extract injections, thyroid tablets, royal jelly capsules, ozone enemas, linseed oil, castor oil enemas, clay packs, laetrile, coffee enemas, and vaccines from the influenza virus. The main problem with the therapy—apart from the fact it doesn't work—is that there is no actual recipe, and it seems that everything that can be sold/included is thrown in the mix.

The therapy was developed by a German physician called Max Gerson, who practiced his cure in New York City until he died in 1959. It is still available and widely promoted as a cure in Mexico.

In 1947, a review of 86 patients by the New York County Medical Society found no evidence of the treatment having any effect on cancer.

In the 80s, at least 13 cancer patients treated with the therapy were admitted to San Diego hospitals with Campylobacter Fetus sepsis, which was attributable to the liver injections. None were cancer free, one died within a week, and five were comatose due to low serum sodium levels.

Numerous other deaths have been attributed to this approach due to the use of coffee enemas.

Ginger

Ginger is obtained from the root of plants in the Zingiber family and is popular in cuisine.

It has been promoted as a cure for cancer with the claim it is 10,000 times more effective than conventional chemotherapy. Yes, 10,000 times more effective.
According to the American Cancer Society, there is no scientific evidence of it having any effect on cancer.

Ginseng
Ginseng is a species of perennial plant, the root of which is promoted for its therapeutic value, which also includes the claim that it can fight cancer.
Various tests have been conducted with all arriving at the same conclusion, that it has no effect on cancer.

Glyconutrients
Glyconutrients is a type of sugar which is extracted from plants. A company called Mannatech repackaged this sugar and marketed it under the brand name Ambrotose, which, it is claimed, promotes cellular health and boosts the immune system.
It's surprising a company is promoting sugar to cure cancer when others are saying sugar feeds cancer cells, but as it doesn't work, it's redundant anyway.
The Memorial Sloan Kettering Cancer Center says there is no evidence of glyconutrients having any effect on cancer.

Goldenseal
Goldenseal (or Hydrastis canadensis) is a herb from the buttercup family which is claimed to cure cancer.
Severe toxic side-effects have resulted in many deaths from this protocol.
There is no evidence of it having any effect on cancer.

Gonzalez Protocol
The Gonzalez Protocol was a regime devised by Nicholas Gonzalez 1947-2015, who based his protocol on the Gerson Therapy treatment.

Nutritional supplements of up to 150 pills per day, that include minerals, vitamins, trace elements, extracts of animal organs such as the thymus and liver of sheep or cows, was used in addition to the Gerson Therapy.
It would seem to me that again another treatment was thrown into the Gerson mix and claimed success in treating cancer patients.
The Memorial Sloan-Kettering Cancer Center has said that the treatment is a type of metabolic therapy that shows no evidence of efficacy.

Grapes
Another diet-based cure that was invented by Johanna Brandt 1876-1964, who claimed that a grape diet could cure cancer.
More recently grapes have been promoted in the form of grape seed extract (GSE).
The American Cancer Society says there is no evidence to confirm that grapes, or GSE, or drinking red wine, has any effect on cancer.

Graviola
Made from the soursop fruit and sold as a dietary supplement with the claim that it cures cancer.
After tests by the US Federal Trade Commission it was found to have no effect on cancer.

Gotu kola
Gotu kola is a swamp plant native to parts of Africa and Asia.
It is sold as a supplement that is claimed to be a cure for cancer.
Scientific tests have confirmed that it has no effect on cancer.

GSE
GSE is a cure based on grape seed extract that follows up on the claim by Johanna Brandt 1876-1964, that a grape diet can cure cancer.
The American Cancer Society says there is no evidence to confirm that grapes, or GSE, or drinking red wine, has any effect on cancer.

Hallelujah Diet
The hallelujah diet is a restrictive biblical diet based on raw food and claimed by its inventor, the Rev George M Malkmus, to have cured his cancer.
It's worth remembering that a lot of people have cured cancers that they never had in the first place. In this case the Rev George M Malkmus never consulted a cancer specialist, but instead relied on nutritionists and chiropractors for his diagnosis. He also confirmed that he never had any biopsies and didn't know if it was even malignant. Just a lump then?
The Hallelujah Diet is unbalanced and can lead to serious deficiencies in the human body that are essential in fighting cancer.

Herbalism
Herbalism is a whole-body approach to promote health, in which substances are derived from entire plants so as not to disturb the delicate chemistry of the plant.
According to Cancer Research UK, there is no evidence that herbal remedies can treat, prevent or cure cancer.

High pH therapy
High pH therapy is the use of caesium chloride, a toxic salt claimed to target cancer cells and cure cancer.
Tests have concluded that the salt has no effect on cancer in the human body, and its use can induce cardiac arrest, hypokalemia (low levels of potassium), arrythmia, and death.

Holistic Medicine
Holistic medicine is a general term for an approach to medicine that includes mental and spiritual aspects. Practitioners believe that the whole person is made up of separate and independent parts, so if one part is not working well, it affects all the other parts.
Treatments include spiritual counselling, massage, acupuncture, advice on diet and exercise, etc.

Practitioners believe that all people have innate healing powers and that the patient is a person, not a disease.
Healing takes a team approach involving the patient and doctor and addresses all aspects of a person's life using a variety of health care practices.
Treatment allegedly involves finding and fixing the cause of the condition, not just alleviating the symptoms.
The American Cancer Society say that available scientific evidence does not support claims that these complementary and alternative methods, when used without mainstream or conventional medicine, are effective in treating cancer or any other disease.

Homeopathy
Invented by Samuel Hahnemann 1755-1843, it is based on the idea like-treats-like, so if say you can't sleep because you have too much caffeine in your system, you administer a homeopathic remedy made from caffeine to cure your sleeplessness. It's only a small amount; similar to dropping a single asprin in the Atlantic Ocean, letting it mix and calling it a cure.
It is said that homeopathy does no harm and has no side effects, which is because all you're really getting is a sugar tablet. If it had a side effect where it killed cancer cells, that would be good, but it don't.
I couldn't find a recognised cancer charity website that didn't say; there is no scientific evidence homeopathy can treat or prevent cancer, or words to that effect.
Please see article on homeopathy before this section for more details.

Hoxsey Therapy
Hoxsey Therapy was invented by a naturopath by the name of Harry Hoxsey and uses a caustic herbal paste for external cancers which is made up of corrosive agents such as arsenic sulphide.
For internal cancers he recommended the use of laxatives, vitamin supplements, douches, and dietary changes.

The caustic herbal paste is a very painful and useless treatment which can cause a lot of other problems.
The treatment for internal cancers includes potassium iodide, red clover, burdock, stillinga root, berberis root, pokeroot, ash bark, buckthoun bark, licorice and red clover, all of which have been found to be useless against cancer cells.
After repeated clashes with the Food and Drug Administration, he was forced to close his clinic in Dallas in the late 50s, however, his chief nurse offered it in Mexico afterwards.
The man himself developed prostate cancer in 1967 and underwent surgery after his therapy proved ineffective.
A review by the Memorial Sloan-Kettering Cancer Center found no evidence that the Hoxsey Therapy was effective as a treatment for cancer.

Hydrastis canadensis

Hydrastis canadensis (or Goldenseal) is a herb from the buttercup family which is claimed to cure cancer.
Severe toxic side-effects have resulted in many deaths from this protocol.
There is no evidence of it having any effect on cancer.

Hydrazine sulfate

Hydrazine sulfate is a chemical compound promoted to cure cancer and also used in the production of agricultural chemicals and rocket fuel.
Tests were conducted by the National Cancer Institute on 243 patients with non-small cell lung cancer, and 266 patients with advanced lung cancer, the results showed nerve damage and a significant reduction in the quality of life accompanied by kidney and liver failure, however, no evidence was found of it having any effect on cancer and in fact was found to increase the incidence of breast, lung, and liver cancers and basal cell carcinoma.

Hyperbaric chamber therapy
Hyperbaric therapy involves the use of pressurised oxygen. The patient is enclosed in a chamber where the oxygen is released on the understanding that cancer can't survive in an oxygen rich environment, which is the opposite of what happens. Cancer cells thrive on oxygen, which is the reason tumours make new vessels that tap into alternative supplies, a process called angiogenesis. In effect, hyperbaric therapy feeds the cells it claims to kill, and that isn't a good thing.

Inonotus obliquus
Inonotus obliquus is more commonly known as chaga mushroom. Originally used as a folk remedy in Siberia and Russia since the 16th century, it is now promoted as Chaga Tea, with the claim that it can cure cancer.
It is widely promoted on the internet and is freely available to purchase.
There is no scientific evidence that it has any effect on cancer, and if used in conjunction with other drugs, can have dangerous effects.

Inositol hexaphosphate
Inositol hexaphosphate is also marketed as IP-6, a vitamin-like substance. It is found in animals and many plants, especially cereals, nuts, and legumes. It can also be made in a laboratory. The claims state it has been used to cure not only cancer, but osteoporosis, Alzheimer's, cardiovascular disease, depression, diabetes, kidney stones, Parkinson's, and probably ingrown toenails, so it's very specific in its use.
On its website www.IP-6.net it lists various websites for you to check, one of them being The American Cancer Society, but when I contacted them, they had never heard of it.
It's interesting to note that although the website has lots of suggestive comments relating to it curing cancer, when you go to a site to purchase it, there are no claims made regarding cancer; it merely says it's for proper function of the body, whatever that means.

A book has been written by Abulkalam M. Shamsuddin, MD, Ph.D, a Professor of Pathology, and it is claimed that he has popularised IP-6 as an anti-cancer tool. Not surprising when you discover that if you go online to buy IP-6, the pills are called, Shamsuddin unique IP-6 with Inositol. I wonder if he has an interest in promoting it as a wonder drug that cures cancer. I wonder if his friends just call him 'Sham' for short. Interestingly, the site selling it makes no claims about using it to treat cancer. Tests on cancer cells in a petri dish confirm that it can slow their replication, but as no conclusive testing has been done on humans, there is nothing to suggest it cures cancer, which is confirmed on the FAQ section of the website where it states; The anticancer effect of Inositol in vivo is relatively week [sic].

Insulin potentiation therapy
Insulin potentiation therapy is the practice of injecting insulin alongside a low dose of conventional chemotherapy drugs in the belief this improves the overall effect of the treatment.
Potentiation is the increase in strength of nerve impulses.
The theory is that by introducing insulin into the chemotherapy regimen, a lower dose of chemotherapy will have the same effect as a higher dose without insulin.
Developed in Mexico by Dr Donato Perez Garcis in the 30s, it was based on the belief that cancer cells consume more sugar and are therefore more sensitive to insulin, so reducing the chemotherapy normally given to 10% will have the same effect. There is no evidence that it has any effect on treatment and reducing the amount of chemotherapy necessary is idiotic.

IP-6 with Inositol
IP-6 with Inositol is a vitamin-like substance. It is found in animals and many plants, especially cereals, nuts, and legumes. It can also be made in a laboratory.
The claims state it has been used to cure not only cancer, but osteoporosis, Alzheimer's, cardiovascular disease, depression,

diabetes, kidney stones, Parkinson's, and probably ingrown toenails, so it's very specific in its use.
On its website www.IP-6.net it lists various websites for you to check, one of them being The American Cancer Society, but when I contacted them, they had never heard of it.
It's interesting to note that although the website has lots of suggestive comments relating to it curing cancer, when you go to a site to purchase it, there are no claims made regarding cancer; it merely says it's for proper function of the body, whatever that means.
A book has been written by Abulkalam M. Shamsuddin, MD, Ph.D, a Professor of Pathology, and it is claimed that he has popularised IP-6 as an anti-cancer tool. Not surprising when you discover that if you go online to buy IP-6, the pills are called, Shamsuddin unique IP-6 with Inositol. I wonder if he has an interest in promoting it as a wonder drug that cures cancer. I wonder if his friends just call him 'Sham' for short. Interestingly, the site selling it makes no claims about using it to treat cancer. Tests on cancer cells in a petri dish confirm that it can slow their replication, but as no conclusive testing has been done on humans, there is nothing to suggest it cures cancer, which is confirmed on the FAQ section of the website where it states; The anticancer effect of Inositol in vivo is relatively week [sic].

Ipe roxo or Ipes
Ipe roxo is another name for Pau d'arco, which is a tea made from the bark of the Tabebuia tree found in a South American rainforest and is claimed to be an ancient Inca Indian remedy. The bark is brewed into lapacho tea and marketed as a cure for cancer.
It was studied in the 70s and found to cause nausea, vomiting, and have the ability to interfere with blood clotting.
No evidence was found of it having any effect on cancer, but when consumed, can be dangerous.

Iscador
Iscador is an extract of mistletoe, which was first proposed by Rudolf Steiner 1861-1925, he believed in the occult and founded the Society for Cancer Research to promote his cure. He claimed the plant had to be harvested when the sun, moon, and planets were in exact alignment.
According to the American Cancer Society, well-designed clinical trials have been carried out and no evidence found to support any claim that mistletoe has any effect on cancer.
The Swiss Society for Oncology also tested it for effectiveness and concluded that it had no effect.

Issels Treatment
Issels Treatment involves the removal of metal fillings from a patient's mouth and a restrictive diet in an attempt to remove traces of metal from the body.
Issels has to make sense as it's a medical fact that there has never been a patient with cancer that hasn't had metal fillings in their teeth. (Yeah, I made that last bit up.)
Cancer Research UK state that there is no scientific or medical evidence to back up the claims made by the Issels website.

JS–114, JS–101
JS–114, JS–101 is a liquid formula containing inositol, nitric acid, sodium sulfite, potassium hydroxide, sulfuric acid, and catechol, that it is claimed cures Alzheimer's disease, multiple sclerosis, diabetes, AIDS, and cancer.
The claim is the mixture can lower the voltage of cells, causing them to digest themselves; a claim that was found to be false.
The ingredients were tested by the National Cancer Institute and found to have no effect on cancer in humans, either separately or combined.

Jim's Juice
Jim's Juice is a liquid formula containing inositol, nitric acid, sodium sulfite, potassium hydroxide, sulfuric acid, and catechol,

that it is claimed cures Alzheimer's disease, multiple sclerosis, diabetes, AIDS, and cancer.
The claim is the mixture can lower the voltage of cells, causing them to digest themselves; a claim that was found to be false.
The ingredients were tested by the National Cancer Institute and found to have no effect on cancer in humans, either separately or combined.

Juice Plus
Juice Plus is a line of dietary supplements made from concentrated fruit and vegetable juice extract.
Brent Wallace is one of the main promotors and his advertising reads: Juice Plus product is the magic ingredient. It works! Massive dose of nutrition killed my cancer!, and there's a video to back it up.
You can read more about Juice Plus at: I'm not convinced – Brent Wallace Juice Plus.
Juice Plus is a dietary supplement, nothing more, it has no effect on cancer.
Memorial Sloan-Kettering Cancer Center cautioned that Juice Plus is being aggressively promoted to cancer patients based on claims of its antioxidant effects, but the supplement can interfere with chemotherapy and should not be considered a substitute for real food.

Juicing
Juicing has been claimed to cure cancer, but nobody knows why. Tests have been done that confirm that some extracted juices are healthier than whole foods, but as far as cancer is concerned, it has no effect.

Kansas Snakeroot Therapy
Kansas snakeroot therapy (also known as echinacea) is a herbal supplement derived from plants in the daisy family.
It is marketed primarily to prevent and lessen the symptoms of cold and flu.

Others sell it as a cure for cancer, but there is no evidence of this anywhere other than in their sales pitch.
In addition, some products have been found to be contaminated with arsenic, lead, and selenium.
According to Cancer Research UK, there is no scientific evidence to show that Kansas Snakeroot Therapy (echinacea) can help treat, prevent, or cure cancer in any way.

Kelley Treatment
Developed in the 1960s by a dentist, William Donald Kelley, the Kelley treatment is similar to Gerson Therapy but with prayer and osteopathic manipulation thrown in for good measure.
The actor, Steve McQueen, used this treatment three months before his death.
It includes vitamin and enzyme supplements, computerised metabolic typing using his Protein Metabolism Evaluation Index (??) which, he claimed, could diagnose cancer before it was clinically apparent, and his Kelley Malignancy Index could detect cancer, growth rate, location, and prognosis.
He was convicted of practicing medicine without a licence in 1970 after a witness testified he had diagnosed lung cancer and prescribed a treatment plan after simply taking a drop of blood from the patient's finger.
It is claimed that his records were analysed by Mr Gonzalez, but no evidence was found to confirm any benefit to cancer patients.
Coffee enemas and up to 150 pills per day were also part of the treatment plan.

Kombucha
Kombucha not only cures cancer, but AIDS as well.
It is a fermented tea that has been found to have adverse side effects such as poisoning, muscle inflammation, and infection.
There has been at least one death attributed to drinking kombucha and it has no effect on either cancer or AIDS.

Kousmine Diet

The Kousmine diet is a restrictive diet devised by Catherine Kousmine (1904–1992) which emphasized fruit, vegetables, grains, pulses, and the use of vitamin supplements.

As with all cancer diets, it simply weakens the patient and can result in death.

There is no evidence to suggest that the diet has any effect on cancer.

Krebiozen

Krebiozen is a mineral oil-based liquid claimed to cure cancer.

Analysis of the oil has proved that it is nothing more than basic mineral oil with a price tag of $170,000 per gram.

The American Cancer Society say there is no evidence of it having any effect on cancer, and the US Food and Drug Administration say it has been linked to several dangerous side effects.

Laetrile

Laetrile is another name for Amygdalin, which is obtained from the pits or seeds of apricots, apples, peaches, red cherries, plums, and other fruits as well as bitter almonds.

It was first patented in the 1950s and was known as Laetrile.

Touted as an alternative cancer treatment in the 60s and 70s, it is banned by the Federal Drugs and Administration due to the fact that when your intestines break it down, it converts into cyanide.

The idea is that cyanide kills the cancer cells, but the reality is that numerous deaths have been attributed to its use.

It was then repackaged as Vitamin B17 in an effort to get around regulations for drugs, but it isn't a vitamin and doesn't act like a vitamin.

There is no vitamin that reduces blood pressure to dangerous levels and induces a coma.

As little as 50 grams of amygdalin, or whatever name they choose to call it, can kill you.

Unsurprisingly, clinics in Mexico still promote it's use, but after analysis by the Food and Drug Administration, some samples were found to have excessive levels of bacteria, and samples had been bulked out with other harmful substances.
Amygdalin has been independently tested on up to 20 animal tumours and found to have no benefit either alone or together with other substances.
In a clinical trial in 1982 by the Mayo Clinic and three other cancer centres, it was administered as recommended to advanced cancer patients for which there was no other treatment available. Out of 178 patients, there was no improvement, but in those still alive after seven months, their tumours had increased, and several patients experienced symptoms of cyanide poisoning and had to stop treatment.
In a US Supreme Court ruling in 1979, it was determined that the general public deserve protection from amygdalin and called it a fraudulent cure.

Laevorotatory
Laevorotatory is another name for Amygdalin, which is obtained from the pits or seeds of apricots, apples, peaches, red cherries, plums, and other fruits as well as bitter almonds.
It was first patented in the 1950s and was known as Laetrile. Touted as an alternative cancer treatment in the 60s and 70s, it is banned by the Federal Drugs and Administration due to the fact that when your intestines break it down, it converts into cyanide. The idea is that cyanide kills the cancer cells, but the reality is that numerous deaths have been attributed to its use.
It was then repackaged as Vitamin B17 in an effort to get around regulations for drugs, but it isn't a vitamin and doesn't act like a vitamin.
There is no vitamin that reduces blood pressure to dangerous levels and induces a coma.
As little as 50 grams of amygdalin, or whatever name they choose to call it, can kill you.

Unsurprisingly, clinics in Mexico still promote it's use, but after analysis by the Food and Drug Administration, some samples were found to have excessive levels of bacteria, and samples had been bulked out with other harmful substances.
Amygdalin has been independently tested on up to 20 animal tumours and found to have no benefit either alone or together with other substances.
In a clinical trial in 1982 by the Mayo Clinic and three other cancer centres, it was administered as recommended to advanced cancer patients for which there was no other treatment available.
Out of 178 patients, there was no improvement, but in those still alive after seven months, their tumours had increased, and several patients experienced symptoms of cyanide poisoning and had to stop treatment.
In a US Supreme Court ruling in 1979, it was determined that the general public deserve protection from amygdalin and called it a fraudulent cure.

Lapacho
Lapacho is another name for Pau d'arco, which is a tea made from the bark of the Tabebuia tree found in a South American rainforest and is claimed to be an ancient Inca Indian remedy.
The bark is brewed into lapacho tea and marketed as a cure for cancer.
It was studied in the 70s and found to cause nausea, vomiting, and have the ability to interfere with blood clotting.
No evidence was found of it having any effect on cancer, but when consumed, can be dangerous.

Larrea Tridentata Therapy
Larrea tridentata is also sold as Chaparral, which is made from leaves and twigs from the creosote bush.
Although it contains biologically active molecules that have been successful in blocking cellular division of cancer cells in a petri dish, it had no effect on cancer cells in the human body.

Several patients (not in any trial) who drank chaparral tea regularly developed kidney cysts, kidney cancer and liver damage.
There is no evidence to show it having any effect on cancer cells in the body.

Light Therapy
Also known as chromotherapy, the use of different coloured light is used which allegedly corresponds to chakras or different organs in the body.
According to the American Cancer Society, chromotherapy or the use of light boxes have no effect on any type of cancer.

Lipid therapy
Lipid therapy is another name for Revici's Guided Chemotherapy, which is another cancer cure linked to acidity in the body.
Despite using the word chemotherapy, it doesn't even fulfil the definition, but does lend credibility to the treatment.
It was invented by Emanuel Revici 1896-1997, who in 1993 had his medical licence permanently revoked by New York State.
Administered by either mouth or injection, it is a chemical mixture that includes lipid alcohol, zinc, iron, caffeine, and various metals.
There is no evidence of it having any effect on cancer and has serious side effects.

Lipoic acid
Lipoic acid is an antioxidant available as a dietary supplement, claimed to be capable of curing AIDS, HIV, and cancer.
It is able to repair oxidative damage and regenerate antioxidants such as vitamin C, E, and glutathione, however there is no evidence of it having any effect on cancer and as a cure is worthless.

Live Blood Analysis

The examination of blood under a microscope to detect and predict cancer. Once detected, dietary supplements are advised that function as treatment.

There is no evidence to show it having any effect on cancer and the practice has been dismissed as quackery by the medical profession.

Live cell therapy

Live cell therapy involves the use of fresh embryonic cells taken from the corresponding organ of an animal and injected into the patient.

The claim is that the recipient's body transports the animal cells to target the organ and repair the cancerous tissue.

The American Cancer Society says that there is no evidence to suggest that this works, and the practice has caused serious side effects and death.

Livingston Wheeler Therapy

A method of locating the Progenitor Cryptocides (a made-up name for something that doesn't exist) and treating cancer by eradicating the bacterium.

There is no evidence to show it having any effect on cancer.

Lorraine Day's 10-step program

A regime devised by Lorraine Day that advises you to give up work, go on a restrictive diet and stop watching television.

I don't think it requires any further explanation as she's obviously not right in the head if she believes giving up television cures cancer.

Macrobiotic Diet

The macrobiotic diet is a restrictive diet based on grains and unrefined foods, which balance the yin and yang foods.

You should eat yin foods for cancers that are due to excess yang, and (surprisingly) yang foods for cancers that are yin, and no, I have no idea how it is determined as only practitioners are gifted in this respect.

The main problem is that some of the suggested diets don't even contain the required amounts of nutrients to survive, even if you're healthy.
In addition, you're not allowed to wear synthetic or woollen clothing next to the skin, bathe/shower in hot water, and you must chew your food a minimum of 50 times.
People using this diet during cancer have died due to malnutrition.
Early on in my treatment, someone suggested this to me and I tried it, but I'd rather have the cancer than try to live on this diet, plus it doesn't work anyway.

Magnetic Therapy
Placing magnets around the body in order to treat illness by interfering with iron in the blood.
Unsurprisingly, no evidence has been found to give this treatment any credibility.

Mandelonitrile beta D gentiobioside/Mandelonitrile beta glucuronide
Mandelonitrile beta D gentiobioside is another name for Amygdalin, which is obtained from the pits or seeds of apricots, apples, peaches, red cherries, plums, and other fruits as well as bitter almonds.
It was first patented in the 1950s and was known as Laetrile.
Touted as an alternative cancer treatment in the 60s and 70s, it is banned by the Federal Drugs and Administration due to the fact that when your intestines break it down, it converts into cyanide.
The idea is that cyanide kills the cancer cells, but the reality is that numerous deaths have been attributed to its use.
It was then repackaged as Vitamin B17 in an effort to get around regulations for drugs, but it isn't a vitamin and doesn't act like a vitamin.
There is no vitamin that reduces blood pressure to dangerous levels and induces a coma.
As little as 50 grams of amygdalin, or whatever name they choose to call it, can kill you.

Unsurprisingly, clinics in Mexico still promote its use, but after analysis by the Food and Drug Administration, some samples were found to have excessive levels of bacteria, and samples had been bulked out with other harmful substances.
Amygdalin has been independently tested on up to 20 animal tumours and found to have no benefit either alone or together with other substances.
In a clinical trial in 1982 by the Mayo Clinic and three other cancer centres, it was administered as recommended to advanced cancer patients for which there was no other treatment available. Out of 178 patients, there was no improvement, but in those still alive after seven months, their tumours had increased, and several patients experienced symptoms of cyanide poisoning and had to stop treatment.
In a US Supreme Court ruling in 1979, it was determined that the general public deserve protection from amygdalin and called it a fraudulent cure.

Mangosteen
Marketed as a superfruit in products such as XanGo Juice, it is a fruit from Southeast Asia that is harvested for its juice and bark. It is promoted as a cure for cancer, but there is no evidence that it has any effect on either the cells in a dish, or cancer in the body.

Marijuana
Marijuana or Cannabis is dried buds from varieties of the cannabis sativa plant.
Also known as pot, grass, weed, hemp, hash, ganja and lots of other names.
It seems to kill cancer cells in a dish, but there aren't enough trials to confirm or deny how successful it is on humans, and there are so many strains and variations, it's going to take time. There seems to be potential, but there is no evidence to suggest it cures cancer.

What I can confirm is that when you are on treatment and have no appetite, marijuana will give you the 'munchies', and you'll eat again, and sometimes it makes the food taste way better than normal, which is great if chemo has taken your taste away.
I can also help with sleep, which again, if you're on chemo and can't sleep, is a good thing.
In some countries, you can get it legally, in others you can't, but I don't know of any country where you can't get some somewhere.
I wouldn't recommend smoking joints filled with tobacco, as that sort of defeats the point, but edibles—where no smoke is generated—would probably be okay; but I'm not recommending it. I can't. Then again, I did use it when I was on chemo and for taste and sleeping it was wonderful when I had access to it.
If you do decide to try it, be sensible.

The Mattei Cancer Cure
The Mattei cancer cure or Electrohomeopathy is a treatment devised by Count Cesare Mattei (1809–1896), who suggested that different "colours" of electricity could be used to treat cancer.
I'm struggling to understand just what colours of electricity are available, but although this cure was popular in the late nineteenth century, it has been described as idiotic by those who actually know about the effect electricity has on the human body, and specifically cancer cells.

Megavitamin therapy
Megavitamin therapy (Orthomolecular medicine) is the use of high doses of vitamins, minerals, amino acids, trace elements and fatty acids claimed to cure cancer.
It is claimed to correct imbalances or deficiencies based on individual biochemistry and the idea that if the body is healthy, then it will kill the cancer itself.
Some vitamins in large doses have been linked to increased risk of cardiovascular disease, development of cancer, and death.

A balanced diet will provide all the necessary vitamins, minerals, etc., necessary, and if a deficiency is detected can be remedied by your consultant.

Metabolic Therapy
Another throw everything-at-it approach with restrictive diets and coffee enemas.
Invented by Hans Alfred Nieper 1928-1998, it recommends amygdalin and vitamins which, he claimed, could re-balance the build-up of toxic substances in the body and cure not only cancer, but arthritis, multiple sclerosis, and loads of other serious illnesses. His methods were discredited as both ineffective and unsafe.

MGN3
MGN3 is another name for Biobran, which is made from breaking down rice bran with enzymes from the Shitake mushroom.
It is claimed to increase the number of natural killer (NK) cells in the blood as NK cells are part of the immune system.
As it has been promoted for a cancer cure for at least twelve years, it's surprising the manufacturers haven't conducted any clinical trials to prove its effectiveness.
There is no evidence to confirm it has any effect on NK or cancer cells.

MMS
MMS is another name for Miracle Mineral Supplement, which is a toxic solution of 28% sodium chlorine in citrus juice, promoted for treating cancer, HIV, malaria, common colds, Parkinson's, autism, acne, AIDS, and other ailments.
Its main use is as an industrial bleach.
Side effects include nausea, vomiting, diarrhoea, symptoms of severe dehydration, renal failure, and other life-threatening conditions.
It was invented by Jim Humble, a former scientologist who promoted it in his 2006 book, The Miracle Mineral Solution of the 21st Century.

It is reported that in August 2009, a woman took it as a preventative for malaria and within 15 minutes she was ill, and 12 hours later was dead.

Modified citrus pectin
Modified citrus pectin is a chemically extracted substance from citrus fruits.
It is marketed as a dietary supplement to treat prostate cancer and melanoma
Cancer Research UK say there is no evidence shown that it has any effect on prostate cancer, melanoma, or any other type of cancer.

Moerman Therapy
Moerman therapy is a highly restrictive diet devised by Cornelis Moerman (1893–1988). Its effectiveness is supported by anecdote only and there is no evidence of its worth as a cancer treatment.

Morado
Morado is another name for Pau d'arco, which is a tea made from the bark of the Tabebuia tree found in a South American rainforest and is claimed to be an ancient Inca Indian remedy.
The bark is brewed into lapacho tea and marketed as a cure for cancer.
It was studied in the 70s and found to cause nausea, vomiting, and have the ability to interfere with blood clotting.
No evidence was found of it having any effect on cancer, but when consumed, can be dangerous.

Moxibustion
Moxibustion is the practice of burning dried-up mugwort near the patient, while using acupuncture or acupressure at the same time
There is no evidence that it has any effect on cancer.

Milk thistle
Milk thistle is a biennial plant that is claimed to have an ability to slow the growths of certain kinds of cancer.
Cancer Research UK say that there is no evidence of it having any effect on cancer of any type.

Miracle Mineral Supplement/Solution

Miracle Mineral Supplement is a toxic solution of 28% sodium chlorine in citrus juice, promoted for treating cancer, HIV, malaria, common colds, Parkinson's, autism, acne, AIDS, and other ailments.

Its main use is as an industrial bleach.

Side effects include nausea, vomiting, diarrhoea, symptoms of severe dehydration, renal failure, and other life-threatening conditions.

It was invented by Jim Humble, a former scientologist who promoted it in his 2006 book, The Miracle Mineral Solution of the 21st Century.

It is reported that in August 2009, a woman took it as a preventative for malaria and within 15 minutes she was ill, and 12 hours later was dead.

Mistletoe

Mistletoe is a plant proposed by Rudolf Steiner 1861-1925, as a cure for cancer and who believed it needed to be harvested when planetary alignment most influenced its potency.

According to the American Cancer Society, well-designed clinical trials have been carried out and no evidence found to support any claim that mistletoe has any effect on cancer.

The Swiss Society for Oncology also tested it for effectiveness and concluded that it had no effect.

Mushrooms

Mushrooms are widely promoted on the internet as a cancer treatment.

Various types are said to have different effects, depending on whether you eat them raw, cook them, smoke them, or use a mushroom extract.

There is no evidence that any type of mushroom or mushroom extract can prevent or cure cancer.

Native American Healing

Native American healing is shamanistic form of medicine traditionally practiced by some indigenous American peoples and which have been claimed as being capable of curing human diseases, including cancer.
The American Cancer Society say that scientific evidence does not support claims that Native American Healing can cure cancer or any other disease.

Naturopathy

Naturopathy is a system of alternative medicine based on a belief in energy forces in the body, and an avoidance of conventional medicine.
It is widely promoted as a treatment for cancer and other ailments.
It's comforting to know that some of the doctors who specialise in naturopathy have studied as much as 20 hours online to obtain the right to call themselves a doctor.

Nerium oleander

Nerium oleander is an extract obtained from one of the most poisonous of commonly grown garden plants and is claimed to be a cure for cancer.
The problem is that even a small amount of oleander can cause death, and there is no evidence of it having an effect on cancer.

Nieper Therapy

A plant and fungus based diet that has so little nutritional value, that people can die of malnutrition from it.
There is no evidence to show it having any effect on cancer.

Nitriloside

Nitriloside is another name for Amygdalin, which is obtained from the pits or seeds of apricots, apples, peaches, red cherries, plums, and other fruits as well as bitter almonds.
It was first patented in the 1950s and was known as Laetrile.
Touted as an alternative cancer treatment in the 60s and 70s, it is banned by the Federal Drugs and Administration due to the fact that when your intestines break it down, it converts into cyanide.

The idea is that cyanide kills the cancer cells, but the reality is that numerous deaths have been attributed to its use.
It was then repackaged as Vitamin B17 in an effort to get around regulations for drugs, but it isn't a vitamin and doesn't act like a vitamin.
There is no vitamin that reduces blood pressure to dangerous levels and induces a coma.
As little as 50 grams of amygdalin, or whatever name they choose to call it, can kill you.
Unsurprisingly, clinics in Mexico still promote its use, but after analysis by the Food and Drug Administration, some samples were found to have excessive levels of bacteria, and samples had been bulked out with other harmful substances.
Amygdalin has been independently tested on up to 20 animal tumours and found to have no benefit either alone or together with other substances.
In a clinical trial in 1982 by the Mayo Clinic and three other cancer centres, it was administered as recommended to advanced cancer patients for which there was no other treatment available.
Out of 178 patients, there was no improvement, but in those still alive after seven months, their tumours had increased, and several patients experienced symptoms of cyanide poisoning and had to stop treatment.
In a US Supreme Court ruling in 1979, it was determined that the general public deserve protection from amygdalin and called it a fraudulent cure.

Noni juice
Noni juice is derived from the fruit of the Morinda Citrifolia tree from Southeast Asia, Australasia, and the Caribbean.
Noni juice has been promoted as a cure for cancer, but The American Cancer Society say there is no evidence of any type to justify this claim.

Oleander
Oleander is an extract obtained from one of the most poisonous of commonly grown garden plants and is claimed to be a cure for cancer.
The problem is that even a small amount of oleander can cause death, and there is no evidence of it having an effect on cancer.

Orgone Accumulator
This one is the best yet.
Orgone is a type of life force discovered by Wilhelm Reich 1897-1957.
Patients sit inside an orgone accumulator, which was also invented by Wilhelm. It's a cupboard like box with an organic lining.
The problem with this cure is that Orgon, is a made-up name. It doesn't exist. It can't accumulate or do anything else as it isn't anywhere to begin with. The whole thing is a scam.

Orthomolecular medicine
Orthomolecular medicine is the use of high doses of vitamins, minerals, amino acids, trace elements and fatty acids claimed to cure cancer.
It is claimed to correct imbalances or deficiencies based on individual biochemistry and the idea that if the body is healthy, then it will kill the cancer itself.
Some vitamins in large doses have been linked to increased risk of cardiovascular disease, development of cancer, and death.
A balanced diet will provide all the necessary vitamins, minerals, etc., necessary, and if a deficiency is detected can be remedied by your consultant.

Oxygen therapy (1)
Oxygen therapy involves the use of a Hyperbaric chamber. The patient is enclosed in a chamber where the oxygen is released under pressure on the understanding that cancer can't survive in an oxygen rich environment, which is the opposite of what happens. Cancer cells thrive on oxygen, which is the reason tumours make new vessels that tap into alternative supplies, a process called angiogenesis.
In effect, hyperbaric therapy feeds the cells it claims to kill.

Oxygen therapy (2)

Oxygen therapy is the practice of injecting hydrogen peroxide, oxygenated blood, or administering oxygen under pressure to the rectum, vagina, or other bodily opening.

As a result of introducing oxygen under pressure to the rectum, there have been numerous deaths.

The American Cancer Society say there is no evidence of this practice having any effect on cancer and can be extremely dangerous.

Panacur c

Panacur c is a dog deworming treatment.

Please see article on dog dewormer before this section for more details.

Pau d'arco

Pau d'arco is a tea made from the bark of the Tabebuia tree found in a South American rainforest and is claimed to be an ancient Inca Indian remedy.

The bark is brewed into lapacho tea and marketed as a cure for cancer.

It was studied in the 70s and found to cause nausea, vomiting, and have the ability to interfere with blood clotting.

No evidence was found of it having any effect on cancer, but when consumed, can be dangerous.

Polarity Therapy

Energy based treatment based on the idea that the positive or negative charge of a person's electromagnetic field has an effect on their health.

The American Cancer Society says that polarity therapy has no effect on cancer or any other disease.

Poly-MVA

Poly-MVA is a dietary supplement created by Merrill Garnett, a dentist turned biochemist in 1931.

It is promoted as a cure for a number of diseases including HIV, AIDS and cancer, however, there is no evidence it has any effect on cancer and can interfere with conventional treatment.
Side effects include blood clots and death.

Protocel
Protocel is a liquid formula containing inositol, nitric acid, sodium sulfite, potassium hydroxide, sulfuric acid, and catechol that it is claimed cures Alzheimer's disease, multiple sclerosis, diabetes, AIDS, and cancer.
The claim is the mixture can lower the voltage of cells, causing them to digest themselves; a claim that was found to be false.
The ingredients were tested by the National Cancer Institute and found to have no effect on cancer in humans, either separately or combined.

Psychic surgery
Psychic surgery does less than nothing, if that's possible.
It is nothing more than a sleight-of-hand confidence trick in which a hidden piece of raw animal entrails is hidden in the hand, then the practitioner pretends to remove a lump of tissue from the body of the patient.

Purasin
Purasin is another name for Amygdalin, which is obtained from the pits or seeds of apricots, apples, peaches, red cherries, plums, and other fruits as well as bitter almonds.
It was first patented in the 1950s and was known as Laetrile.
Touted as an alternative cancer treatment in the 60s and 70s, it is banned by the Federal Drugs and Administration due to the fact that when your intestines break it down, it converts into cyanide.
The idea is that cyanide kills the cancer cells, but the reality is that numerous deaths have been attributed to its use.
It was then repackaged as Vitamin B17 in an effort to get around regulations for drugs, but it isn't a vitamin and doesn't act like a vitamin.

There is no vitamin that reduces blood pressure to dangerous levels and induces a coma.
As little as 50 grams of amygdalin, or whatever name they choose to call it, can kill you.
Unsurprisingly, clinics in Mexico still promote its use, but after analysis by the Food and Drug Administration, some samples were found to have excessive levels of bacteria, and samples had been bulked out with other harmful substances.
Amygdalin has been independently tested on up to 20 animal tumours and found to have no benefit either alone or together with other substances.
In a clinical trial in 1982 by the Mayo Clinic and three other cancer centres, it was administered as recommended to advanced cancer patients for which there was no other treatment available. Out of 178 patients, there was no improvement, but in those still alive after seven months, their tumours had increased, and several patients experienced symptoms of cyanide poisoning and had to stop treatment.
In a US Supreme Court ruling in 1979, it was determined that the general public deserve protection from amygdalin and called it a fraudulent cure.

Purple Coneflower Therapy
Purple coneflower therapy (also known as echinacea) is a herbal supplement derived from plants in the daisy family.
It is marketed primarily to prevent and lessen the symptoms of cold and flu.
Others sell it as a cure for cancer, but there is no evidence of this anywhere other than in their sales pitch.
In addition, some products have been found to be contaminated with arsenic, lead, and selenium.
According to Cancer Research UK, there is no scientific evidence to show that echinacea can help treat, prevent, or cure cancer in any way.

Quercetin
Quercetin is a plant-based dietary supplement that is claimed to cure cancer.
Due to its antioxidant effect, it can interfere with conventional treatment and can exacerbate certain cancers, such as breast cancer, causing the tumours to increase.
It has also been proven to induce blood clots, both to the heart and brain, which can result in death.
The American Cancer Society say there is no evidence of it preventing or curing cancer and can increase both the size and number of tumours present.

Rauvolfia serpentine
Rauvolfia serpentine is a plant used in herbal remedies that is claimed to cure cancer.
When tested by the American Cancer Society, it was found to have many dangerous side effects that actually increase the risk of developing cancer.

Red clover
Red clover is a European species of clover, claimed to cure cancer.
There is no evidence of it having an effect on cancer cells, or cancer in the human body.

Revici's Guided Chemotherapy or Revici's Cancer Control
Revici's Guided Chemotherapy is another cancer cure linked to acidity in the body.
Despite using the word chemotherapy, it doesn't even fulfil the definition, but does lend credibility to the treatment.
It was invented by Emanuel Revici 1896-1997, who in 1993 had his medical licence permanently revoked by New York State.
Administered by either mouth or injection, it is a chemical mixture that includes lipid alcohol, zinc, iron, caffeine, and various metals.
There is no evidence of it having any positive effect on cancer and has serious side effects.

Rick Simpson Oil RSO

Mr Simpson had skin cancer and discovered that by rubbing oil made from marijuana on the lesions, they fell off after only days. It also cures a variety of other diseases as well.

The oil has been independently tested by numerous research facilities and found to have no effect on cancer.

Please see main article on Rick Simpson Oil RSO before this section for more details.

Rife Frequency Generator

The Rife frequency generator was invented by Royal Raymond Rife, an American scientist, in the 1930s.

The machine produces a very low electromagnetic wave similar to radio waves but undetectable to the human ear. The theory is that if the electromagnetic waves vibrate at a specific frequency, they can break up the cancer cells, as all cells have a frequency, and if you can match that frequency, they can be destroyed. The problem is it doesn't work.

There are two problems with this invention, the first one being the guy was trying to do good when he invented it. He didn't set out to make a machine that didn't work.

The second problem is that even though it doesn't work, it does sound very plausible, and many people have capitalised on the idea and sold machines that ruin people's lives.

Claims are made that the machines can cure cancer, asthma, HIV, AIDs, brain tumours, hiccups, ingrown toenails, think of anything and these machines can fix it.

Unfortunately, they do nothing except empty your bank account and put your life at risk.

Rocket fuel treatment

Rocket fuel treatment is another name for Hydrazine sulfate, a chemical compound promoted to cure cancer.
Tests were conducted by the National Cancer Institute on 243 patients with non-small cell lung cancer and 266 patients with advanced lung cancer, the results showed nerve damage and a significant reduction in the quality of life accompanied by kidney and liver failure, however, no evidence was found of it having any effect on cancer.

RSO Rick Simpson Oil

Mr Simpson had skin cancer and discovered that by rubbing oil made from marijuana on the lesions, they fell off after only days.
It also cures a variety of other diseases as well.
The oil has been independently tested by numerous research facilities and found to have no effect on cancer.
Please see main article on RSO Rick Simpson Oil before this section for more details.

Safe-guard Canine Dewormer

Safe-guard Canine Dewormer is a dog deworming treatment.
Please see article on dog dewormer before this section for more details.

Sampson Root Therapy

Sampson root therapy (otherwise known as Echinacea) is a herbal supplement derived from plants in the daisy family.
It is marketed primarily to prevent and lessen the symptoms of cold and flu.
Others sell it as a cure for cancer, but there is no evidence of this anywhere other than in their sales pitch.
In addition, some products have been found to be contaminated with arsenic, lead, and selenium.
According to Cancer Research UK, there is no scientific evidence to show that echinacea can help treat, prevent, or cure cancer in any way.

Saw palmetto
Saw palmetto is a type of palm tree found in the south-eastern United States, the extracts of which are promoted as a cure for prostate cancer.
The American Cancer Society say that there is no evidence of it having any effect on cancer.

Seasilver
Seasilver is a dietary supplement made from plant extracts.
It was aggressively promoted by two US companies as a cure for every type of cancer, which lead to the prosecution of the owners According to the Memorial Sloan-Kettering Cancer Center, there is no evidence of it having any effect on cancer.

Silybum Marianum
Silybum marianum is obtained from the Milk thistle, a biennial plant that is claimed to have an ability to slow the growths of certain kinds of cancer.
Cancer Research UK say that there is no evidence of it having any effect on cancer of any type.

Serenoa repens
Serenoa repens is also known as Saw palmetto which is a type of palm tree found in the south-eastern United States, the extracts of which are promoted as a cure for prostate cancer.
The American Cancer Society say that there is no evidence of it having any effect on cancer.

Shark cartilage
Based on the belief that as sharks can't get cancer, ingesting ground shark skeleton must make you immune as well and can cure existing cancers. The problem is, sharks do get cancer, even in their cartilage.
Numerous studies have been carried out since I. William Lane PhD, author of the book Sharks Don't Get Cancer, made the claim, but since the premise is flawed, no evidence has been found to confirm his theory.
It has no effect on cancer.

Sheridan's Formula
Sheridan's Formula is a liquid formula containing inositol, nitric acid, sodium sulfite, potassium hydroxide, sulfuric acid, and catechol, that it is claimed cures Alzheimer's disease, multiple sclerosis, diabetes, AIDS, and cancer.
The claim is the mixture can lower the voltage of cells, causing them to digest themselves; a claim that was found to be false.
The ingredients were tested by the National Cancer Institute and found to have no effect on cancer in humans, either separately or combined.

Snakeroot
Snakeroot is derived from Rauvolfia serpentine, a plant used in herbal remedies that is claimed to cure cancer
When tested by the American Cancer Society, it was found to have many dangerous side effects that actually increase the risk of developing cancer.

Sodium bicarbonate
Sodium bicarbonate is promoted as a cure for cancer based on the theory that cancer is a fungus and is always white; both of which are wrong.
Treatment is most commonly administered by direct injection into a tumour, which can lead to death.
At its most basic, it's a treatment based on an incorrect assumption, and tests have concluded that the claims are false.

Soursop fruit
Soursop fruit was sold as a dietary supplement with the claim that it cures cancer. It's a fruit people, it doesn't curc cancer.
After tests by the US Federal Trade Commission it was found to have no effect on cancer.

Strychnos nux-vomica
Strychnos nux-vomica is a tree from Asia, the bark of which contains strychnine, which is a highly toxic alkaloid used as a pesticide to kill rodents.

There is no evidence of it having any effect on cancer, however, there have been deaths linked to its use.

Substance X

Substance X is another name for Krebiozen, which is a mineral oil-based liquid claimed to cure cancer.

Analysis of the oil has proved that it is nothing more than basic mineral oil with a price tag of $170,000 per gram.

The American Cancer Society say that there is no evidence of it having any effect on cancer, and the US Food and Drug Administration say it has been linked to several dangerous side effects.

T-UP

T-UP is a product made from concentrated aloe.

It is promoted as a cure for cancer that you either drink or inject into the bloodstream or directly into a tumour.

As a result of several cancer patients dying from this treatment, it is not available in the UK and is illegal in the USA.

Other than the claims by the alternative practitioners offering the treatment, there is no evidence to show it having any effect on cancer.

Taheebo

Taheebo is another name for Pau d'arco, which is a tea made from the bark of the Tabebuia tree found in a South American rainforest and is claimed to be an ancient Inca Indian remedy.

The bark is brewed into lapacho tea and marketed as a cure for cancer.

It was studied in the 70s and found to cause nausea, vomiting, and have the ability to interfere with blood clotting.

No evidence was found of it having any effect on cancer, but when consumed, can be dangerous.

Tapioca

Tapioca is derived from the cassava plant, which is a woody shrub from South America that is rich in carbohydrate and also produces cyanide to deter animals from eating it.

The aim is to introduce it to the cancer cells with the aim of causing them to commit suicide; unfortunately, it can lead to cyanide poisoning.
Although research has been carried out on rats, there was insufficient evidence to conduct human trials.
It has no effect on cancer cells other than in a petri dish.

Trifolium pratense
Trifolium pratense is another name for Red clover, which is a European species of clover, claimed to cure cancer.
There is no evidence of it having an effect on cancer cells, or cancer in the human body.

Trimethylbicyclonitramineoheptane chloride
Trimethylbicyclonitramineoheptane chloride or 714X, is a mixture of chemicals marketed as a cure for cancer and other serious diseases.
It was developed by Gaston Naessens from France and is made using camphor in a chemical reaction with ammonia and sodium chloride.
Banned in the US by the Food and Drug Administration, it has been tested and found to have no effect on cancer.
The main ingredient in the potion is water.
In 1989 Naessens was arrested and charged with murder after a patient using 714-X died after refusing conventional treatment, but although arrested, he never went to trial and was acquitted.

Ukrain
Ukrain is made from chelidonium majus, a member of the poppy family promoted for its ability to treat cancer.
According to the American Cancer Society, available scientific evidence does not support claims that celandine is effective in treating cancer.

Uncaria tomentosa
Uncaria tomentosa is a woody vine found in the tropical jungles of South and Central America, which is promoted as a cure for cancer.

It has been tested and found to have no effect on cancer, however, its use does have some serious side effects which include death.

Urine therapy or Urotherapy

In urine therapy, patients are told that by drinking their urine or having it introduced into the body by way of enema, is a cure for cancer.
There are no curative properties in urine to show it having any effect on cancer.

Venus flytrap

Venus flytrap is a carnivorous plant from which the extract is promoted as a cure for skin cancer.
According to the American Cancer Society, there is no scientific evidence that it has any effect on cancer.

Vitacor

Vitacor is claimed to be a cancer cure that is widely promoted on the internet.
Invented by Matthias Rath, it is a type of vitamin supplement that is said to ensure cellular health. He has claimed his treatment can reverse AIDS, HIV, diabetes, cardiovascular disease, cancer, etc.
Mr Rath has been involved in many court cases regarding his claims and illegal trials on AIDS patients in South Africa.
Cancer Research UK say there is no evidence of his treatment having any effect on cancer.

Vitamin B17

Vitamin B17 is another name for Amygdalin, which is obtained from the pits or seeds of apricots, apples, peaches, red cherries, plums, and other fruits as well as bitter almonds.
It was first patented in the 1950s and was known as Laetrile.
Touted as an alternative cancer treatment in the 60s and 70s, it is banned by the Federal Drugs and Administration due to the fact that when your intestines break it down, it converts into cyanide.
The idea is that cyanide kills the cancer cells, but the reality is that numerous deaths have been attributed to its use.

It was then repackaged as Vitamin B17 in an effort to get around regulations for drugs, but it isn't a vitamin and doesn't act like a vitamin.
There is no vitamin that reduces blood pressure to dangerous levels and induces a coma.
As little as 50 grams of amygdalin, or whatever name they choose to call it, can kill you.
Unsurprisingly, clinics in Mexico still promote its use, but after analysis by the Food and Drug Administration, some samples were found to have excessive levels of bacteria, and samples had been bulked out with other harmful substances.
Amygdalin has been independently tested on up to 20 animal tumours and found to have no benefit either alone or together with other substances.
In a clinical trial in 1982 by the Mayo Clinic and three other cancer centres, it was administered as recommended to advanced cancer patients for which there was no other treatment available. Out of 178 patients, there was no improvement, but in those still alive after seven months, their tumours had increased, and several patients experienced symptoms of cyanide poisoning and had to stop treatment.
In a US Supreme Court ruling in 1979, it was determined that the general public deserve protection from amygdalin and called it a fraudulent cure.

Walnuts
Walnuts are edible seeds of any tree of the genus juglans, the hulls of which are said to cure cancer by killing the parasites that cause it in the first place.
A small number of cancers have been linked to parasites as potential causes of cancer of the bile ducts, and to a lesser extent, bladder cancer, however, The American Cancer Society have tested walnuts for their effectiveness and found no evidence that they remove parasites or have any effect on cancer.
Even if they did remove the parasites after a cancer had developed, a further treatment would be needed to treat the cancer.

Wheatgrass
Wheatgrass is claimed to shrink cancer tumours.
The American Cancer Society says that scientific evidence does not support claims that wheatgrass or the wheatgrass diet can cure or prevent cancer.

Wild yam
The roots of the wild yam are made into creams and dietary supplements that are claimed to prevent and cure cancer.
Scientific tests have proved that wild yam has no preventative or curative effects on cancer and is completely ineffective.

XanGo Juice
XanGo Juice is made from the Mangosteen fruit from Southeast Asia that is harvested for its juice and bark.
It is promoted as a cure for cancer, but there is no evidence that it has any effect on either the cells in a dish, or cancer in the body.

Zoetron Therapy
An electromagnetic device that emits a weak field that is claimed to kill cancer cells.
Patients visited a clinic in Mexico and paid $15,000+ for the treatment.
In 2005, criminal charges were brought against the owners for making false claims.
There is no evidence that electromagnetic fields have any effect on cancer cells.

"Sometimes they say no, it can't be done, but no doesn't listen."
~ Lawrence Wray

And finally

If you'll indulge me?

This life is amazing when you think of the things that happen.

My dad was a very clever man, but he always claimed he wasn't. Without a doubt, he was one of life's workers (unlike me) and never held himself above anybody else. I don't think anyone would have argued when he said he wasn't educated as it was a fact. He left school at thirteen and started his first job; however, he was well educated in the ways of life and had an easy-going attitude.

I remember he was always making up poems, telling jokes and singing. When Dana won the Eurovision Song Contest in 1970 with 'All Kinds of Everything', he sang it for the rest of his life, along with songs by Jim Reeves, Johnny Cash, and any other singalong songs of the time.

Living in Northern Ireland—which at that time was segregated into 'The Protestants' and 'The Catholics'—he drove a taxi and didn't care which side called him or who he drove, they were just people to him, and although he was a Protestant, he was called 'Gerry', which was considered to be a Catholic name at the time, and which occasionally caused confusion. He didn't care if you were tall or short, fat or skinny, clever or stupid, Protestant or Catholic, black or white; to him, you were just another companion on life's journey. If you would listen to his poems or share a joke, he was one happy guy.

He worked all hours driving his taxi and the business expanded. More taxis appeared, then he built a petrol station, before starting a bus company. I suspect it was something of a revelation to him that he was wealthy, but as long as he had a packet of ciggies or (later) tobacco for his pipe, he had a smile on his face. He was wealthy in his mind with no regard for the money.

The thing that made me proudest of my dad (and there were a lot of things) was the fact he drove a bus for a Special Care School for kids where he picked them up from their houses in the morning and delivered them back home in the afternoon. Even though we had drivers who could have drove this route, it was his, and nobody else was allowed to drive *his kids*. He loved his work, and he loved the kids. Protestant and Catholic kids would be on the bus and he'd sing all the way there and back, and they joined in. Some of the parents complained when their Protestant kids started singing 'Danny Boy', which was incorrectly assumed to be a Catholic song, and others complained when their Catholic kids started singing 'The Sash', which was correctly assumed to be a Protestant song.

One morning, he stopped outside a house to collect one of the children and the parents rushed out. I remember him saying he thought something was very wrong, but they told him their little girl—one who had never uttered a word her whole life—had started to sing the previous evening. Of course, it had to be 'The Sash', and, inevitably, she was a Catholic, but I don't suppose the parents gave any thought as to what the tune was; they were just so happy their little girl had uttered her first words.

The first word she ever spoke in her life was made possible by my dad being my dad. Not caring what anyone thought as long as he was able to get the kids to smile and join in the fun.

My dad did that. No degrees and no formal education. Doctors said it couldn't be done. Psychologists and therapists had tried and failed. Experts in their field had given up.

So, do miracles happen or is it just a matter of never giving up?

Lots of people have been given a terminal diagnosis and survived, including me.

Years later, after he had retired, we were walking through a shopping centre when a guy—who obviously had Down's Syndrome—ran up to my dad and threw his arms around him. It was emotional, and they both cried, but even after all the years had passed, he still remembered singing in the bus on the way to and from the school.

I've done a lot of things in my life; some big, some small, some good and some bad, but I'll never come close to this one thing my dad did.

Why am I telling you this? Because everyone had given up trying. She couldn't talk and never would, yet… she did.

I have a hope this book helps at least one person in their fight against cancer; that I'll have made a difference, then I'll have done at least one thing right, and also, if he's looking down, he'll have a little smile on his face.

When you're given the death sentence that is cancer, don't give up. Keep fighting.

Acknowledgements.

Tim Minchin

I'd like to thank Tim Minchin for allowing me to use his quote. I contacted him by email and received a very nice reply and his full support in doing anything that helps cancer sufferers.

"*You know what they call alternative medicine that's been proved to work? - Medicine.*" ~ Tim Minchin

For those of you who know him, you already know just how good he is, and for those of you who haven't had the pleasure yet, please pay a visit to YouTube and see just what a genius he is, or even better, go to a live performance.

Stephen Fry

When I contacted Stephen about using his quote, he was exceptionally helpful as already mentioned in the Celebrities and Cancer section.

"*Alternative medicine people call themselves "holistic" and say it's the "whole" approach. Well, if it's the whole approach, let it be the mind as well. Use logic, use sense, use the incredible five wits you were given by creation.*" ~ Stephen Fry

Ricky Gervais

Mr Gervais is a hard man to pin down, but eventually his agent said that Ricky wished me well with the book and anything that he had said that helped could be used.

"*You don't see faith healers working in hospitals in the same way that you don't see psychics winning the lottery every week.*" ~ Ricky Gervais

When I initially tried to contact him, he was on tour, so it was entirely understandable that I didn't receive an immediate reply. Having watched him live and seen his most recent video, I'm surprised he has the energy for anything else anyway. Again, if you haven't seen his performance on Netflix in 'Humanity', make a point of watching it, you won't be disappointed.

Mr G is a talented dude and his series 'After Life' on Netflix explores what happens to those left behind after cancer has struck, but, of course, with a comedy twist, but even so, bring tissues. (update: Season 3 will be coming 14th January 2022)

And now, the end is near

Frank Sinatra sang, My Way.
'And (a) now, the end is near, and so I face the final curtain.'

Me? Oh, hell no.

I'm the one who set fire to the damned curtain, then turned around and walked the other way.

Stuff the final curtain nonsense.

Not far now, so I'd like to ask two favours.

The first one is: **Don't let cancer define you.**

Some people go through life after having had cancer and it's like, 'I had cancer, I will never recover.' or 'I had cancer. I can no longer do the things I used to do.'

'I had cancer', is nothing more than an excuse; the clue is in the word, 'had'.

Yes, I concede, I do have some problems after cancer, but I'd rather have the problems than be dead. None of the problems are so severe that the alternative is better.

Be happy you survived.

Give yourself time.

Think about what you've gone through and where you are now.

Appreciate life and get on with it.

Other people have gone on to do great things after cancer. Some write books, some do Ironman triathlons, or fun runs or half marathons or full marathons, or swim the channel, or jump out of planes, or raise money for charity, etc.

Others who went through exactly the same experience, lie in the house because they had cancer. They started off with a 'poor me' attitude and having beat cancer they still have a 'poor me' attitude. It's no way to live—if you could even consider it living.

Cancer is not an excuse.

If anything, having beat cancer is a reason to grab life by the balls and claim everything as yours.

Be a cancer survivor.

You can say, "I am a warrior."

Be the winner I know you are.

Come out stronger with the realisation that you've beat one of the hardest things on earth and as a result, you're a lot stronger than mere mortals.

As I've said already, you've got a superpower, so treat it as that and not a crutch, not an excuse.

And the second favour is: **Pay it forward.**

If you hear about someone just diagnosed, help them.

Give them a call.

Offer your experience.

Honestly, it will be appreciated.

Okay, so it's the end, finally

It's hard to know how to finish a book... to write the very last word. Books usually end with... well... 'The End', but that's pretty boring.

What I will say to you, Dear Reader, is 'Thank You' for having stuck with me and reading through some of my rants.

Hopefully, I've motivated you to participate in your own cure.

Hopefully, you've learnt something helpful.

Hopefully, you'll avoid all the mistakes I made.

But, I would ask you to remember one thing—and it's me being selfish (which as you know I am)—and that is, there is nothing worse than watching somebody die, simply because they didn't try; so… don't let that be you, and yes, that should be in block capitals, DON'T LET THAT BE YOU.

Fight like your life depends on it. It does.

Always ask for help.

You have to participate in your own cure.

Tomorrow will be better.

My very best wishes.

Lawrence

CANCEROLOGY

Printed in Great Britain
by Amazon

78312583R00289